Prevention and Treatment of Complications in Proctological Surgery

Mario Pescatori

Prevention and Treatment of Complications in Proctological Surgery

With contributions from:

Bernardina Fabiani
Vlasta Podzemny
Lorenzo Carlo Pescatori

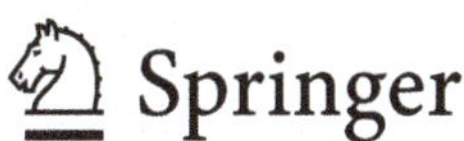

Mario Pescatori, MD, FRCS, EBSQ
Coloproctology Unit
Ars Medica Hospital
and La Sapienza University
Rome, Italy

Contributors:

Bernardina Fabiani, MD
Department of Surgical Clinic II
La Sapienza University
Umberto I Hospital, Rome, Italy
Illustrations

Vlasta Podzemny, MD
Editorial Office
Techniques in Coloproctology
Springer-Verlag, Milan, Italy
Revision of chapters 1, 2 and 8

Lorenzo Carlo Pescatori, MS
Department of Gastroenterology
La Sapienza University
S. Andrea Hospital, Rome, Italy
Bibliography

Foreword by:

Stanley M. Goldberg, MD
FACS, Hon. FRACS (Aust), Hon. FRCS (Eng), Hon. AFC (Fr), Hon. FRCPS (Glasg), Hon. FRSM (Eng), Hon. FPCS (Phil), Hon. FRCS (Edin), Honoris Causa (Lleida), Hon. SAS (Spain), Hon. JSS (Japan)

The drawings published in this volume are the author's

ISBN 978-88-470-2076-4 ISBN 978-88-470-2077-1 (eBook)

DOI 10.1007/978-88-470-2077-1

Library of Congress Control Number: 2011934755

9 8 7 6 5 4 3 2 1 2011 2012 2013 2014

Cover design: Ikona S.r.l., Milan, Italy
Typesetting: Graphostudio, Milan, Italy

Springer-Verlag Italia S.r.l. – Via Decembrio 28 – I-20137 Milan
Springer is a part of Springer Science+Business Media (www.springer.com)

Foreword

It is always a compliment and an honor to be asked to write a Foreword to a book. I am especially pleased to do so for "Prevention and Treatment of Complications in Proctological Surgery," by Professor Mario Pescatori.

The book's content is arranged in an orderly and comprehensive manner. I especially enjoyed the fact that in each of the chapters the author included his own experience in the management of complications. Moreover, the fact that this book has a single author has resulted in a uniformity of style besides allowing the relevant aspects of some of the cases to be referred to in multiple chapters.

The chapters on hemorrhoids were particularly interesting since this is the first textbook that discusses in great detail the complications of the PPH procedure. Every colon and rectal surgeon in the world will profit by reading this excellent chapter.

Fistula surgery is undergoing a transformation, with the increasing use of sphincter-saving techniques. The chapter on fistula includes a brief description of the new operation which involves ligating the fistula tract in the intersphincteric space. This is the only new textbook that I know of that has included this technique in the management of this condition.

As might be expected in a book of this nature, some of its recommendations will be considered controversial, but this does not detract from the book. Lastly, the references are very up to date.

Best of all, the book epitomizes Professor Pescatori's lifetime career in the demanding field of colorectal surgery. The progress made during his many years in practice is reflected in the text of this book.

Minneapolis, August 2011 Stanley M. Goldberg

Preface

According to the literature, one out of every four patients undergoing surgery for colorectal disease develops complications, some of which are fatal. This is especially hard to accept when a benign, minor pathology is involved. A colleague of mine lost the first patient that he operated on, due to complications following a simple hemorrhoidectomy. His despair can easily be imagined.

Morbidity and mortality conferences are of the utmost importance for the surgical staff. Experience in the management of complications is not well described in the literature. As a young surgeon, I found *Complications in Surgery*, by Artz and Hardy, to be particularly helpful but to the best of my knowledge nothing similar has been published recently, at least nothing specifically addressing complications in coloproctological surgery. Thus, after working as a surgeon for many years, including the past 30 in coloproctology, I would like to fill this gap, at least in part, by sharing my experience in the prevention and management of surgical complications. To narrow the scope of this volume, I have not included abdominal procedures or pediatric operations.

The most important (and self-evident) recommendation an experienced surgeon can make is that operations should be performed only when they are necessary. Good surgeons are good doctors who also know how to operate. They are "good" because they cure many patients, not because they operate on many patients. Moreover, it is fairly often the patients themselves who obstinately insist on surgery and see it as a miracle cure. For many of them, it is easier to expect that surgery will provide a rapid solution rather than to modify ingrained poor eating habits or confront psychosomatic problems. However, both of these are often the cause of immunosuppression, which physically weakens the patient, making him or her more susceptible to surgical complications.

The following remark, made by Sir Alan Parks early in the 1980s regarding ileo-anal reservoirs, has made a lasting impression on my professional career, "In order to perform these operations well it is essential to know how to deal with the complications." What he meant was that some operations are frequently associated with complications, and a good surgeon knows how to handle them. When I assisted (so to speak) the famous surgeon in performing a posterior plication of the pelvic floor to treat fecal incontinence, I was lucky in a certain sense. I saw him accidentally open the patient's rectum but I also saw how he sutured it. Since then, each time I perform a post-anal repair, I remember his scissors moving quickly on the posterior mesorectum and I slow down, to avoid the same complication; but if it ever occurred, I would know what to do in order to correct the problem. Surgeons must always be ready to fix a mistake, since mistakes can happen regardless of the surgeon's degree of experience. However, just like the athlete who has suffered a setback in a competition, the important thing is to recover lost ground.

More recently, Steve Wexner noted that surgical success in treating rectovaginal fistulae can be defined as the ability to cure the patient with a second or third operation, since disease persists after the first procedure in 50% of patients. Accordingly, this book also addresses re-operations.

Of equal importance to the surgical procedure itself is the pre- and postoperative evaluation. The aim of a particular operation must be well defined, which implies the ability to recognize the real causes of a patient's symptoms; otherwise a hidden concomitant pathology, like the submerged part of an iceberg, will sink the surgical ship. As I have emphasized in this volume, this is especially true of patients with obstructed defecation.

What dangers lie in wait during surgery? What can the surgeon do before, during, and after an operation to prevent complications? When faced with a complication, whether early or late, how can we treat it? These are among the many issues discussed in the book you are about to read, which I have chosen to write in a colloquial and practical rather than an academic style. The text and the case reports are accompanied by numerous photographs and illustrations. To encourage the reader's interactive involvement, I have described several procedures step by step, including not only what to do but also what not to do. Each chapter ends with a section called "Unforgettable Complications," which also discusses, where relevant, the medical-legal issues.

While it is certainly the case that one learns best from one's own mistakes, it is my sincere hope that the reader is able to profit from my many years of experience, as reflected in a reduced number of failures and improved surgical results.

Rome, August 2011 Mario Pescatori

Acknowledgements

I wish to thank Mrs. Caterina De Bono, secretary of my Coloproctology Unit, as well as Antonella Cerri, Paola Capponi, Elisa Geranio and Corinna Parravicini of Springer-Verlag Italia for their valuable help.

Two expert colorectal surgeons, Dr. Paola De Nardi, from the University Hospital San Raffaele, in Milan, Italy, and Dr. Ines De Stefano, from the Civil Hospital in Orbassano, Italy, made useful suggestions for improving the text. I am grateful to Marina Fiorino who kindly helped with the editing of the text.

Finally, thanks are due to my co-workers for their assistance in the ward and in the theatre.

Without their valuable cooperation, this book could not have been written.

Mario Pescatori

Contents

01 Anal Fissure 1

1.1 Introduction 1

1.2 Early and Late Complications After Partial Internal Sphincterotomy 1

1.3 Anal Incontinence 1

1.4 What Should Be Done if Incontinence Develops? 6

1.5 Anal Sepsis 7

1.6 Suture Dehiscence 8

1.7 Tricks of the Trade 9

1.8 An Unforgettable Complication 10

Summary 12

Suggested Readings 12

02 Hemorrhoids 15

2.1 Introduction 15

2.2 Surgical Complications After Manual Hemorrhoidectomy (Ferguson and Milligan-Morgan Procedures): Live from the Operating Room 15

2.3 THD/DGHAL and Mucopexy (Doppler-guided, Laser-assisted) 20

2.4 Stapled Hemorrhoidopexy (PPH) 22

2.4.1 Hemorrhage 23

2.4.2 Other Complications 23

2.4.3 Chronic Proctalgia and the Post-defecation Pain Syndrome 26

2.4.4 Retained Staples and Bleeding Granulomatous Polyps 27

2.4.5 Retropneumoperitoneum, Pneumoperitoneum, Pneumomediastinum, and Cervical Emphysema 28

2.4.6 Rectal Inclusion Cysts 30

2.4.7 Total Obliteration of the Rectal Lumen 30

2.4.8 Rectal Diverticulum or Rectal Pocket Syndrome 30

2.4.9 Rectovaginal Fistulae 31

2.4.10 Trauma to the Penis in Passive Anal Sex 32

2.4.11 Dysplasia and Cancer 32

2.4.12 Retro-rectal Hematoma 32

2.4.13 Hemoperitoneum 33

2.4.14 Dehiscence of the Rectal Suture and Rectal Lacerations with Hemorrhage and/or Pelvic Sepsis ... 33
2.4.15 Rectal Perforation and Pelvic Sepsis ... 34
2.4.16 Thrombosis of the Inferior Vena Cava ... 35
2.5 Complications After Other Operations ... 35
2.5.1 Semi-open or Semi-closed Hemorrhoidectomy ... 35
2.5.2 Farag Suturing of Internal Hemorrhoids ... 35
2.5.3 Hussein's Manual Hemorrhoidopexy ... 35
2.5.4 Whitehead-Rand Hemorrhoidectomy ... 35
2.5.5 Parks' Submucosal Hemorrhoidectomy ... 37
2.5.6 Coagulation of Hemorrhoids ... 38
2.6 Treating the Complications ... 38
2.6.1 Pain ... 38
2.6.2 Urinary Retention ... 39
2.6.3 Hemorrhage ... 39
2.6.4 Fecaloma ... 39
2.6.5 Thrombosed External Hemorrhoids ... 39
2.6.6 Anal or Rectal Stenosis ... 40
2.6.7 Anal Fissure ... 41
2.6.8 Abscess or Fistula ... 41
2.6.9 Skin Tags ... 41
2.6.10 Anal Incontinence ... 42
2.6.11 Severe Anal Sepsis ... 42
2.6.12 Fournier's Gangrene ... 43
2.6.13 Particular Complications after PPH ... 44
2.7 Tricks of the Trade ... 44
2.8 Two Unforgettable Complications ... 48
2.8.1 Case Number One ... 48
2.8.2 Case Number Two ... 48
Summary ... 49
Suggested Readings ... 50

03 Anal Abscesses and Fistulae ... 57
3.1 Introduction ... 57
3.2 Postoperative Bleeding ... 57
3.3 Iatrogenic Fistula ... 58
3.4 Persisting or Early Recurrent Local Sepsis ... 58
3.5 Suture Dehiscence and Non-healing Wounds ... 60
3.6 The Prevention of Postoperative Anal Incontinence ... 64
3.7 The Management of Postoperative Anal Incontinence ... 71
3.8 Complications After Surgery for Hidradenitis Suppurativa ... 74
3.9 Tricks of the Trade ... 74
3.10 An Unforgettable Complication ... 77
Summary ... 79
Suggested Readings ... 80

04 Rectovaginal Fistulae ... 85
4.1 Introduction ... 85
4.2 Types of Operations and Postoperative Complications ... 86

4.3 Bleeding and Dyspareunia ... 88
4.3.1 Bleeding ... 88
4.3.2 Dyspareunia ... 88
4.4 Local Sepsis and Suture Dehiscence ... 88
4.5 Re-interventions ... 90
4.6 Drains ... 90
4.7 Fecal Incontinence ... 90
4.8 An Unforgettable Complication ... 92
Summary ... 95
Suggested Readings ... 95

05 Sacrococcygeal Pilonidal Sinus ... 99
5.1 Introduction ... 99
5.2 Types of Operations ... 99
5.3 Postoperative Bleeding ... 99
5.4 Local Sepsis and Suture Dehiscence ... 101
5.5 The Prevention of Local Sepsis ... 101
5.6 The Treatment of Local Sepsis and Suture Dehiscence ... 102
5.7 Sinus Pilonidalis Associated with Anal Fistula or Abscess ... 103
5.8 An Unforgettable Complication ... 104
Summary ... 106
Suggested Readings ... 106

06 Tumors of the Rectum and Anus ... 109
6.1 Introduction ... 109
6.2 TEM or Transanal Endoscopic Mucosectomy ... 109
6.3 Transanal Submucosal Excision According to Parks: "Live Surgery" ... 111
6.4 Other Transanal Techniques ... 114
6.4.1 Through the Rigid Sigmoidoscope ... 114
6.4.2 Using an endoGIA or a Urologic Resectoscope ... 114
6.5 Non-transanal Local Excision ... 114
6.5.1 The York-Mason Procedure ... 114
6.5.2 Kraske Operation ... 114
6.5.3 Intersphincteric Resection ... 115
6.6 Complications Following Surgery for Anal Tumors ... 115
6.7 Two Unforgettable Complications ... 115
6.7.1 Case Number One ... 115
6.7.2 Case Number Two ... 117
Summary ... 118
Suggested Readings ... 118

07 Anal Condylomata and Anorectal Stricture ... 121
7.1 Introduction ... 121
7.2 Complications After Surgery for Anal Condylomata ... 123
7.3 Complications After Surgery for Anal Stricture ... 124
7.4 Complications After Surgery for Rectal Stricture ... 126
7.5 "Live Surgery:" The Prevention of Postoperative Complications After Anoplasty ... 127

7.6 A Trick of the Trade 130
7.7 An Unforgettable Complication 130
Summary 132
Suggested Readings 133

08 Obstructed Defecation (OD) and Related Diseases 135
8.1 Introduction 135
8.2 Our Relevant Complications Following Surgery for Obstructed Defecation 139
8.3 Postoperative Complications After Internal Delorme 141
8.4 Anal Incontinence Following Surgery for Rectocele and Rectal Internal Mucosal Prolapse 144
8.5 The Prevention of Postoperative Incontinence 145
8.6 The Treatment of Postoperative Incontinence 146
8.7 Postoperative Complications After STARR and Transtar 147
8.8 Other Operations for Rectocele Using a Transanal Stapler 152
8.8.1 Circular Stapler 152
8.8.2 Linear Stapler 152
8.9 Postoperative Complications After Rectocele Repair Using Prosthetic Meshes 153
8.10 Complications After Surgery for Anismus or a Non-relaxing Puborectalis Muscle 153
8.11 Operating on a Patient with Solitary Rectal Ulcer Syndrome (SRUS) and Obstructed Defecation 155
8.12 Two Unforgettable Complications 156
8.12.1 Case Number One 156
8.12.2 Case Number Two 157
Summary 159
Suggested Readings 160

09 Fecal Incontinence 165
9.1 Introduction 165
9.2 Complications During and After Post-anal and Total Pelvic Floor Repair: "Live Surgery" 165
9.3 Anterior Levatorplasty 169
9.4 Sphincter Reconstruction 169
9.5 Sacral Neuromodulation 171
9.5.1 Radiofrequency Energy 172
9.6 Dynamic Graciloplasty and Gluteoplasty 172
9.6.1 Graciloplasty 172
9.6.2 Gluteoplasty 172
9.7 Artificial Sphincter 173
9.8 Bulking Agents 174
9.9 Puborectalis Sling and Silicone Ring 175
9.9.1 Puborectalis Sling 175
9.9.2 Silicone Ring 175
9.10 Trick of the Trade 175
9.11 Unforgettable Complications 175
9.11.1 The First Five 175
9.11.2 The Last One 176

Summary ... 178
Suggested Readings ... 178

10 External Rectal Prolapse ... 183
10.1 Introduction ... 183
10.2 Postoperative Complications in Our Series ... 183
10.3 "Live Surgery": The Prevention of Complications After a Delorme-Rehn Operation ... 184
10.4 Complications After the Altemeier Procedure (Perineal Proctosigmoidectomy) ... 188
10.5 Complications After Other Procedures ... 191
10.5.1 Transperineal Rectopexy with the Prosthesis Fixed to the Sacrum and Posterior Levatorplasty ... 191
10.5.2 Transvaginal Sacrospinous Rectopexy ... 191
10.5.3 Manual Transanal Rectal Prolapse Excision ... 191
10.6 Circular Stapled Transanal Prolapsectomy ... 191
10.7 Transanal Rectal Prolapsectomy Using the Contour Stapling Device ... 192
10.8 Cauterization-Plication According to El-Sibai and Shafik ... 193
10.9 An Unforgettable Complication ... 193
Summary ... 195
Suggested Readings ... 195

Subject Index ... 197

1 Anal Fissure

1.1 Introduction

The definition, incidence, and conservative treatment of anal fissure have been adequately discussed elsewhere as have the other pathologies covered in this volume; thus, with few exceptions, these topics are not discussed here. This leaves more space for the real theme of this book: the prevention and cure of complications associated with surgical therapy for proctological disease.

However, a few comments must be made regarding the pathogenesis of anal fissure. Crohn's disease may be at the root of anal fissure. In an Italian multicentric study on this subject (Pescatori et al., 1995), in 19% of the cases the first sign of Crohn's disease was anal fistula or fissure. In diabetic patients or those suffering from empty sella syndrome with hypopituitarism and growth hormone (which is involved in scar tissue formation) deficiency, the surgical wound will heal with difficulty thus, the smaller the wound, the better.

A few remarks must also be made concerning treatment. Anal fissure is more often than not associated with anal hypertonia. In these patients, it makes sense to perform an internal sphincterotomy, but not in others since the procedure can cause hypotone and therefore anal incontinence.

1.2 Early and Late Complications After Partial Internal Sphincterotomy

The complications are listed in Table 1.1.

Table 1.1 Early and late complications after partial internal sphincterotomy in 417 patients (adapted from Pernikoff et al., 1994)

Early complications	Number of cases
Soiling	30
Flatus incontinence	15
Rectal bleeding	11
No wound healing	7
Fecal urgency	5
Fecal impaction	4
Fecal incontinence	4
Anal pruritus	2
Anal pain	1
Late complications	
Soiling	22
Flatus incontinence	14
Rectal bleeding	7
Fecal urgency	5
Fecal incontinence	2
Mucorrhea	2
Fecal impaction	2
Anal pain	1

1.3 Anal Incontinence

I intentionally use the term "anal incontinence"and not "fecal incontinence." After sphincterotomy, it is uncommon for a patient to suffer from fecal incontinence, although he/she may be troubled by gas or mucus incontinence. Usually, incontinence, which occurs in up to 4 out of 10 patients (almost 37%), is temporary; but in rare cases it is permanent. Out of 111 patients who developed anal incontinence after undergoing surgery for anal fissure at the Mayo Clinic, only one had severe incontinence at one month, although this impressive result may have been due to the highly skilled treatment available at that famous hospital.

Among patients treated elsewhere, the incidence of severe incontinence after sphincterotomy is 1-8%. A study by Khubchandani, an American surgeon who works in Allentown, Pennsylvania, opened our eyes to this problem and was the stimulus for treatments such as chemical sphincterotomy, which includes the use of nitroglycerin, calcium channel blockers, and other substances. Alternatively, botulinum toxin A (Botox) can be injected into the internal sphincter. The article was published in 1989; since then, surgeons have become more likely to operate only on patients with chronic fissure and/or those who were not cured with the non-invasive methods mentioned above.

At the end of 2010, the abstract of a study conducted in the UK by Conaghan and Farouk was published. Over a period of 7 years, the two colorectal surgeons used diltiazem cream to treat 462 patients suffering from anal fissure; those who were not cured (84) were treated with Botox and fissurectomy. There were very few cases (17) of recurrence. Most were treated with fissurectomy and Botox again or anoplasty. Internal sphincterotomy was necessary in only four patients.

The current trend in anal fissure surgery is to avoid sphincterotomy because of the risk of incontinence. However, in 2008, a meta-analysis of the trials comparing internal sphincterotomy and Botox found that the two procedures were associated with similar rates of incontinence and other complications (Sajid et al., 2008).

In another study (Pescatori et al., 2002), my group reported that 3 years after sphincterotomy 13% of the patients suffered from incontinence. All except one were multiparous women over 50 years of age who had had vaginal deliveries. These results allow the identification of a high-risk category of patients. These women have a descending perineum and occult lesions of the external anal sphincters that can be seen on perineal ultrasonography or on transanal ultrasonography with a rotating probe. In these cases, it is advisable to perform a minimal rather than a standard sphincterotomy to prevent incontinence, i.e., the incision made in the internal sphincter should extend only along the full length of the fissure and not as far as the dentate line. It is also important to inform the patient about the risks associated with the procedure before she signs the informed consent form!

Can the type of internal sphincterotomy performed play a role in the development of incontinence? Yes, of course. Incontinence is more severe after posterior sphincterotomy (Poisson, 1977; Orsay et al., 2004). The reason is anatomical: posteriorly, between the internal and external sphincters, there is a weak, triangular-shaped area that consists of loose tissue, which can be the site of soiling. Laterally, the external sphincter rests directly on the internal sphincter and tends to form a barrier against soiling (Fig. 1.1). Posterior sphincterotomy also seems to be associated with a greater degree of postoperative pain and slower wound healing than lateral sphincterotomy (Abcarian, 1980).

According to some authors, incontinence (soiling) is even more severe after Notaras' closed sphincterotomy (Arroyo et al., 2004; Wiley et al., 2004), because with the closed method it is harder to control the extent of the sphincterotomy so that it is often longer than absolutely necessary. However, both the complications associated with the closed and open procedures and their incidences are similar, according to Altomare et al., who compared the two techniques (2005). On the other hand, Wiley, cited above, reported three complications after open sphincterotomy (one case of sepsis and two cases of pain) but only one (pain) after closed sphincterotomy.
An overview of the effects of internal sphincterotomy on anal continence will help us to understand why some surgeons believe that this procedure is no longer the gold standard for the surgical treatment of anal fissure, and why some of them (for example, Conaghan and Farouk) only perform internal sphincterotomy in 2% of their patients.

Some of the data are perplexing. For instance, Farouk (cited above), who now hardly ever performs internal sphincterotomy, reported that the rate of incontinence after the procedure was only 2%. Two authors from important institutions (one from the Mayo Clinic), both with large case series and many years of follow-up, reported extremely discordant data regarding incontinence: 8% vs.

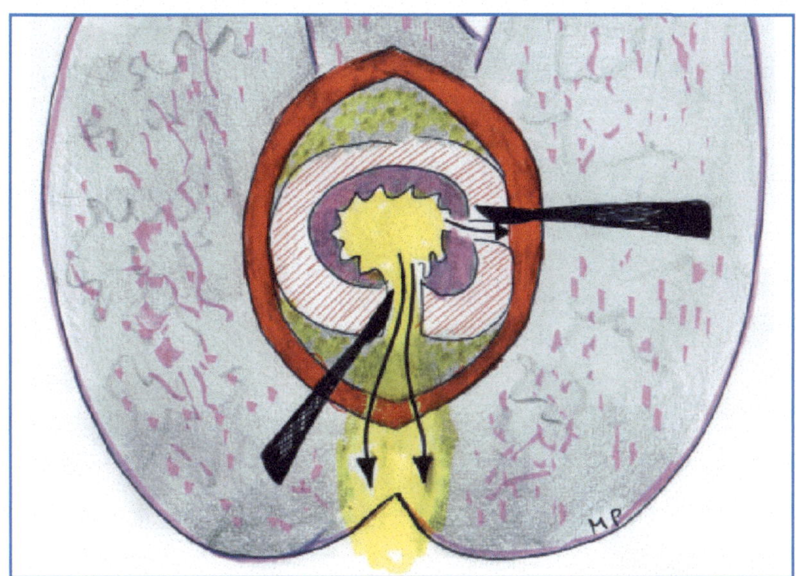

Fig. 1.1 The patient is in the lithotomy position. During posterior sphincterotomy, a triangle of minor resistance is created because of the anatomical relationships between the internal sphincter (*pink*) and the superficial portion of the external sphincter (*red*). The minor resistance area may cause fecal and mucous soiling (*arrows*). By contrast, when lateral internal sphincterotomy is carried out, the internal sphincter is protected by the close connection with the external sphincter. Accordingly, posterior internal sphincterotomy for fissure is more likely to cause postoperative anal incontinence than the lateral procedure

45%. Evidently, there is incontinence in which gas is occasionally passed and incontinence in which there is a loss of control over defecation. The same is true for sphincterotomy: on the one hand, one can make an incision over a distance equal to the length of the fissure and, on the other, an incision up to the dentate line or beyond. An example of the former was described by the Turkish surgeon Bulent Mentes, who reported only 1.1% incontinence with this limited approach.

From this point of view, the study conducted by the Spanish surgeon Garcia-Granero and his colleagues (2009) is highly informative, since incontinence rates were presented with respect to the extent of sphincterotomy, as measured by transanal ultrasonography.

In discussing the relationship between sphincterotomy and incontinence, it likewise needs to be pointed out that cutting the internal sphincter of a patient with anal hypertonia is a very different matter than cutting the internal sphincter of a patient who is already incontinent.

Another important issue is follow-up results, which may vary depending on whether the patient is followed by the operating surgeon or by another surgeon, and whether the follow-up is done by phone, by mail, or by outpatient visits.

And, of course, there are also differences among patients. If the surgeon performs a sphincterotomy in a patient with hypertonia but fails to determine whether that patient is introverted, anxious or tense, then his or her psychoneuromuscular status will probably cause persistence or recurrence of anal spasm. This, combined with hard feces that have been trapped for a long while in spastic sigmoid colon, can lead to fissure recurrence. These concepts, supported by the observations of our psychologist, were originally covered in a chapter I wrote, together with Mattana, on anal fistulae for a book on coloproctology (Springer, 2008). However, that section was deleted by the editors of the book prior to publication, which is evidence of how little attention is paid to the holistic approach. Miliacca, Gagliardi, and I recently (2009) wrote about the use of the "draw-the-family" test in patients with benign anorectal disease. The test, which is simple, useful, and well accepted by patients, may help to identify individuals whose psychological profile puts them at risk of disease persistence/recurrence. The reader is advised to explore this fascinating aspect of coloproctology in greater detail.

The data in Table 1.2 should be read critically and the studies mentioned should be consulted individually.

A more comprehensive appreciation of the problem of anal fissure would be a quality of life analysis, but few of the studies listed took this aspect into consideration. In my experience, incontinence after sphincterotomy performed only in patients with hypertonia and very often measured based on manometry results, as reported by

Table 1.2 Continence problems after lateral internal sphincterotomy

Author	Year	Number of cases	Follow-up (months)	Continence problems (%)
Khubchandani	1989	1355	NR	35
Pernikoff	1994	500	72	9[a]
Kanellos	1998	27	23	38[b]
Farouk	1998	183	2	2
Nyam	1999	585	72	45
Hasse	2004	209	>3	21
Hyman	2004	35	1.5	8.6[c]
Parellada	2004	27	24	45[d]
Casillas	2005	298	51	7
Mentes	2005	244	12	1
Garcia-Granero	2009	140	21	29
Hancke	2010	30	70-94	47[e]

NR, not reported.
[a]Fecal incontinence: 0.5%.
[b]Fecal incontinence: 5%; half of the patients also underwent hemorrhoidectomy.
[c]Deterioration of quality of life was found only in 2.9%.
[d]Fecal soiling and gas incontinence but no incontinence for liquid or solid stool.
[e]All patients had gas and mucus incontinence.

Pescatori et al. (1991) (5% incontinence) and Rosa et al. (2007) (0.4% incontinence), is not relevant here, as there is not much risk associated with made to measure sphincterotomy.

It is of course important to know how to perform alternative procedures. Before discussing the most common of these procedures, I will mention one that was recently proposed by an Italian group (Lolli et al., 2010), in which centrifuged adipose tissue is injected in order to stimulate tissue regeneration, based on the fact that fat contains stem cells. The eight patients who underwent this treatment had no complications aside from moderate hematoma (two patients) at the donor site (the hypogastric area).

The frequently used alternatives to internal sphincterotomy include excision of the fissure plus anoplasty. According to Hancke et al. (2010), this operation should be routinely performed as it minimizes the risk of incontinence. However, I do not agree. While in my experience there was indeed no case of incontinence among the 21 patients who underwent fistulectomy plus anoplasty, another complication occurred three times: partial wound dehiscence - and these were not patients with hypertonia. Thus, I doubt that long-term fistula recurrence can be avoided in patients with hypertonia without sphincterotomy or at least Botox injections.

In a study (described in an abstract in 2010) comprising 217 patients who underwent fissurectomy plus anoplasty and 60 who underwent only fissure excision, the French surgeon Bouchard and colleagues reported ten complications: three cases of infection, three of urinary retention, and one of fecaloma. That is a very low number, although the authors did not mention dehiscence, and further conclusions can only be drawn once the full study is published. Nonetheless, I mention their data here because, as far as I know, it is the largest case series of patients who underwent anoplasty for anal fissure. The authors also remarked that the patients who recovered most rapidly were those who had been treated by anoplasty and fissurectomy.

A prudent way to maintain continence is to associate fissure excision with chemical sphincterotomy, performed with the calcium channel blocker diltiazem, for instance. This is an alternative to fissurectomy and Botox injections. Arthur et al. (2008) compared the two methods and noted two cases of incontinence, albeit slight and temporary, with the second alternative.

A report by Patti et al. on the effects of fissurectomy and anoplasty on continence in patients without anal hypertonia was published in 2010. The study population consisted of 16 female patients in whom conservative therapy had failed.

Five of them had gas or mucus incontinence for two months postoperatively (but one had already been incontinent before surgery). After one year, only two of these patients still had complaints. Evidently, the operation did not have any serious negative effects. It should be noted that the same surgeons who removed the fissure also removed the hypertrophied papilla, if there was one. After a prospective trial, published in Techniques in Coloproctology in 2005, Gupta concluded that when the papilla has been removed healing is more rapid, even if an internal sphincterotomy has been performed. The surgical wound in such cases is a bit larger, but this is necessary. The sentinel hemorrhoid, is a different story. In an older study, Vafai and Mann (1981), at St. Mark's Hospital, recommended that the sentinel hemorrhoid not be removed because this would cause more postoperative pain (Fig. 1.2).

For a more precise, literature-based analysis of the risks associated with the different procedures, the reader is advised to consult the guidelines of the American Society of Colon and Rectal Surgeons (ASCRS), published by Orsay et al. in 2004.

Other American surgeons avoid performing internal sphincterotomy because of the risk that these patients will become incontinent (Pelta et al., 2007). In over 100 cases, Pelta and colleagues performed only a lay-open of the small tract corresponding to the fissure and removed the hypertrophic papilla. After a year, there were three recurrences and no changes in preoperative continence status.

Perhaps a word of encouragement is required here for readers who are now hesitant about performing a sphincterotomy to treat anal fissure, given the risk of incontinence as a postoperative complication. Najarian et al. (all expert surgeons on Billingham's team), after a survey among American colorectal surgeons, wrote in Colorectal Disease (2005): "The type of anal incontinence that most frequently develops after internal sphincterotomy for anal fissure is incontinence to gas. Incontinence to liquid or solid stool is only found in 2% of patients. Incontinence after sphincterotomy is rare." This statement appeared only in an abstract, whose title is reassuring for proctologists reluctant to change their operative strategies: "Fear, facts, or beliefs? The myth of incontinence after sphincterotomy"

Another reassuring study was conducted in Australia and presented at the Congress of the ASCRS five years later (McMurrick et al., with the well-known Polglase as senior author, 2010). Out of 228 patients who underwent sphincterotomy, not a single one developed permanent incontinence. The study is fairly reliable, more so than that of Billingham, cited above, because more patients (70%) completed the authors' questionnaire.

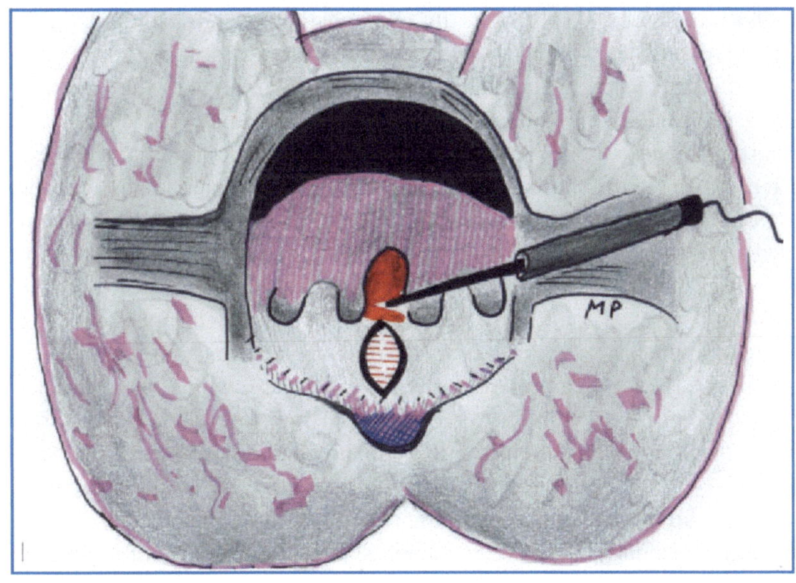

Fig. 1.2 Excision of the hypertrophic anal papilla (*red*), proximal to the chronic fissure (*dotted line*), anal verge, hemorrhoid, and "sentinel" skin tag (*purple*). The patient is in the lithotomy position and an anal retractor has been positioned

1.4 What Should Be Done if Incontinence Develops?

In this situation it is a good idea to wait because the problem is often temporary. If it persists, there are two options: a) inject bulking agents (PTQ, Solesta, Coaptite, Gate Keeper or Durasphere) into the defect in the internal sphincter; b) perform transanal electrostimulation (even at the patient's home) or electrostimulation of the posterior tibial nerve. Sphincteroplasty is rarely necessary. It is possible to reconstruct either just the internal sphincter or, if required, the external sphincter as well.

But what about preoperative anal hypertonia and its evaluation? Ideally, manometry should be performed and the pressure in the anal canal, the so-called resting tone, which is due in large part (80%) to the internal sphincter, about to be partially divided, should be recorded. If an ultrasound machine with a rotating probe, but not a polygraph, is at hand, the diameter of the internal sphincter can be measured. A diameter of < 2 mm indicates anal hypertonia (Fig. 1.3). However, it must be kept in mind that this parameter is unreliable if the patient is not young and does not have constipation due to obstructed defecation. With the passage of time and prolonged straining on defecation, the internal sphincter thickens and the relationship between sphincter diameter and spasm becomes less accurate. Alternatively, a careful digital rectal examination can be made with the index finger, as my colleagues and I demonstrated in a prospective study (1996) of anal hypertonia.

In summary, the best options are: standard sphincterotomy in patients with marked hypertonia, minimal sphincterotomy in patients with slight hypertonia or at high risk (not only elderly multiparous women, but also patients with diarrhea or those with prior anal surgery), and no sphincterotomy in patients with normal anal tone.

What operation can be performed to treat the last category of patients? There are two options: a) excision of the fissure and anoplasty; b) excision of the fissure and injection of Botox. Note that neither option involves internal sphincterotomy.

When dividing the internal sphincter, attention must be paid to avoid cutting the subcutaneous part of the external sphincter. While this may not seem to be a problem, since the internal sphincter is whitish and the external one is pink, in elderly multiparous patients, patients suffering from constipation, or those with pudendal nerve damage, the striated muscle of the external sphincter, especially the distal part, becomes dystrophic and therefore as pale as the smooth muscle of the internal sphincter (Fig. 1.4). An ultrasound study conducted at St. Mark's Hospital showed that it is possible to mistake the external for the internal sphincter. In some patients who had undergone what was intended to be an internal sphincterotomy, what had actually been cut was the subcutaneous part of the external sphincter!

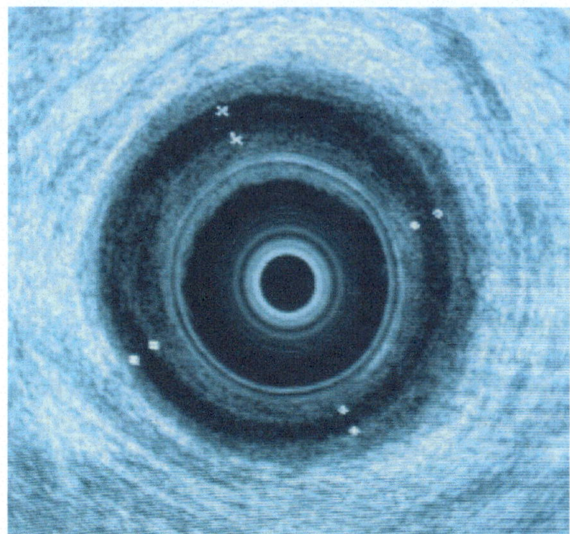

Fig. 1.3 Internal sphincter size measurement (hypoechoic ring) using transanal ultrasonography with a rotating probe. Two of the four diameters are < 2 mm, indicating mild hypertonia. The patient is in Sims position and has a recurrence of a fissure

A final question: Does anal stretch still have a role in the treatment of anal fissure? This was the procedure that was used for decades. When I was in England, in 1976, I visited Sheffield hospital and observed Professor Duthie, the fastest but also a highly competent surgeon (he performed a Billroth II in 45 min!). His last case of the day was a patient with an anal fissure, which he treated by forceful stretch, inserting four fingers into the patient's anus. This procedure has since been abandoned by specialists because it can cause incontinence in up to 50% of patients (Jensen et al., 1984). Speakman et al. showed, by means of transanal

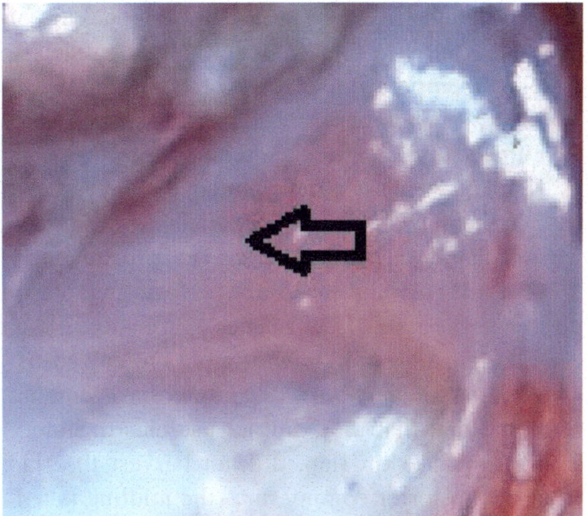

Fig. 1.4 In a multiparous or elderly woman with pudendal neuropathy and sphincter dystrophy, the distal part of the external sphincter (*arrow*) may be as pale as the internal one, thus misleading the surgeon so that, instead of performing an internal sphincterotomy, he/she cuts the subcutaneous part of the external sphincter

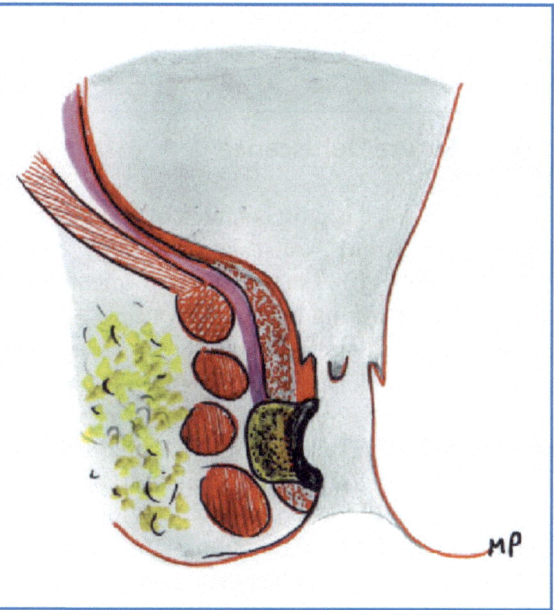

Fig. 1.5 Anal fissure with abscess

ultrasound, that there were anal lesions after anal stretch (1991). I have performed it only twice.

Together with Luigi Brusciano, I evaluated cases of successful pneumatic dilatation (published in 2005, with Renzi as first author). Walfisch and Silberstein (1998) and Boschetto et al. (2004) also reported positive results after this procedure. However the English surgeons Collins and Lund (2007) are rather skeptical about its positive effect.

Some experts, for instance Giuseppe Dodi, recommend digitoclasia, a "gentle" version of anal stretch in which only two fingers are used. The procedure can be performed in an outpatient setting with the patient under local anesthesia. There are no wounds or bleeding, and the patient can go home immediately. However, one thing is certain: anal stretch should not be performed in high-risk patients (those with a deficient internal sphincter).

1.5 Anal Sepsis

A good way to begin the management of these patients is to rule out the presence of anal sepsis before surgery. Fissures that have become abscesses should be diagnosed before or during the operation so that the abscess can be properly drained.

If the patient is immunosuppressed, diabetic, or careless about anal hygiene, or if wound healing is delayed, an abscess may form, most commonly in the lower left lateral intersphincteric region or the perianal region, and may lead to fistula formation (Fig. 1.5). This necessitates treatment with antibiotics, curettage of the wound in an outpatient setting, or even re-operation.

The development of sepsis might also be related to the technique used. If the first incision is made in the lower part of the anal canal instead of the upper border or the perianal skin, or if the mucosa of the anal canal is cut during a closed sphincterotomy, it will be more difficult for the patient to keep a wound that is "inside" the anus clean and to disinfect it with sitz baths. If good hemostasis is not achieved, a hematoma can form and become infected. If, after sphincterotomy, the entire surgical wound is sutured, this might facilitate the development of endoanal sepsis.

And, after anoplasty, is sepsis a frequent occurrence? While we might expect that it is, since there are sutured wounds in the anal canal, the problem is of minor importance. Sepsis developed in only 2 out of 16 patients in the above-cited study conducted by Patti et al., in which anoplasty was performed with a sliding skin flap, and in only 3 out of 54 patients after Y-V anoplasty (dehiscence presumed to be due to sepsis) in a case series of Chambers et al. (2010).

1.6 Suture Dehiscence

Suture dehiscence is most common in patients with diabetes or Crohn's disease. In these cases, Yakovlev et al. (2011) suggest to perform a temporary sacral nerve stimulation.

In perianal wounds, a suture breakdown is not particularly problematic; the wound is small (it should not be > 1-2 cm) and will heal by secondary intention. The only shortcut possible is to use catgut (which is often not available) or Vicryl Rapid which gives way if sepsis develops underneath so that the pus can drain off. Moreover, Nelson (2005) demonstrated that, among the surgical wounds made in treating anal fissure, the lateral internal sphincterotomy wound heals best and the most quickly.

We now shift the discussion to sutures of the mucosal or, more frequently, cutaneous flap used in anoplasty. As mentioned earlier, a small dehiscence of this suture occurred in 3 out of 21 of my patients. Fortunately, there was only a slight dehiscence (involving 2-3 stitches) and there were no significant consequences, except for delayed wound healing (Fig. 1.6). The wounds did not become chronic and the fissures did not recur. The same problem was seen in 2 of the 16 patients of Patti et al. (already cited) but neither patient had to undergo re-operation. However, one of the 3 patients of Chambers et al. (cited above) who developed suture dehiscence required re-operation.

Kundall et al. (2003) reported that hyperbaric oxygen therapy is effective for patients with surgical wounds that do not heal with any other treatment.

Can the method used to perform anoplasty influence the risk of dehiscence? Probably it can, even though I do not know of any randomized trials on this subject. Various authors have emphasized the fact that they did not use electrocautery to prepare the skin flap, did not harvest the flap from the posterior commissure (the midline is less well vascularized), and did remove the underlying fibrotic tissue (in order to place the sutures in healthy tissue). These are elementary principles of plastic surgery and I adhere to them as well.

There was no anal stenosis after anoplasty in my patients but it has been described in the literature. This is one of the dangers associated with a large dehiscence. Patients at risk should be advised to perform self-dilatation at home, for instance with Dilatan from Sapimed.

If the wound persists, wound healing agents, such as oil-based VEA, Colostrum, Vulnamin, Abound, Cicatrene, or Fitostimoline, should be prescribed. If there is also anal hypertonia, which may slow down or impede healing, it can be treat-

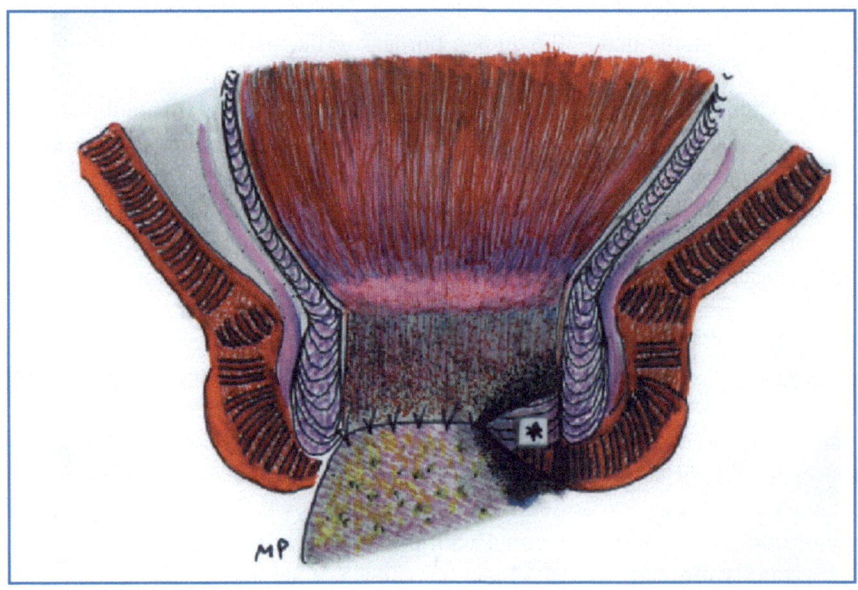

Fig. 1.6 Partial dehiscence of cutaneous anoplasty (*asterisk*) after excision of a chronic fissure in a patient without anal hypertonia. The anorectal ring is *pink*. Cutaneous flap detachment from the epithelium of the high anal canal reveals the underlying sphincteric fibers

ed with Antrolin, a calcium channel blocker and analgesic, or Rectogesic (active ingredient: nitroglycerin); these are creams for topical use. Dermatrans and similar medications, i.e., patches that release nitrates that cause vasodilatation and relax the sphincter, can also be used but they should not be given to patients who are hypotensive, on vasodilating drugs, or who are pregnant. The main side effect is headache. In cases of hypertonia and subacute stenosis, anal dilators such as Dilatan can be prescribed.

One more thing to note, not about skin flaps but about the skin incision in sphincterotomy, is that it heals more slowly if made posteriorly (Saad and Omer, 1992) because, as mentioned above, the blood supply to this area is very limited.

1.7 Tricks of the Trade

This is the first Tricks of the Trade section. Some of these tricks will already be familiar to the reader, others will seem to be self-evident, but in any case they are worth mentioning. In addition, please be aware that in the journal Techniques in Coloproctology of which I am the Editor-in-Chief (www.springerlink.com) there is also a Tricks of the Trade section, to which one's own tricks can be submitted. Consult the Instructions for Authors regarding online contributions.

As for tricks related to anal fissures:

1. The risk of intraoperative bleeding can be kept to a minimum during internal sphincterotomy. Instead of dividing the muscle with scissors or electrocautery, rest the tip of the (very narrow, blunt) forceps on the distal edge of the sphincter and then ask the instruments nurse to touch the forceps with the electrocautery device. Dissection will occur gradually and with only minimal bleeding (Fig. 1.7).
2. Another tip for obtaining good hemostasis: If after internal sphincterotomy the dissection margins bleed, avoid becoming obsessed with coagulating because the end result might be ischemia, necrosis, and ulceration of the epithelium of the anal canal and thus an endoanal wound that is very slow to heal. Instead, first try this: use your finger to exert pressure on the area; then infiltrate the area with adrenaline, with or without a needle.
3. If the fissure is deep and has hard thick margins and you are concerned that simple curettage is not sufficient to remove it or that it might contain neoplastic cells, use scissors or electrocautery to obtain removal and, if necessary, send the specimen for histological analysis. If the patient has anal hypertonia or if you have decided to proceed with an internal sphinctero tomy anyway, try to avoid a lateral sphincterotomy, although it is commonly performed,

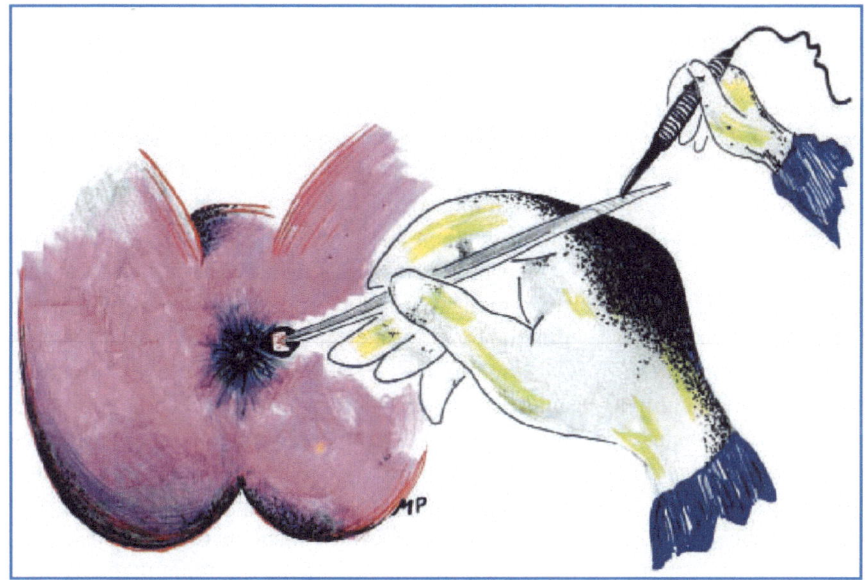

Fig. 1.7 Electrocauterization "transferred" to the clamp used to perform a hemostatic lateral internal sphincterotomy. Direct electrocauterization by the electrocautery tip is more likely to cause intraoperative bleeding

because this will result in a second surgical wound, thus preventing the patient's unproblematic recovery. In these cases, I perform a posterior sphincterotomy at the point where the fissure has been excised and the internal sphincter exposed. The wound is then covered with anoplasty using the Arnoux or the Martin technique, just barely lowering the mucosa of the distal rectum. Or better yet, to avoid the risk of ectropion of the mucosa, the epithelium of the proximal part of the anal canal can be used to cover the surgical defect. It is advisable to perform this repair because otherwise, as mentioned earlier, there is a less resistant triangular area which might cause soiling. This trick is especially helpful in patients with Crohn's disease or diabetes, since their wounds heal less easily and two surgical wounds are obviously a bigger problem than one. However, this approach is not recommended for patients who already had soiling preoperatively since it will aggravate their problems with incontinence. But, as repeatedly stated in this chapter, in the patient with anal hypotone, it is better to avoid sphincterotomy in the first place.

1.8 An Unforgettable Complication

Now for the first in a series of striking postoperative complications that I have observed in my career, after performing anorectal and pelvic floor surgery. Each one is presented as an interactive exercise. Halfway through, the reader is asked: What happened next? Why did the complication occur? What would you have done?

Note: After nearly all of these complications, there is a drawing that sums up the dynamics of the situation and the treatment. I would suggest that, if you choose to participate in the exercise, do not look at the drawing until you have finished reading the case report; otherwise you will obviously discover ahead of time how the problem was solved.

The patient in our first unforgettable complication was a psychologically stable 47-year-old woman suffering from chronic constipation, proctalgia, and moderate rectal bleeding.

Her general practitioner found that she had an anal fissure, which was treated with an analgesic cream containing cortisone. As this was unsuccessful, the patient decided to consult with a specialist, who after digital rectal examination diagnosed an internal mucosal prolapse of the rectum. The woman was operated on a few days later, undergoing a stapled transanal rectal resection (STARR). Neither proctoscopy, nor manometry, nor transanal ultrasound was performed preoperatively.

A week later, the patient developed a high fever and abdominal pain, and was found to have suture dehiscence and anal stenosis. A few months later, she sought a new surgeon and came to me. She had obstructed defecation, tenesmus, and rectal bleeding. The results of the various diagnostic tests revealed, among other things, retained staples, some of which were floating in the lumen of the rectum. I therefore decided to operate and found a fistula and a rectal diverticulum, both results of the earlier dehiscence, as well as a rectal stenosis.

So, what would you do at this point?

I laid open the fistula and diverticulum, removed the staples, and performed an anoplasty (Figs. 1.8 and 1.9).

The patient improved for a few months but then had a recurrence of intense proctalgia, with the pain occurring upon defecation, which had a very negative effect on her quality of life. Boccasanta et al. (2004) reported that 20% of patients who undergo STARR develop painful defecation. Since my patient refused a temporary colostomy, I suggested a period of total parenteral nutrition at home so that her intestine could recover and she would have as few bowel movements as possible. With this approach, the pain was indeed greatly reduced. Follow-up visits included the extraction of a staple from her rectum. However, after 3 months, when she had resumed a normal diet, the severe pain returned. Over a year has passed and the patient is still suffering from proctalgia—all of this the result of an improperly treated anal fissure.

Nonetheless, STARR is not useless for treating anal fissures. In Correspondence recently published in the British Journal of Surgery, German authors reported the healing of a concomitant anal fissure in some patients who underwent STARR for obstructed defecation linked to other causes. The patients probably had anal hypertonia that was corrected by dilatation with the 36-mm circular anal

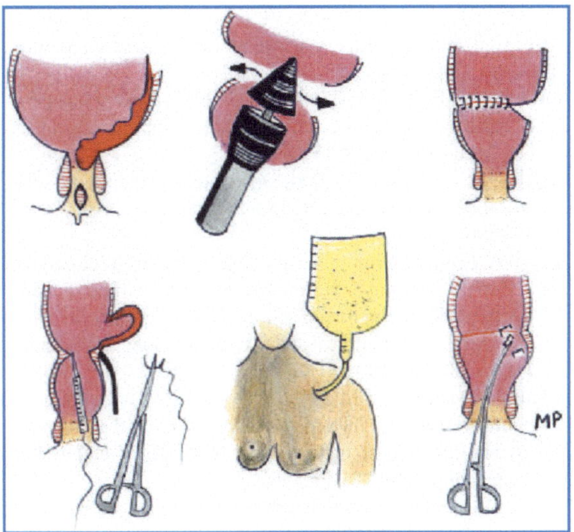

Fig. 1.8 STARR was performed in this patient with anal fissure, to treat a rectal internal mucosal prolapse. This resulted in rectal suture dehiscence (*top*) followed by a stricture stenosis, a rectal diverticulum, and fistula (*black, bottom left*). After a course of home parenteral nutrition, the wounds healed but the patient still suffers from severe chronic proctalgia despite removal of the staples

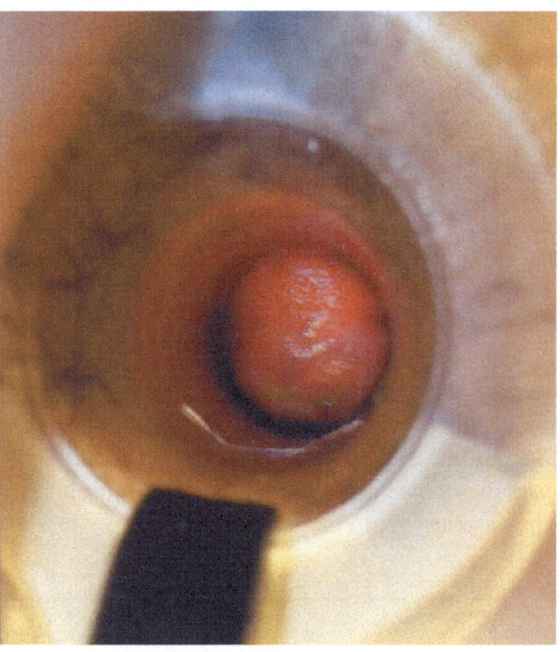

Fig. 1.9 a This patient, in the Sims position, was treated for a recurrence of a rectal internal mucosal prolapse

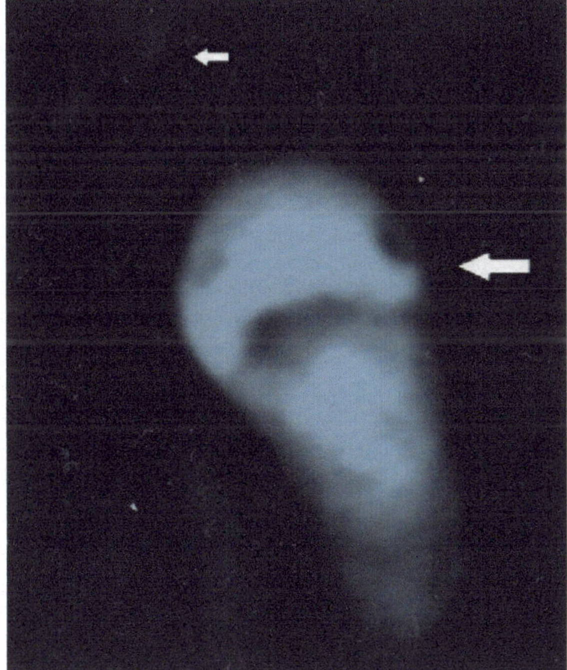

Fig. 1.9 b Sagittal magnetic resonance imaging. The patient had severe proctalgia and had undergone a STARR procedure one year earlier. In the high portion of the rectovaginal septum, a round area of activity indicates abscess or inflammation (*large arrow*). *Small arrow*: sacrococcyx

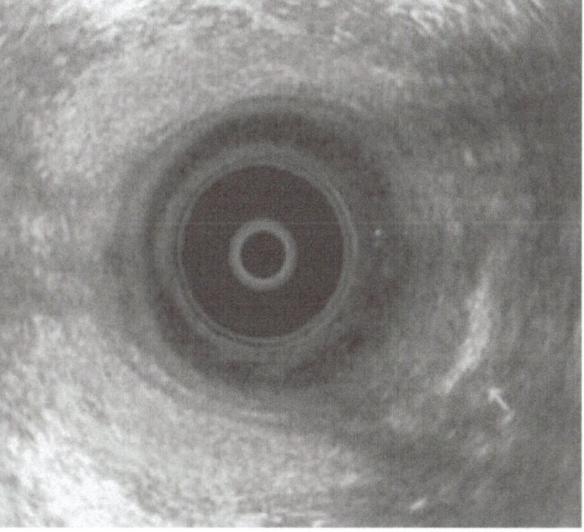

Fig. 1.9 c Transanal ultrasonography with a rotating probe in a patient in the Sims position. Anteriorly (*arrow*), just above the puborectalis muscle, the hyperechogeneic area indicates the retained staples and postoperative fibrosis. During rectal exploration, the patient had pain in this area

dilator (CAD), as if a mini anal stretch had been performed. In any case, however, treating an anal fissure with STARR is like using a Kalashnikov to kill a mosquito that is buzzing around your house: the insect will be eliminated, but a big hole will be left in the wall. That is what happened to the patient above. The rectal wall gave way, due to the trauma caused by the surgery, and the result was a dehiscence followed by a fistula and diverticulum. The cure was worse than the disease.

Just as the patient's ill health has continued so does her law suit against the first surgeon, whom she is suing for a rather large amount in damages. Since offense is the best form of defense, this surgeon has blamed me for the patient's problems. The case has yet to be decided.

Summary

Local sepsis and hemorrhage are rare after surgery for anal fissure. The most common complication is incontinence, usually gas and mucus incontinence, but it is seldom either severe or permanent, except after anal divulsion. It is advisable to avoid internal sphincterotomy unless the patient has anal hypertonia, and to perform only a limited sphincterotomy if the patient has hypertonia and deficient sphincters. Elderly or multiparous women as well as individuals suffering from diarrhea are high-risk patients.

Fissurectomy with injections of Botox and simple laying-open of the fissure are the two procedures associated with the least risk of incontinence.

Delayed wound healing and anal sepsis can occur, especially in patients with diabetes or Crohn's disease, and in those who undergo fissure excision and anoplasty. Suture dehiscence can be a complication of the latter procedure.

Suggested Readings

Abcarian H (1980) Surgical correction of chronic anal fissure: results of lateral internal sphincterotomy vs. fissurectomy-midline sphincterotomy. Dis Colon Rectum 23:31-36

Aigner F, Conrad F (2008) Fissurectomy for treatment of chronic anal fissures. Dis Colon Rectum 51:1163

Algaithy ZK (2008) Botulinum toxin versus surgical sphincterotomy in females with chronic anal fissure. Saudi Med J 29:1260-1263

Altomare DF, Rinaldi M, Troilo VL et al (2005) Closed ambulatory lateral internal sphincterotomy for chronic anal fissures. Tech Coloproctol 9:248-249

Altomare DF, Binda GA, Canuti S et al (2011) The management of patients with primary chronic anal fissure: a position paper. Tech Coloproctol 15 (in press)

Argov S, Levandovsky O (2000) Open lateral sphincterotomy is still the best treatment for chronic anal fissure. Am J Surg. 179:201-202

Arroyo A, Pérez F, Serrano P et al (2004) Open versus closed lateral sphincterotomy performed as an outpatient procedure under local anesthesia for chronic anal fissure: prospective randomized study of clinical and manometric long term results. J Am Coll Surg 199:361-367

Arthur JD, Makin CA, El-Sayed TY et al (2008) A pilot comparative study of fissurectomy/diltiazem and fissurectomy/botulinum toxin in the treatment of chronic anal fissure. Tech Coloproctol 12:331-336

Badejo OA (1984) Outpatient treatment of fissure-in-ano. Trop Geogr Med 36:367-369

Baraza W, Boereboom C, Shorthouse A et al (2008) The long-term efficacy of fissurectomy and botulinum toxin injection for chronic anal fissure in females. Dis Colon Rectum 51:239-243

Boccasanta P, Venturi M, Stuto A et al (2004) Stapled transanal rectal resection for outlet obstruction: a prospective, multicenter trial. Dis Colon Rectum 47:1285-1296

Boschetto S, Giovannone M, Tosoni M et al (2004) Hydropneumatic anal dilation in conservative treatment of chronic anal fissure: clinical outcomes and randomized comparison with topical nitroglycerin. Tech Coloproctol 8:89-92

Brisinda G, Cadeddu F, Mazzeo P et al (2007) Botulinum toxin A for the treatment of chronic anal fissure. Expert Rev Gastroenterol Hepatol 1:219-228

Brown CJ, Dubreuil D, Santoro L et al (2007) Lateral internal sphincterotomy is superior to topical nitroglycerin for healing chronic anal fissure and does not compromise long-term fecal continence: six-year follow-up of a multicenter, randomized, controlled trial. Dis Colon Rectum 50:442-448

Cerdán FJ, Ruiz de León A, Azpiroz F et al (1982) Anal sphincteric pressure in fissure-in-ano before and after lateral internal sphincterotomy. Dis Colon Rectum 25:198-201

Chambers W, Sajal R, Dixon A (2010) V-Y advancement flap as first-line treatment for all chronic anal fissures. Int J Colorectal Dis 25:645-648

Cho DY (2005) Controlled lateral sphincterotomy for chronic anal fissure. Dis Colon Rectum 48:1037-1041

Collins EE, Lund JN (2007) A review of chronic anal fissure management. Tech Coloproctol 11:209-223

Conaghan P, Farouk R (2010) Anal fissure healing and sphincter preservation can be successfully achieved in most patients with chronic anal fissure. ASCRS Meeting Abstracts, Dis Colon Rectum 53:587

Cundall JD, Gardiner A, Laden G et al (2003) Use of hyperbaric oxygen to treat chronic anal fissure. Br J Surg 90:452–453

Elsebae MM (2007) A study of fecal incontinence in patients with chronic anal fissure: prospective, randomized, controlled trial of the extent of internal anal sphincter division during lateral sphincterotomy. World J Surg 31:2052-2057

Farouk R, Monson JR, Duthie GS (1997) Technical failure of lateral sphincterotomy for the treatment of chronic anal fissure: a study using endoanal ultrasonography. Br J Surg 84:84-85

Favetta U, Amato A, Interisano A et al (1996) Clinical, manometric and sonographic assessment of the anal sphincters. A comparative prospective study. Int J Colorectal Dis 11:163-166

Favetta U, Amato A, Interisano A et al (1994) Comparative evaluation of anal resting tone and sphincter relaxation by means of digital exploration, anorectal manometry and anal ultrasound. Tech Coloproctol 3:14-15

Filingeri V, Gravante G (2005) A prospective randomized trial betwen subcutaneous lateral internal sphincterotomy with radiofrequency bistoury and conventional Parks' operation in the treatment of anal fissures. Eur Rev Med Pharmacol Sci 9:175-178

Garcea G, Sutton C, Mansoori S et al (2003) Results following conservative lateral sphincteromy for the treatment of chronic anal fissures. Colorectal Dis 5:311-314

García-Granero E, Sanahuja A, García-Botello SA et al (2009) The ideal lateral internal sphincterotomy: clinical and endosonographic evaluation following open and closed internal anal sphincterotomy. Colorectal Dis 11:502-7

Giordano P, Gravante G, Grondona P et al (2009) Simple cutaneous advancement flap anoplasty for resistant chronic anal fissure: a prospective study. World J Surg 33:1058-1063

Goligher JC (1965) An evaluation of internal sphicterotomy and simple sphincter-stretching in the treatment of fissure-in-ano. Surg Clin North Am 45:1299-1304

Gupta PJ (2005) A study of suppurative pathologies associated with chronic anal fissures. Tech Coloproctol 9:104-107

Gupta PJ, Kalaskar S (2003) Removal of hypertrophied anal papillae and fibrous anal polyp increases patient satisfaction after anal fissure surgery. Tech Coloproctol 155-158

Hancke E, Rikas E, Suchan K et al (2010) Dermal flap coverage for chronic anal fissure: lower incidence of anal incontinence compared to lateral internal sphincterotomy after long-term follow-up. Dis Colon Rectum 53:1563-1568

Herold A, Lehur PA, Matzel KE, O'Connell PR (2008) Coloproctology (series: European Manual of Medicine). Springer, pp 45-51

Jensen SL, Lund F, Nielsen OV et al (1984) Lateral subcutaneous sphincterotomy versus anal dilatation in the treatment of fissure in ano in outpatients: a prospective randomised study. Br Med J 289:528-530

Kang GS, Kim BS, Choi PS et al (2008) Evaluation of healing and complications after lateral internal sphincterotomy for chronic anal fissure: marginal suture of incision vs. open left incision: prospective, randomized, controlled study. Dis Colon Rectum 51:329-333

Katsinelos P, Papaziogas B, Koutelidakis I et al (2006) Topical 0.5% nifedipine vs. lateral internal sphincterotomy for the treatment of chronic anal fissure: long-term follow-up. Int J Colorectal Dis 21:179-183

Khubchandani IT, Reed JF (1989) Sequelae of internal sphincterotomy for chronic fissure in ano. Br J Surg 76:431-434

Kiyak G, Korukluoğlu B, Kuşdemir A et al (2009) Results of lateral internal sphincterotomy with open technique for chronic anal fissure: evaluation of complications, symptom relief, and incontinence with long-term follow-up. Dig Dis Sci 54:2220-2224

Leong A (2005) Internal sphincterotomy versus rotation flap to treat chronic anal fissures. Asian J Surg 28:192

Leong AF, Seow-Choen F (1995) Lateral sphincterotomy compared with anal advancement flap for chronic anal fissure. Dis Colon Rectum 38:69-71

Libertiny G, Knight JS, Farouk R (2002) Randomised trial of topical 0.2% glyceryl trinitrate and lateral internal sphincterotomy for the treatment of patients with chronic anal fissure: long-term follow-up. Eur J Surg 168:418-421

Liratzopoulos N, Efremidou EI, Papageorgiou MS et al (2006) Lateral subcutaneous internal sphincterotomy in the treatment of chronic anal fissure: our experience. J Gastrointestin Liver Dis 15:143-147

Lolli P, Malleo G, Rigotti G (2010) Treatment of chronic anal fissures and associated stenosis by autologous adipose tissue transplant: a pilot study. Dis Colon Rectum 53:460-466

Lubowski D (2008) Topical therapy is first line treatment for chronic anal fissure because of the risk of incontinence with sphincterotomy. Dis Colon Rectum 51:1157-1158

Lysy J, Israeli E, Levy S et al (2006) Long-term results of "chemical sphincterotomy" for chronic anal fissure: a prospective study. Dis Colon Rectum 49:858-864

Maturanza M, Maritato F, Costanzo A et al (1997) Combined outpatient surgical-cryotherapeutic treatment of anal fissures. Our experience. Minerva Chir 52:393-395

McMurrick P, Polglase A, Binns K et al (2010) Prospective Comparison Of Sphincterotomy Vs Botox Injection For Anal Fissure. ASCRS Meeting Abstracts, Dis Colon Rectum 53:588

Menteş BB, Ege B, Leventoglu S et al (2005) Extent of lateral internal sphincterotomy: up to the dentate line or up to the fissure apex? Dis Colon Rectum 48:365-370

Menteş BB, Güner MK, Leventoglu S et al (2008) Fine-tuning of the extent of lateral internal sphincterotomy: spasm-controlled vs. up to the fissure apex. Dis Colon Rectum 51:128-133

Menteş BB, Irkörücü O, Akin M et al (2003) Comparison of botulinum toxin injection and lateral internal sphincterotomy for the treatment of chronic anal fissure. Dis Colon Rectum 46:232-237

Menteş BB, Tezcaner T, Yilmaz U et al (2006) Results of lateral internal sphincterotomy for chronic anal fissure with particular reference to quality of life. Dis Colon Rectum 49:1045-1051

Miliacca C, Gagliardi G, Pescatori M (2010) The 'Draw-the-Family Test' in the preoperative assessment of patients with anorectal diseases and psychological distress: a prospective controlled study. Colorectal Dis 12:792-798

Mishra R, Thomas S, Maan MS et al (2005) Topical nitroglycerin versus lateral internal sphincterotomy for chronic anal fissure: prospective, randomized trial. ANZ J Surg 75:1032-1035

Mousavi SR, Sharifi M, Mehdikhah Z (2009) A comparison between the results of fissurectomy and lateral internal sphincterotomy in the surgical management of chronic anal fissure. J Gastrointest Surg 13:1279-1282

Nelson R (2005) Operative procedures for fissure in ano. Cochrane Database Syst Rev 18:CD002199

Orsay C, Rakinic J, Perry WB et al (2004) Practice parameters for the management of anal fissures (revised). Dis Colon Rectum 47:2003-2007

Ortiz H, Marzo J, Armendariz P et al (2005) Quality of life assessment in patients with chronic anal fissure after lateral internal sphincterotomy. Br J Surg. 92:881-885

Pascual M, Parés D, Pera M et al (2008) Variation in clinical, manometric and endosonographic findings in anterior chronic anal fissure: a prospective study. Dig Dis Sci 53:21-26

Patti R, Famà F, Barrera T et al (2010) Fissurectomy and anal advancement flap for anterior chronic anal fissure without hypertonia of the internal anal sphincter in females. Colorectal Dis 12:1127-1130

Pelta AE, Davis KG, Armstrong DN (2007) Subcutaneous fissurotomy: a novel procedure for chronic fissure-in-ano. a review of 109 cases. Dis Colon Rectum 50:1662-1667

Pérez-Miranda M, Robledo P, Alcalde M et al (1996) Endoscopic anal dilatation for fissure-in-ano: a new outpatient treatment modality. Rev Esp Enferm Dig 88:265-272

Pernikoff BJ, Eisenstat TE, Rubin RJ et al (1994) Reappraisal of partial lateral internal sphincterotomy. Dis Colon Rectum 37:1291-1295

Pescatori M, Ayabaca SM, Cafaro D (2002) Tailored sphincterotomy or fissurectomy and anoplasty? Dis Colon Rectum 45:1563-1564; author reply 1564

Pescatori M, Interisano A, Basso L et al (1995) Management of perianal Crohn's disease. Results of a multicenter study in Italy. Dis Colon Rectum 38:121-124

Pescatori M, Maria G, Anastasio G (1991) "Spasm related" internal sphincterotomy in the treatment of anal fissure. Coloproctology 13:20-22

Pescatori M, Mattana C (2008) Fissures. In: Coloproctology, Herold A, Lehur P-A, Matzel KE, O'Connell PR Eds; pp 45-51

Poisson J (1997) Anal fissure. Can J Surg 20:417-421

Ram E, Alper D, Stein GY et al (2005) Internal anal sphincter function following lateral internal sphincterotomy for anal fissure: a long-term manometric study. Ann Surg 242:208-211

Renzi A, Brusciano L, Pescatori M et al (2005) Pneumatic balloon dilatation for chronic anal fissure: a prospective, clinical, endosonographic, and manometric study. Dis Colon Rectum 48:121-126

Renzi A, Izzo D, Di Sarno G et al (2008) Clinical, manometric, and ultrasonographic results of pneumatic balloon dilatation vs. lateral internal sphincterotomy for chronic anal fissure: a prospective, randomized, controlled trial. Dis Colon Rectum 51:121-127

Rosa G, Lolli P, Piccinelli D et al (2005) Calibrated lateral internal sphincterotomy for chronic anal fissure. Tech Coloproctol. 9:127-131; discussion 31-32

Saad AM, Omer A (1992) Surgical treatment of chronic fissure in ano: a prospective randomized study. East Afr Med J 69:613-615

Sajid MS, Vijaynagar B, Desai M et al (2008) Botulinum toxin vs glyceryltrinitrate for the medical management of chronic anal fissure: a meta-analysis. Colorectal Dis 10:541-546

Simkovic D, Smejkal K, Hladík P (2000) Assessment of sphincterotomy results in patients treated for anal fissure. Rev Esp Enferm Dig 92:399-404

Speakman CT, Burnett SJ, Kamm MA et al (1991) Sphincter injury after anal dilatation demonstrated by anal endosonography. Br J Surg 78:1429-1430

Srinivasaiah N, Laden G, Duthie GS et al (2008) The long-term efficacy of fissurectomy and botulinum toxin injection for chronic anal fissure in females. Dis Colon Rectum 51:1589

Usatoff V, Polglase AL (1995) The longer term results of internal anal sphincterotomy for anal fissure. Aust N Z J Surg 65:576-578

Vafai M, Mann CV (1981) Closed lateral internal anal sphincterotomy without removal of sentinel pile for fissure-in-ano. Coloproctology 3:91-93

Walfisch S, Silberstein E (1998) Balloon anal dilatation for anal fissure. Tech Coloproctol 2:73–75

Wiley M, Day P, Rieger N et al (2004) Open vs. closed lateral internal sphincterotomy for idiopathic fissure-in-ano: a prospective, randomized, controlled trial. Dis Colon Rectum 47:847-852

Yakovlev A, Karasev SA, Dolgich OY (2011) Sacral nerve stimulation: a novel treatment of chronic anal fissure. Dis Colon Rectum 54:324-327

Yucel T, Gonullu D, Oncu M et al (2009) Comparison of controlled-intermittent anal dilatation and lateral internal sphincterotomy in the treatment of chronic anal fissures: a prospective, randomized study. Int J Surg 7:228-231

Zbar AP, Pescatori M (2004) Functional outcome following lateral internal anal sphincterotomy for chronic anal fissure. Colorectal Dis 6:210-211

2 Hemorrhoids

2.1 Introduction

Although only a limited number of surgical procedures to treat anal fissure have been described in the literature, many surgical procedures are available to treat hemorrhoids. We know that there are also many possible complications of hemorrhoid surgery. Early complications include hemorrhage; somewhat later there may be abscess formation, and over the long-term incontinence (Hall and Goldberg, 2003).

I think it is best to first cover the most commonly performed operations. According to the Annual Report of the Italian Society of Colo-Rectal Surgery (Società Italiana di Chirurgia Colo-Rettale, SICCR), published in Techniques in Coloproctology by Occelli and Bruni, there are two well-established methods (the Milligan-Morgan and the Ferguson procedures), one that is gaining in importance (transanal hemorrhoidal dearterialization/Doppler-guided hemorrhoidal artery ligation, THD/DGHAL), and another that is becoming slightly less popular (the procedure for prolapse and hemorrhoids, PPH). The complications associated with the two well-established procedures and with THD are on the whole well-known, whereas PPH/stapled hemorrhoidopexy can cause unusual problems that are sometimes severe and are therefore discussed here separately.

In comparing the problem of fissure with that of hemorrhoids, surgeons (especially in Italy) tend to forget one thing that the two conditions have in common: only rarely is surgical treatment necessary, perhaps in only one out of ten cases if not even less often. And clearly, the more we operate, the greater the risk of complications.

In this chapter, instead of making a list of complications and commenting on them, as in the previous chapter, we discuss their prevention and/or their causes during surgery. For practical purposes, we shall start with the latter.

2.2 Surgical Complications After Manual Hemorrhoidectomy (Ferguson and Milligan-Morgan Procedures): Live from the Operating Room

Let's imagine we are at the operating table, faced with a case that is not simple: a 60-year-old multiparous woman with fourth-degree hemorrhoids, (i.e., irreducible ones) that have an external fibrotic component (Fig. 2.1). We have decided to perform a hemorrhoidectomy, which, as shown by various meta-analyses, is the most radical operation in a proctologist's repertoire.

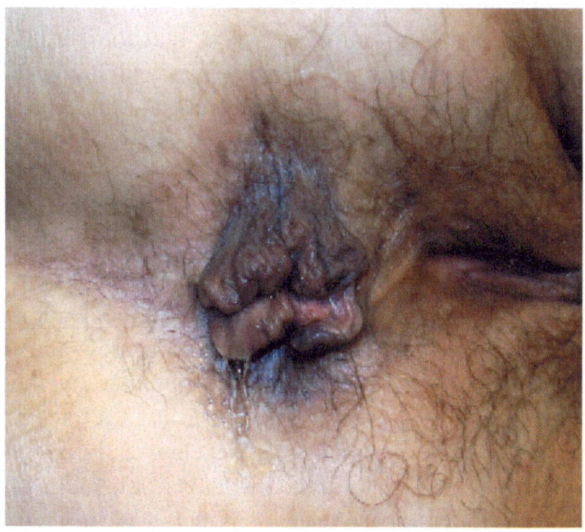

Fig. 2.1 Hemorrhoids with fibrotic external tissue

Before proceeding, it is necessary to insert one comment about preoperative antibiotic prophylaxis. While some excellent surgeons do not use it, it is definitely necessary in cardiopathic and immunodepressed patients. Cases of Fournier's gangrene after hemorrhoidectomy have been reported. Although very rare, this complication can lead to abdominoperineal resection of the rectum.

Assume that we are performing a Ferguson procedure not only because that is what I do most often, but also because Jóhansson and Påhlman (2006) reported that continence is better after a Ferguson than after a Milligan-Morgan procedure, and our patient already has deficient anal sphincters.

Does the patient's position have an effect on the complication rate? The only difference is that if the patient is in the *jack-knife* position the hemorrhoids are usually "deflated" such that no blood runs into the operative field, which simplifies the work of the surgeon and the surgical team.

Before the operation begins, we must consider the preparation by the anesthetist. The patient is awake, which means that she has been given spinal anesthesia, placing her at greater risk of urinary retention after surgery. We therefore caution the anesthetist not to give the patient large volumes of intravenous fluids. (If the patient was an elderly man with prostate problems it would be essential that he receive minimal fluids). The first surgical move that we make is one that can easily cause damage, i.e., insertion of the anal retractor (as this is a Ferguson procedure and assessing the rectum is never a bad idea), since we know that the patient has weak sphincters due to her age and multiple deliveries. To avoid stretching the muscle fibers and thereby damage the continence mechanism, it is best to use an instrument that does not overly dilate and is not too wide (< 32 mm), such as a Fansler, Ferguson, or Sapimed Beak dilator (Fig. 2.2). Some surgeons prefer the 36-mm circular anal dilator (CAD) used on PPH. It should be noted that even if the patient were a young male with a narrow anus, we could damage (lacerate) the sphincter by the excessively energetic insertion of a large retractor. It is therefore essential that we choose the right instrument and perform the maneuver delicately. If a Milligan-Morgan procedure is being performed, an anal retractor is not needed.

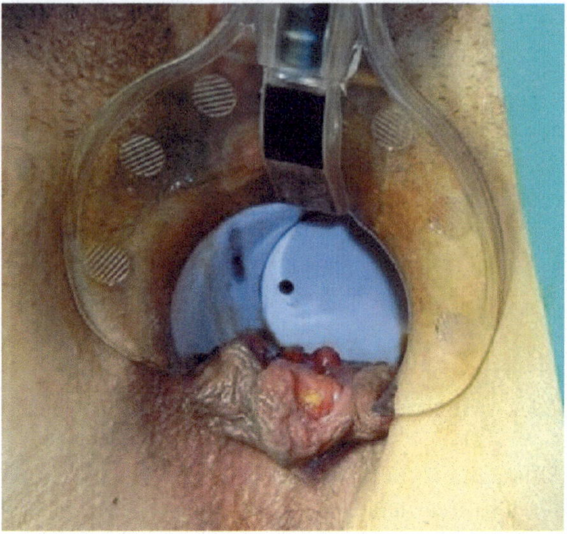

Fig. 2.2 Ferguson's hemorrhoidectomy with the patient in the lithotomy position. The anal retractor used to prevent sphincter trauma should not be too large. A Beak dilator (Sapimed) was used in this case

We now make the surgical incision. If the patient is in the lithotomy position, we do not start at the anterior hemorrhoid as this will cause blood to fill the operative field. The incision, especially in the Ferguson procedure, should be sufficiently long and in a narrow V-shape, extending to the perianal skin; otherwise, after suturing, there will be unaesthetic "dog's ears," which will result in painful swelling. A cold scalpel is used to avoid skin burns, which could facilitate suture dehiscence and cause pain.

Next we identify the internal sphincter (obviously this is also done in the Milligan-Morgan procedure), so that we can avoid injury to it during excision of the hemorrhoidal nodules. Note: Some surgeons, when performing the Ferguson procedure, place a Kelly under the hemorrhoid and cut the tissue from above. While this is a quick method that prevents bleeding, I do not use it because it does not provide a good view of the internal sphincter proper. In fact, with the Kelly one might even inadvertently pinch the sphincter.

We are now ready to excise the nodules. This may be done with scissors, a cold scalpel or electrocautery, Ultracision (the ultrasonic scalpel), a laser (infrequently used now), or radiowaves.

If we are performing a Milligan-Morgan and not a Ferguson procedure, LigaSure could certainly be used. In fact, a Milligan-Morgan with LigaSure appears to be associated with fewer postoperative problems. In a review published in Colorectal Disease in 2010, Milito et al. evaluated randomized prospective trials (including SICCR: LigaSure vs. traditional Milligan-Morgan, Ferguson, and PPH). The results regarding postoperative complications after using LigaSure were: less pain than after traditional hemorrhoidectomy and the same level of patient satisfaction as after PPH. In particular, a trial of PPH vs. LigaSure demonstrated that postoperative pain is the same after these two procedures (Kraemer et al., 2005). However, it should be noted that with LigaSure the hemorrhoids are removed, so that the procedure is more radical than stapled hemorrhoidopexy. LigaSure is not associated with a lower risk of bleeding – there is no statistically significant difference between the procedures – nor is it associated with a faster, uneventful recovery.

The comparison made by Fareed et al. (2009) between LigaSure and Ferguson hemorrhoidectomy showed that LigaSure is associated with fewer postoperative pain and less problematic recovery. The complications that occur after Ligasure are listed in Table 2.1.

Continuing our operation: During dissection of the hemorrhoids there will be bleeding, especially if scissors are used or a cold scalpel. Since the less blood the better, we could proceed slowly and coagulate the hemorrhoidal plexus as we go. I use a maneuver (described in "Tricks of the Trade", below) to reduce intraoperative bleeding which seems to work well and was also mentioned in the chapter on anal fissure. With the tip of a pair of forceps, I touch the tissue, as is done using an electrocautery device, to excise the pile. At the same time, the instruments nurse touches the other end of the forceps with the electric scalpel.

Obviously, in a Ferguson procedure it is less essential at this phase to obtain hemostasis because one can count on the suture – in part, a hemostatic suture – that will later close the surgical wound. However, it is still important to avoid cutting the underlying fibers of the internal sphincter or else postoperatively there may be soiling (Fig. 2.3).

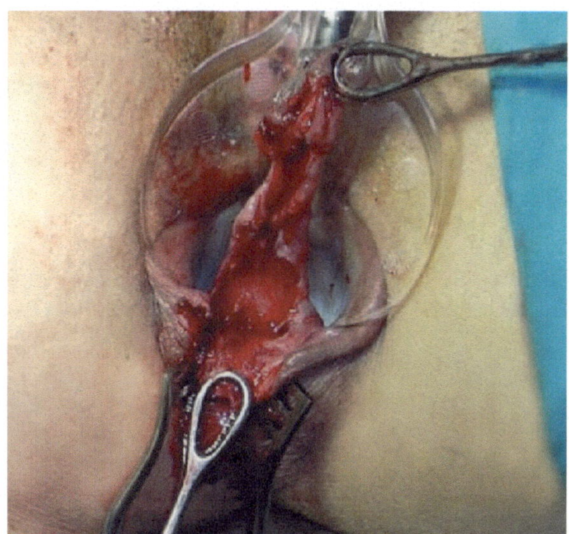

Fig. 2.3 Ferguson's hemorrhoidectomy with the patient in the lithotomy position. Hemorrhoid excision can be extended a few centimeters upward if there is a concomitant rectal internal mucosal prolapse. A report by Gaj and Trecca (2005), based on a study carried out at the Italian coloproctology units, showed that a concomitant rectal internal muocosal prolapse is present in about one-third of hemorrhoid patients. To reduce the risk of postoperative anal incontinence, the internal sphincter should be identified to avoid its damage, as shown in the figure

Now we reach the apex of the hemorrhoid. If there is no prolapse of the internal mucosa of the rectum we can stop here; otherwise it is necessary to extend the dissection upwards for 1-3 cm (Fig. 2.4). Should the hemorrhoidal peduncle be ligated? Consider that a peduncle is not always present. If one performs a Milligan-Morgan procedure with diathermy using the technique of Lentini or Phillips (2009), coagulation is sufficient. If a traditional Milligan-Morgan or Ferguson procedure is

Table 2.1 Percentage of complications in various case series after hemorrhoidectomy with LigaSure

	Luo, 2010 Colorect Dis n = 207	Wang, 2006 World J Surg n = 42	Kraemer, 2005 Dis Colon Rectum n = 25	Chung, 2003 Dis Colon Rectum n = 30
Urinary retention	0	2	1	1
Severe rectal bleeding	6	1	1	1
Anal stenosis	0	2	-	-
Severe constipation	0	3	-	-

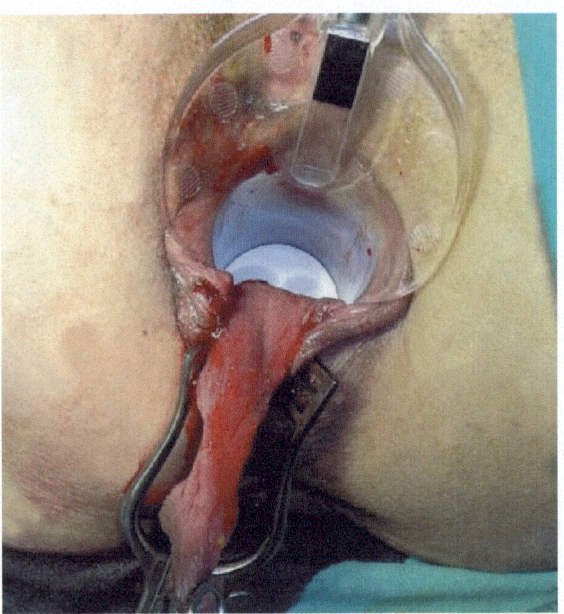

Fig. 2.4 Hemorrhoid excision can be extended above the anorectal ring if there is a rectal internal mucosal prolapse

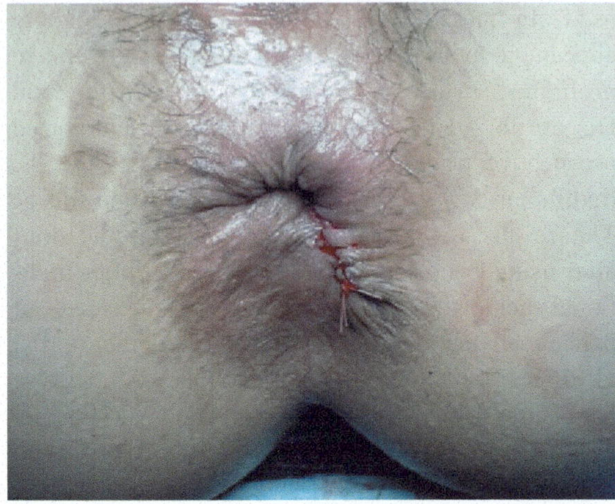

Fig. 2.5 Vicryl Rapid is used to allow the spontaneous drainage of an incidental hematoma or seroma, thus preventing local sepsis

being performed, then a transfixing stitch, normally of 2/0 Vicryl, is appropriate. After having tied the thread, be careful not to pull excessively before it is cut to avoid bleeding due to tissue laceration.

Exeresis has now been completed. In a Ferguson procedure, it would have been less extensive, to avoid the risk of anal stenosis. Note that the Ferguson procedure should not be a "sutured Milligan-Morgan," as this will result in traction between the sutures such that the risk of both dehiscence and, later, anal stenosis will increase. Dehiscence after a Ferguson procedure, or, more often, failure of the wound to heal after a Milligan-Morgan, especially when accompanied by anal spasm, can give rise to a chronic anal fissure. In addition, the wound may not heal if the patient has undiagnosed anal cancer, is immunodepressed, suffers from diabetes, Crohn's disease, or a bacterial superinfection, or is undergoing chemotherapy. The treatment for this patient population is discussed later in the chapter.

At this point in a Milligan-Morgan procedure, extreme care must be taken regarding hemostasis and wound edges, to minimize the risk of postoperative bleeding. In a Ferguson procedure, the first step at this point would be suturing.

Is the risk of hemorrhage necessitating re-operation associated less with closed (Ferguson) than with open (Milligan-Morgan) hermorrhoidectomy? In almost all randomized prospective trials comparing the two techniques, no difference was determined. But, as seen in a table compiled by Hall and Goldberg, in the book edited by Northover and Longo "Reoperations in Colorectal Surgery", published in 2003, after the Ferguson procedure the incidence of re-operation due to hemorrhage varied between 0 and 1.3% (0.06% in a multicenter study of 34 cases conducted by Rosen et al., 0.04% in a study by Korosok on Ferguson hemorrhoidectomy in an outpatient setting (2005), while after Milligan-Morgan hemorrhoidectomy the incidence was higher, ranging from 1% to 1.8%.

This is the reason why, in the past 15 years, I have mostly performed closed hemorrhoidectomy; indeed, there did seem to be a lower incidence of severe postoperative bleeding. Since in two out of ten cases the patient was sent home after one hour, I have a greater sense of security with closed hemorrhoidectomy, knowing that there will not be much bleeding. (This may be purely psychological, as I have not done any statistical analyses to see whether in my patients, the reduction in bleeding is significant).

Returning again to our operation: What suture material should be used for the surgical wound after a Ferguson procedure? To reduce the risk of postoperative sepsis, it is best to use catgut (if available) or Vicryl Rapid (Figs. 2.5 and 2.6). Nivatvongs, at the Mayo Clinic, observed that

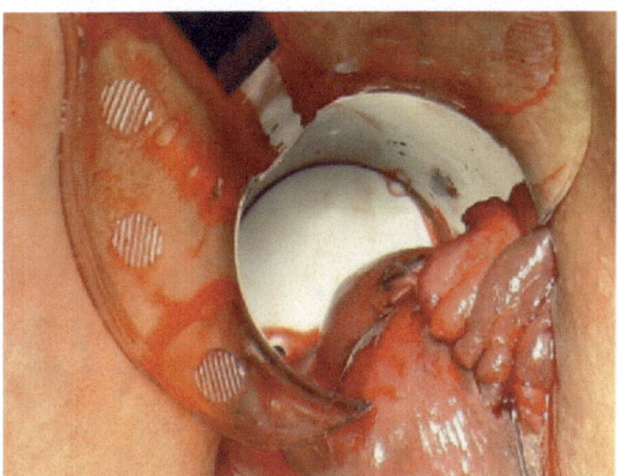

Fig. 2.6 Completed suture of the surgical wound after Ferguson hemorrhoidectomy

Vicryl Rapid is reabsorbed faster than standard vicryl and gives way if an infected hematoma has formed, permitting drainage of the infected site. The data in the literature suggest that suture thickness has an effect on pain (Khubchandani, 2005, among others). It is better to use 4/0 or 5/0 sutures than 2/0 or 3/0. The degree of tension on the sutures should not be excessive, to avoid tissue laceration, but a small amount of tension is needed to help obtain good hemostasis. Also, rather than suturing the skin over the entire length of the surgical wound, it may be better to leave ~0.5 cm open distally, allowing better drainage of secretions.

However, there are no evidence-based rules. I usually suture the whole wound but in my experience, in one out of three cases at least one stitch in the final centimeters gives way. This occurs in 25% of cases, according to Jóhansson and Påhlman (2006). According to Carapeti et al. (1999), the incidence is 60%; however, in the UK, the Milligan-Morgan procedure, not the Ferguson procedure, is firmly established.

If hemostasis is unsatisfactory or there is blood leaking from the suture line, we may want to continue with the same suture thread or turn back towards the high part of the anal canal and towards the peduncle, as some surgeons do. While this is a reasonable strategy, care must be taken to avoid placing tension on the sutures in the other nodules, causing loss of tissue in the anal canal, and provoking lacerations followed by fibrosis and then stenosis.

We are now ready to move on to the other nodules, using the same expertise. In a Milligan-Morgan procedure, it is commonly known that bridges of skin and mucosa must be left intact. If they are not large enough, the patient may develop anal stenosis. If there are hemorrhoids under the bridges, so-called accessory hemorrhoids, they could be left alone, as these nodules may regress over time. If this does not turn out to be the case, then if the nodules are internal an elastic ligature can be applied, or if they are external the patient can be re-operated on in an outpatient setting. There is also an alternative maneuver (which I learned 30 years ago at St. Mark's Hospital): Place stitches in a U-shaped formation starting from the distal rectum, catching the residual hemorrhoid at the muco-cutaneous bridge, right above the dentate line (resulting in less postoperative pain), and then returning to the distal rectum. This hemorrhoidopexy makes the nodule ischemic.

At this point, the operation is nearly completed. Now we must make two decisions regarding postoperative pain. The first is whether to insert a hemostatic tampon. The answer is no, unless it is a soft Spongostan tampon. The second is whether to inject Botox into the internal sphincter, as recently recommended by Patti et al. (2005); however, this is useless in patients with anal hypertonia (which is possible in a male, improbable in a female). Hypertonia increases the likelihood of postoperative pain. An alternative is the application of nitroglycerin cream, which relaxes the muscle.

And what if we had performed an internal sphincterotomy? Although years ago I did just that, in patients who on preoperative manometry had anal hypertonia, I stopped after reading an article by Khubchandani (2002), describing the risk of incontinence associated with this maneuver.

The operation is now finished and in my opinion we have done everything possible to prevent complications. But, before proceeding to THD/DGHAL mucopexy and the Doppler-guided hemorrhoid laser procedure (HeLP), the reader should be reminded of some of the data from the literature. Table 2.2 is a review of the risk of incontinence after the most commonly used hemorrhoidectomy procedures.

Table 2.2 Incontinence after hemorrhoidectomy. A literature review (from Ommer et al., 2008)

Author	Year	Operation	Incontinence (%)
Read	1982	Milligan-Morgan	4
Mc Connell	1983	Parks	0.5
Athanasiadis	1986	Parks	4
Konsten	2000	Milligan-Morgan	20
Ho	2000	Milligan-Morgan	2
Kirsch	2001	Milligan-Morgan	0
Johansson	2002	Milligan-Morgan	8
Ebert	2002	Milligan-Morgan	1
Hetzer	2002	Ferguson	0

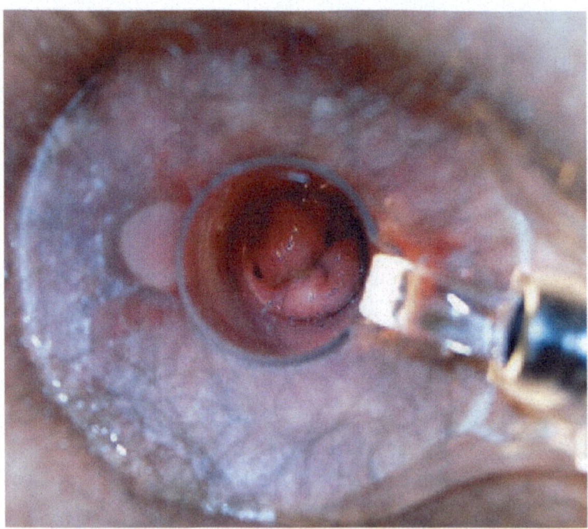

Fig. 2.7 Proctoscopy shows the hemorrhoidal cushions. After hemorrhoidectomy, anal incontinence, if any, is likely to be determined by internal sphincter injuries. According to Hall and Goldberg (2003), anal incontinence is not due to the loss of the hemorrhoidal cushions, because they become abnormal in patients with hemorrhoidal disease

Let me add to this the data from a recent multicenter French study (Soudan et al., 2010), presented at the Congress of the American Society of Colon and Rectal Surgeons (ASRCS). The authors did not observe a single case of incontinence in their 631 patients at one year after hemorrhoidectomy. They had performed 220 Milligan-Morgan procedures and 396 hemorrhoidectomies with anoplasty.

That publication also listed a few other postoperative complications. Early complications, occurring in 7.6% of patients, consisted of 10 cases of rectal bleeding, 13 of urinary retention, 5 of local sepsis, and 7 of fecaloma. Late complications occured at a rate of 8%: 23 cases of anal stenosis, 7 of anal abscess, 3 of delayed wound healing, and 2 of skin tags. According to the authors, the morbidity rate was extremely low because all of the procedures were performed by specialists.

As can be expected, in an emergency hemorrhoidectomy, which is usually indicated for patients with thrombosed hemorrhoids who fail to respond to topical or systemic treatment, there will be more complications, incontinence among them (Rasmussen et al., 1991).

Fistulas are very rare and in general are due to sepsis or associated with Crohn's disease. Those that form after the Ferguson procedure may be iatrogenic, caused by an excessively deep suture that reaches the intersphincteric space (Hall and Goldberg, 2003).

I shall end this section by referring to the data from a clinical and endosonographic study performed by Lindsey et al. (2004). Out of 29 patients who came to their attention for continence problems after Milligan-Morgan hemorrhoidectomy, 26 had lesions of the internal sphincter that could be identified on transanal ultrasound examination. In half of these cases, the sphincter was thinner than normal and in the other half there was some fragmentation of the sphincter. It is interesting to note that 12 of the 15 women with postoperative incontinence were found to have obstetric lesions of the external sphincter. These results imply that extreme care is needed when operating on hemorrhoids in a woman with a history of multiple vaginal deliveries, because she might have subclinical lesions that become acute due to the surgical procedure. Furthermore, they show that incontinence after hemorrhoidectomy is associated especially with sphincter lesions. According to Hall and Goldberg (2003), the loss of anal cushions (Fig. 2.7), does not seem to affect continence to any significant degree because they have become abnormal in patients with hemorrhoids.

2.3 THD/DGHAL and Mucopexy (Doppler-guided, Laser-assisted)

I have performed very few of either of these procedures but to the best of my knowledge I have read what has been written about them, in addition to talking and working with colleagues who have performed quite a few.

These techniques are basically minimally invasive, especially THD/DGHAL, and somewhat less so with mucopexy, also called "recto-anal repair." In mucopexy, a continuous suture is used that partly obliterates and partly raises the hemorrhoidal nodule, sometimes accompanied by concomitant internal mucosal prolapse of the rectum (Fig. 2.8).

In general, the more developed the hemorrhoids, the more extensive and the greater the risk of complications, which are, however, mostly not serious. Out of the 100 adverse events reported to Luigi Basso, who directs the SICCR Observatory of Emerging Technology, four occurred after THD (vs. 2 after LigaSure procedures and 49 after PPH).

Dal Monte et al. (2007) reported only 23 complications among 330 patients (ca. 7%) including 7 cases of bleeding (4 early and 3 late), with one reoperation. Other complications were thrombosed hermorrhoids (5), submucosal rectal hematoma (4), fissures (2), urinary retention (2), and hematuria (1). Unusually, in two cases the needle was left in the sutured tissue.

Forrest et al. (2010) observed postoperative pain and a need for analgesia in only 5% of their 77 patients, but their study was not very rigorously performed, although it has the merit of being a single-center study.

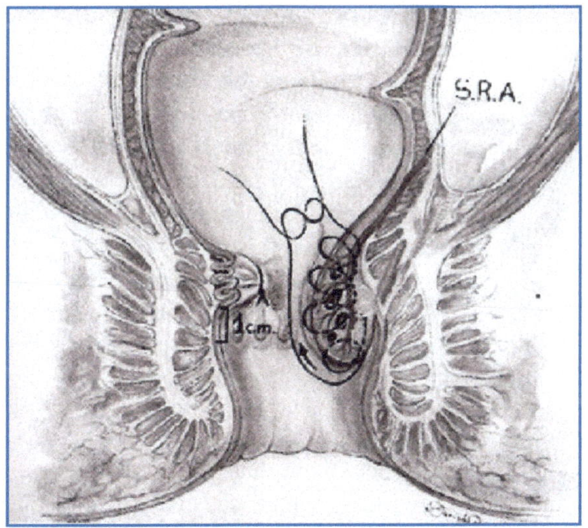

Fig. 2.8 Mucopexy scheme after ligation of the hemorrhoidal vessels, guided by Doppler-ultrasonography. *S.R.A.*, Submucosal rectal anopexy (from Dal Monte et al., 2007)

A more detailed SICCR study (but as it was multicentre some data may have been underestimated), with Infantino as first author, was published in Colorectal Diseases at the end of 2010. One severe hemorrhage and three cases of hemorrhoidal thrombosis were reported in the 114 patients who underwent THD, often with mucopexy, for third-degree hemorrhoids. Postoperative analgesia was required by 30% of these patients.

It is logical to think that the deeper the mucopexy, the more stitches will be needed (an average of 7 per patient) to interrupt the branches of the hemorrhoidal arteries, and the greater the risk of postoperative pain, especially since in the muscular layer of the rectum there are proprioceptive neurons. However, in the case series of Wilkerson et al. (2009), involving 113 patients who underwent DGHAL without mucopexy, 83% did not complain of any postoperative pain.

On the other hand, in a study conducted by Theodoropoulos et al. (2008) in which 147 patients underwent DGHAL, mucopexy, manual hemorrhoidectomy, and minimal mucocutaneous excision for third- or fourth-degree hemorrhoids, 70% of the patients had postoperative pain and requested analgesia. According to the authors, the pain was more often linked to hemorrhoidopexy than to mucopexy. The reason is obvious: if sutures are placed at the level of the hemorrhoids they come into contact with the nerves of the anal canal, especially in cases of fourth-degree hemorrhoids. The article did not mention other complications but it did provide a table with the results of 22 studies on this subject. It is worth consulting.

If THD with mucopexy is performed to treat fourth-degree, nonfibrotic hemorrhoids, the number of complications increases. In a very recent study, by Ratto and Giordano (2011), 8% of the patients had complications of thrombosed hemorrhoids, 6% had rectal bleeding, 14% had urinary retention, and 11% had tenesmus (Table 2.3). As perhaps expected, these results have been rejected by some authors. For example, Sergio Larach and his group in Orlando, Florida (2011, unpublished study) maintain that hemorrhoidal artery ligation (HAL) is associated with the same low number of complications as HAL with mucopexy.

Faucheron et al. (2011) strongly support the use of HAL/rectoanal repair (RAR) Doppler liga-

Table 2.3 Complications after THD in 1195 patients (total 18.5%) (from Giordano et al., 2009; the first author is a consultant for the company which manufactures the THD device)

Complications	%
Pain on postoperative day 1	18.5
Rectal bleeding	12.6
Fever	4.3
Thrombosed hemorrhoids	1.8
Anal fissure	0.8
Urinary retention	0.7
Anal incontinence	0.4
Proctitis	0.2
Fecaloma	0.1

tion and mucopexy for the treatment of fourth-degree hemorrhoids, as shown by their study of 100 patients, 84% of whom were discharged home on the same day as the operation. The incidence of early complications (pain, rectal bleeding, and thrombosed hemorrhoids) was only 9%, and that of late complications (hemorrhage, urgency, thrombosis, and anal fissure) 4%. Only nine recurrences were observed in almost 3 years, but eight patients requested skin tag removal under local anesthesia. These are good results considering the advanced stage of the disease, the low degree of invasiveness of the technique, the length of follow-up, small number of adverse events, and short hospital stay.

Table 2.3 is taken from an important review article and summarizes the complications after THD.

As shown in the table, there were not many complications, which supports the truly minimally invasive aspect of the procedure. One item does stand out, however: the incidence of postoperative pain, which is not exactly negligible compared to the 0 reported by Eu's group in Singapore (where mucopexy is not performed). The same holds true if the incidence is compared with the 2% reported by Szmulowicz et al. (2010) in Cleveland, Ohio (where mucopexy is certainly performed).

Altomare et al., in a multicenter Italian study presented at the ASCRS in 2010, compared THD plus mucopexy to PPH in patients with third-degree hemorrhoids, so that this study is similar to the one from Singapore. The authors confirmed that patients have less postoperative pain after THD.

Recently (Giamundo et al., 2011), a different method for treating hemorrhoids was proposed, using Doppler ultrasound to identify the hemorrhoidal arteries and a laser probe to occlude them via a special proctoscope, with necrosis extending for a depth of 0.5 cm. This procedure can be performed in an outpatient setting and does not require anesthesia. Only three out of 30 patients complained of postoperative pain; four had slight intraoperative bleeding, requiring the use of hemostatic sutures in two cases. This is the hemorrhoid laser procedure (HeLP) and is truly minimally invasive as well as thoroughly effective, provided the patient does not have marked hemorrhoidal prolapse.

Treatment of the various complications is described later in the chapter. Next we look at PPH which, as already noted, can cause unusual problems, some of which may be very serious.

2.4 Stapled Hemorrhoidopexy (PPH)

For the sake of variety, the material in this section is presented somewhat differently. We first look at the usual complications that occur after PPH, then at the unusual, more interesting ones (i.e., those which are never, or almost never described after hemorrhoidectomy).

The list of usual complications is a long one, reflecting the intense interest in stapled hemorrhoidopexy in the literature for at least a decade. Nowadays it is used less often because various meta-analyses have shown that it is associated with a greater recurrence of hemorrhoids than is the case with hemorrhoidectomy, although it may also have been the complications discussed in the following section that led surgeons to use PPH with moderation. For surgeons still performing PPH, the information provided in this section should help to reduce the complication rate. In the immediate postoperative period, one in four patients develops complications (Knight et al., 2008), but if complications can be avoided, PPH is an ideal procedure. The absence of surgical wounds in the anal canal greatly reduces, sometimes even to zero, the incidence of postoperative problems, including those that cause frequent complaints in hemorrhoidectomy patients.

2.4.1 Hemorrhage

Hemorrhage necessitating re-operation occurs in 2-5% of cases, and hemorrhage requiring the patient to be admitted to the hospital so that hemostasis can be obtained in up to 8% (note that, according to Guenin et al. (2005), the incidence is only 0.4%). Knight et al. (2008) reported severe hemorrhage in 5.9% of their 695 patients.

The risk of severe bleeding is greatly reduced if a manual suture is made on the staple line. There have been sensational cases in which the stapler cut but did not "sew," i.e., stapler malfunction.

A woman I saw as an outpatient, who had been operated on in Scotland, underwent a Hartmann procedure because of severe bleeding after PPH. Six years after stoma reversal, she had to be operated on again, for hemorrhoids. However, to my best knowledge, none of the meta-analyses based on prospective randomized trials comparing PPH and hemorrhoidectomy demonstrated that hemorrhage occurs more frequently after stapled hemorrhoidopexy. In a systematic review (one step below a meta-analysis), Laughlan et al. (2009) maintained that there is less bleeding after PPH. The data for this study were prepared by the company that produces the staplers.

According to Brown et al. (2006), who had to re-admit four out of 52 patients who underwent PPH in day surgery because they developed severe bleeding, two factors reduce the risk of this complication: use of the PPH03 stapler, which provides better hemostasis, and maximum tightening of the stapler's closing mechanism before "firing" the staples.

A more modern variant of the procedure is laparoscopic-assisted PPH, proposed by Bozdag et al. (2008). This approach provides better visibility but increases the risk of hemorrhage, as reported in 5 out of 18 patients (27.8%). Note that one-third of these procedures were performed by residents, and only one of the patients, with severe bleeding, had to undergo re-operation.

Regarding re-operations after PPH, Brusciano et al. (2004) pointed out that if a patient who underwent stapled hemorrhoidopexy is re-operated on, the risk of postoperative bleeding increases.

Finally, a Brazilian trial of a new device for PPH deserves mention (Regadas, 2005). Bleeding that was not severe was observed by the authors in 11% of their 85 patients, with perianal hematoma occurring in 3.5%.

2.4.2 Other Complications

Regarding anal stenosis, the results of a prospective trial, conducted by Senagore et al. (2004), comparing PPH and Ferguson hemorrhoidectomy, supported use of the Ferguson procedure (although without statistical significance). The rate of stenosis was 0 after Ferguson hemorrhoidectomy vs. 2.6% after PPH. Two retrospective studies reported stenosis after PPH in 1.6-8.8% of cases (Ng, 2004; Oughriss, 2005); however only 1.4% of the patients with stenosis required surgery (Ng, 2006) (Fig. 2.9).

Incontinence is always mild and may be due to small lesions of the internal sphincter, which the group of Seow-Choen identified with transanal ultrasound using a rotating probe. These findings were not confirmed in a similar study conducted by Altomare et al. and Gravié et al. (2005) reported the occurrence of soiling in 10% of their patients at one-year follow-up after PPH. Knight et al. (2008) reported only 1.1% soiling in their case series. Giordano et al. (2009), in their meta-analysis, also found 1.1% soiling after PPH vs. 2.6%

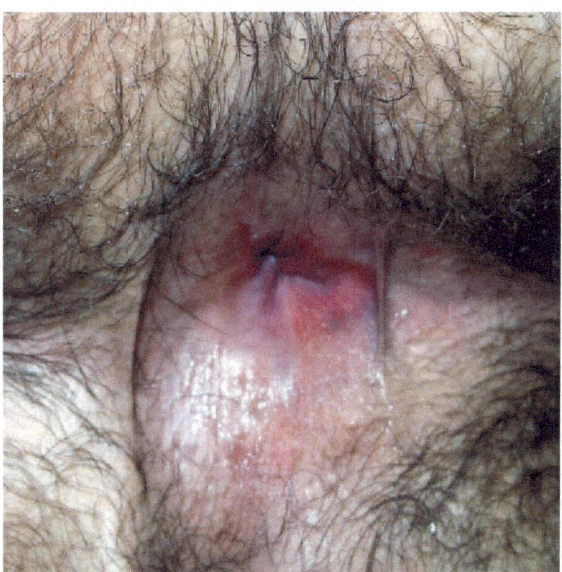

Fig. 2.9 Anal stenosis after Milligan-Morgan hemorrhoidectomy

after hemorrhoidectomy, but the difference was not statistically significant.

According to Carriero et al. (2001), there was no case of fecal incontinence among their 127 patients who underwent PPH with the Lone Star retractor system using small elastic stay hooks, which provides better exposure of mucosal-hemorrhoidal prolapse and does not traumatize the sphincters.

Pigot et al. (2006) concluded that hemorrhoid removal with PPH, i.e., making the purse-string further down and letting the suture fall into the anal canal, results in a greater risk of incontinence (Fig. 2.10).

Anal fissure is rare after PPH: 0.2% in Slawik's (2007) series and 0.9% in that of Knight et al. (2008); it may be due to trauma to the endoanal epithelium during insertion of the stapler. It is a rare complication according to both studies but was 2.8% in the meta-analysis performed by Giordano et al. (2009), i.e., similar to the 2.3% after hemorrhoidectomy.

Urinary retention has no association with the surgical technique used but is linked to other factors. In a multicenter English study (Knight et al., 2008) on complications after PPH, it was the most frequent one (2.8%). Spinal anesthesia, age (> 50 years), sex (M>F), endovenous fluids, the number of hemorrhoidal nodules removed (> 1), pre-existing urinary problems, and anal tampons after surgery all increase the risk of urinary retention (Toyonaga et al., 2006).

Abscesses and anal fisulas are rare, with an incidence of 0-3% in various case series (Hetzer et al., 2002; Senagore et al., 2004; Ortiz et al., 2005; Huang et al., 2007).

There are no alarming reports in the literature about early postoperative pain, except for an article by surgeons at St. Mark's Hospital (Cheetham et al., 2000), who reported that they had to interrupt a trial on PPH vs. hemorrhoidectomy because of seven cases of severe postoperative proctalgia among the 12 patients who had undergone stapled hemorrholidopexy.

In Singapore, a prospective study was performed comparing postoperative pain in a total of 54 PPH and THD patients, all with third-degree hemorrhoids (Ong et al., 2010). In the first week after surgery, less pain was reported in the THD group (0 vs. 3 patients) and patient satisfaction was greater.

In defense of PPH, it should be emphasized that the surgeons in Singapore do not routinely perform hemorrhoidopexy with a stapler but rather hemorrhoidectomy with a stapler, so that the procedure is more radical, i.e., the purse-string is set lower than in standard PPH and the suture is thus located in

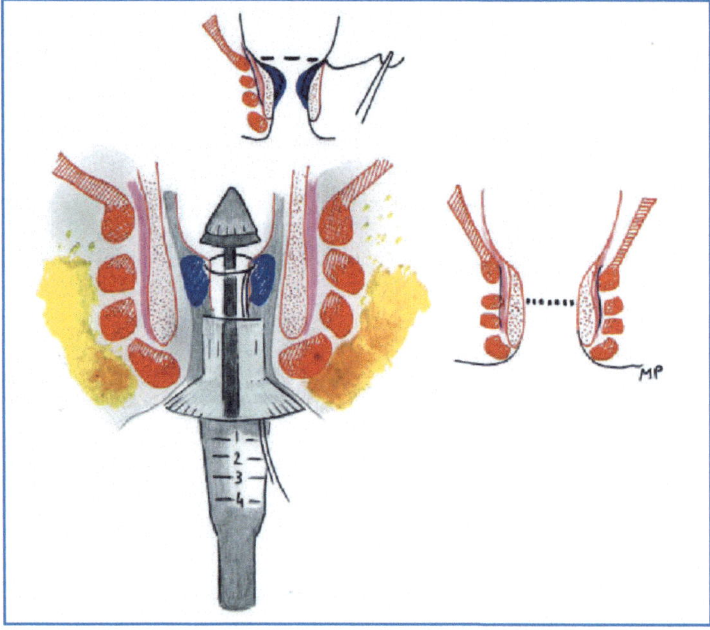

Fig. 2.10 Stapled hemorrhoidectomy (not - pexy). Part of the hemorrhoids (in *blue*) is excised. A "Purse-string" suture is placed 1-2 cm above the anorectal ring, with the suture in the anal canal

the upper part of the anal canal. Accordingly, their patients presumably have more postoperative pain than after a standard PPH. However, only 1.6% of patients had pain severe enough to warrant re-admission (Ng et al., 2006).

In Singapore, or elsewhere, pain can occur even after stapled hemorrhoidopexy. Several authors have suggested solutions to the problem beyond administering the usual analgesia. In a recent article, Imbelloni et al. (2008) maintained that a bilateral pudendal nerve block is effective in reducing pain after hemorrhoidectomy (not after PPH). In 2009, Tegon et al. suggested that local administration of opioids at the end of a hemorrhoidectomy procedure can reduce postoperative pain. Similar strategies or treatments might help in the rare cases of intense pain after stapled hemorrhoidopexy.

In theory, anal spasm should not be the main cause of pain after PPH. The sphincter muscles do not usually remain hypertonic after dilatation with a 36-mm CAD. However, there is a syndrome of painful defecation after PPH (discussed further on) in which pain resolves after treatment with nifedipine p.o., because the drug relaxes the internal sphincter. In these patients (Thaha et al., 2005), the sphincter was hypertonic on postoperative manometry, whereas this was not the case in the patients studied by Phillips' group in a well-received article published in Lancet (2000), which caused an uproar among PPH advocates. Thaha's patients had pain on defecation, while Phillips et al.'s patients had pain all the time. All of these patients had been operated on with the same technique, as verified by Nystrom, an expert in PPH and one of Phillips' coauthors. Thus, the reason for this and other such discrepancies is unclear. Perhaps the endings of the pudendal nerves, irritated by the staples, and not the spastic internal sphincter caused the pain after stapled hemorrhoidopexy.

The reader might ask why I have not mentioned the most obvious cause of pain after PPH: staples erroneously placed in the anal canal instead of the rectum. If the purse-string is made lower than it should be, i.e., on the anorectal ring instead of the distal rectum, that certainly explains the postoperative pain. The technique itself should not be blamed.

Nevertheless, there are over 5000 successful cases, i.e., with only minimal pain, a score of 3 on the visual analog scale (VAS, which ranges from 0 to 10), and all of them reported by the group of Eu and Ng, in Singapore. In all 5000 cases, the purse-string was positioned just above the anorectal ring, and the staples were in the anal canal, so that the procedure was a radical hemorrhoidectomy rather than a hemorrhoidopexy.

Clearly, there is still much to be understood regarding several aspects of pain after surgery for hemorrhoids, and especially after PPH.

There are fewer problems with secretions, pruritus ani, and delayed wound healing after PPH than after hemorrhoidectomy, as shown by various meta-analyses (e.g., Tjandra and Chan, 2007). This means that the recovery period after PPH is shorter and less unpleasant than after manual hemorrhoidectomy. Only 1.6% of patients operated on by Knight et al. (2008), 58% for third-degree and 42% for fourth-degree hemorrhoids, suffered from pruritus ani postoperatively.

Scar formation after PPH is less problematic than after hemorrhoidectomy for two reasons: first, because a double suture is often used, i.e., additional stitches are placed over the initial stitches to obtain good hemostasis, and second because the surgical wound after resection of mucosal prolapse is not surrounded by the internal sphincter, preventing the interruption of scar formation by any muscle spasms that may occur.

Defecation urgency and tenesmus are not rare and occur in 3-25% of patients in various case series. In a survey of surgeons of the ASCRS, the rate rises to over 40%, leading Khubachandani to entitle a recent article (2009) "Is there a PPH syndrome?" It is important to note that almost half of the surgeons in the USA who perform PPH answered, "Yes it does," but added that they continued to perform the procedure, as done by the group of Basdanis in Grece, who also described the PPH syndrome two years later in the same journal. Evidently they do not consider this syndrome to be a major problem.

Moreover, it is clearly the case that there is also a "post-manual-hemorrhoidectomy syndrome," which consists of anal pain or discomfort for days or even weeks, secretions, pruritus, slight rectal bleeding, slow wound healing, etc. Yet we continue to perform hemorrhoidectomy; in fact, experts claim that it is the gold standard for the treatment of hemorrhoids (see the meta-analysis by Nisar et al., 2004). According to John Northover of St. Mark's Hospital, the best operation for hemorrhoids is " the operation one knows how to perform best.". The attitudes cited in this and the previous paragraph clearly dispute the claims for evidence-based medicine.

According to the meta-analysis performed by Giordano et al. (2009), the risk of tenesmus is significantly higher after PPH than after hemorrhoidectomy (13.9% vs. 0, p < 0.001). The problem is caused by the fact that the rectal reservoir is smaller after mucosectomy and fibrosis forms around the staples, which can disturb or chronically stimulate nerve endings. These nerve endings lead to the pudendal nerves and then on to the brain via the spinal cord, arriving in areas of the cortex and subcortex that light up on dynamic MRI (Bittorf et al., 2006).

The rectum has an adaptive reflex that allows the postponement of defecation, by adapting to the bolus of stool so that the stimulus to defecate disappears for quite a while. This does not occur if staples or fibrosis alter the path of the reflex. The result is defecation urgency, i.e. the need to "run" to the bathroom. The treatment for severe cases of urgency is not simple. It consists of staple removal and muco-mucosal re-anastomosis of the rectum, a rather invasive procedure.

2.4.3 Chronic Proctalgia and the Post-defecation Pain Syndrome

This syndrome occurs in 2-3% of patients, according to Ravo et al. (2002), Thaha (2005), and Knight et al. (2008). The pain can be associated with tenesmus due to fibrosis around the staples, which is very hard to cure, and/or to reactive hypertonia of the internal sphincter, which can be successfully treated with 20 mg of nifedipine p.o. bid. However, little can be done to prevent this type of pain since in PPH the staples have to be "fired." It may be that if the purse-string is made higher up, while avoiding removal of most of the smooth muscle of the rectum during excision of the mucosal cylinder, the staples remain further from the vulnerable nerve endings.

Lacerda-Filho et al. (2009) successfully used gabapentin and amitriptylline to treat neuropathic pain after PPH. In this section, we go back a step and consider pain in the first few postoperative days.

Early preoperative pain is not as severe after PPH as after hemorrhoidectomy, which was the basis for the initial success of the new technique. A large majority of the prospective studies on PPH compared PPH and Milligan-Morgan hemorrhoidectomy. The meta-analysis of Tjandra and Chan (2007) examined 25 trials; in 20 of them, the hemorrhoidectomy was a Milligan–Morgan procedure.

While I used the Ferguson procedure in 7 out of 10 cases, I also have 15 years of experience with PPH. (My group reported the first stapled rectal mucosectomy, in 1997, in Techniques in Coloproctology: see www.ucp-club.it/medici_articolo.asp). In those of my patients who underwent Ferguson hemorrhoidectomy (and who were on analgesics), there was very little or no pain and certainly not more pain than experienced by patients who underwent stapled hemorrhoidectomy. However, I have not confirmed this observation in a comparative study, although the postoperative VAS, which we administered for a few years 24-48 hours after surgery, was usually < 4 (on a scale of 0-10).

Based on their randomized prospective trial, Ho and Ho (2006) compiled a table in which VAS results after PPH and Ferguson hemorrhoidetomy were compared; the scores did not differ significantly. Comparisons of the Ferguson and Milligan-Morgan procedures showed that the former is associated with less pain and faster wound healing (You et al., 2005) as well as better anal continence (Johansson et al., 2006).

According to Guenin et al. (2005), who performed 514 Ferguson hemorrhoidecomies, the procedure should be considered the gold standard in the treatment of hemorrhoids because it is associated with very few postoperative complications (3.4%): severe incontinence in only 1% and recovery or improvement in 94.6% of patients at 4.7 years after surgery.

An advantage of PPH is the recovery period, as the absence of wounds in the anal canal allows a quicker recovery and an earlier return to work. However Giordano's meta-analysis (2009) cited several randomized trials reporting a ten-fold lower recurrence after hemorrhoidectomy for third-degree hemorrhoids than after PPH. Mattana et al. (2007) reported a seven-fold lower recurrence after hemorrhoidectomy for fourth-degree hemorrhoids. Another meta-analysis found that overall, (without considering hemorrhoid grade), there was a greater chance of recurrence after PPH than after hemorrhoidectomy: 5.7:1 (Tjandra and Chan, 2007).

But what does recurrence have to do with complications? The answer is that the fear of complications (postoperative pain after surgery for hemorrhoids, or, as discussed in Chap. 3, stool incontinence after surgery for anal fistula) induces patients to seek new, expensive methods of treatment—especially in the case of PPH for patients with hemorrhoids and of fistula plug for those with anal fistula. In the literature, disease persistence or recurrence after either of these procedures is reported to be as high as 50%. If these procedures are rejected (as has already been the case with cryo- and laser therapy for hemorrhoids and with artificial bowel sphincters) in favor of those with a better curative effect, the lack of attention paid to the correct indications for these latter procedures and to the long-term results may lead to more serious problems. Nevertheless, as can well be appreciated, when given the opportunity to try a new procedure, we are eager to determine its efficacy and thus to use it as often as possible.

2.4.4 Retained Staples and Bleeding Granulomatous Polyps

Bleeding granulomatous polyps can occur concomitantly with other lesions that are due to retained staples floating in the rectum. Both cause rectal bleeding, and sometimes pain. It should be noted that pain is a frequent cause of re-operation after PPH. In the cases series of Brusciano et al. (2004) it reached 11% at one year after surgery.

Removing a retained staple detected on digital rectal examination, proctoscopy, CT scan or endoanal ultrasound examination (Fig. 2.11) may seem to be a trivial maneuver, but to avoid rectal bleeding and laceration the staple should be grabbed with a long Kelly clamp and the wound briefly coagulated with diathermy. The staple can thus be removed from the tissue without adverse consequences (Fig. 2.12).

Drummond and Wright (2007) reported the case of a patient with recurrent rectal bleeding due to retained staples which could be felt on digital rectal examination. In my opinion, it is better not to remove the staples unless it is clear that they are causing pain

Fig. 2.11 a Retained staples in a patient with chronic proctalgia, in whom a stapled hemorrhoidopexy was performed 10 years before. Transanal ultrasonography with a rotating probe shows staples located above the anorectal ring, posteriorly (*arrows*). The patient is in the Sims position

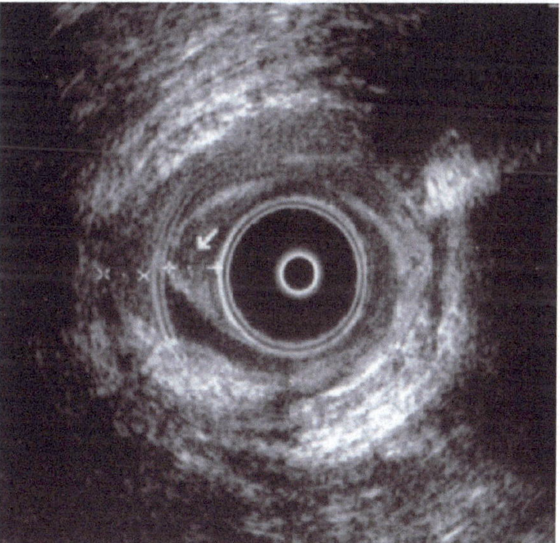

Fig. 2.11 b Symptoms (pain, rectal bleeding, and constipation) are also due to an incomplete relaxation of the puborectalis muscle during defecation. As shown by the markers (*left*), muscle opening is only 4.9 mm, instead of > 10 mm. There is a concomitant rectal internal mucosal prolapse (mixed echogenicity area 6.1 mm long) and a relapsing persistent hemorrhoid, posteriorly, shown by markers (*right*). This is a typical case in which symptom recurrence after PPH is linked to constipation because of forced straining at defecation against the muscle, which does not properly relax

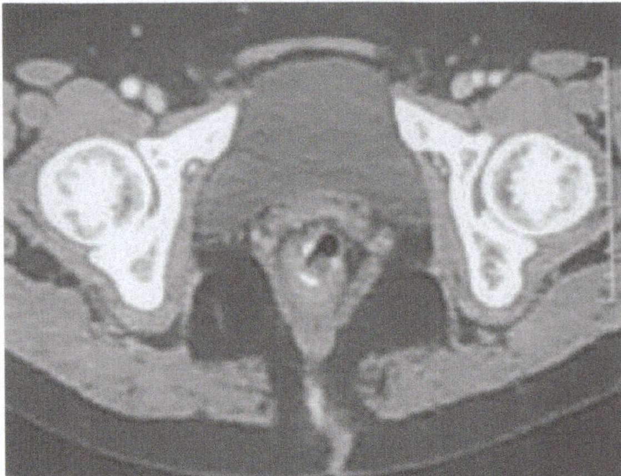

Fig. 2.12 a CT-scan in a patient with rectal bleeding, obstructed defecation, and proctalgia 2 years after PPH. CT-scan shows the hyperintense retained staples

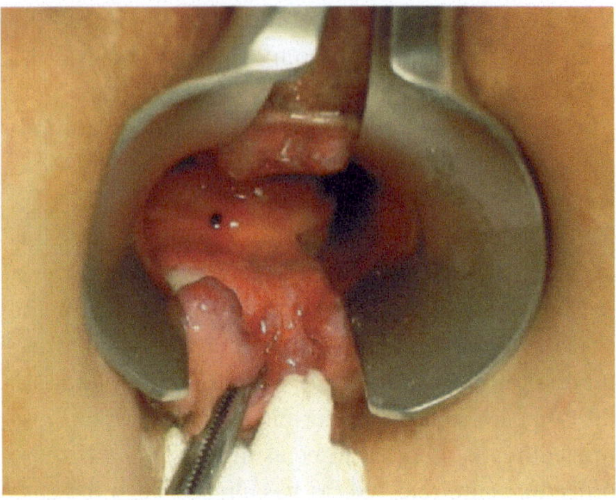

Fig. 2.12 b One of the retained staples is visible in the rectal lumen. The patient is in the lithotomy position

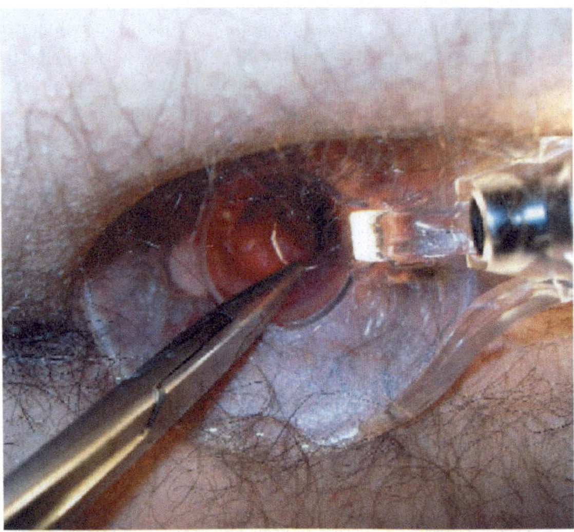

Fig. 2.12 c Staples can be removed using a Kelly to transmit diathermy, aimed at preventing tissue laceration and subsequent bleeding

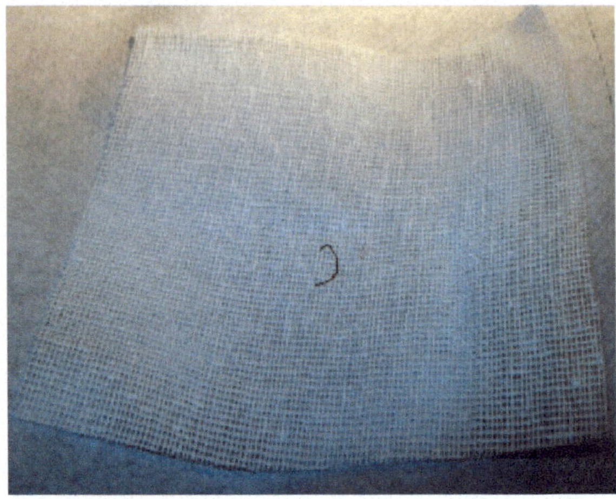

Fig. 2.12 d Removed staple

and bleeding. Fondran et al. (2006) reported that 11% of their 82 PPH patients had late rectal bleeding due to an inflammatory polyp. In all cases, the bleeding resolved after the polyp was removed (Fig. 2.13).

2.4.5 Retropneumoperitoneum, Pneumoperitoneum, Pneumomediastinum, and Cervical Emphysema

Cervical emphysema is manifested as subcutaneous crepitus and a bitonal voice. Various cases have been described in the literature, for example, by Maw et al. (2002), and Filingieri and Gravante (2005). They were usually due to dehiscence of the staple line and air entry (Fig. 2.14). Only one of the authors who observed this complication had to fashion a colostomy; otherwise, conservative therapy (the patient supine, antibiotics, and intravenous fluids) is generally effective.

The same complication has been observed after TEM and after transanal full- thickness excision of a large rectal adenoma (Basso and Pescatori, 2003). Air insufflation during intraoperative colonoscopy may contribute to its development.

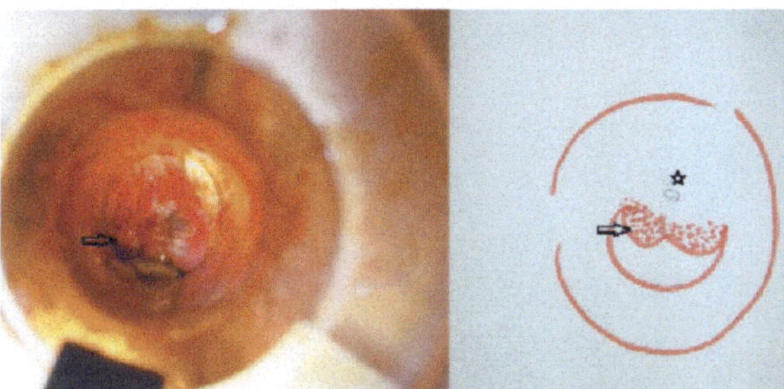

Fig. 2.13 a Patient with rectal bleeding and proctalgia after PPH: granulomatous polyp (*arrow*) and removed staple (*star*)

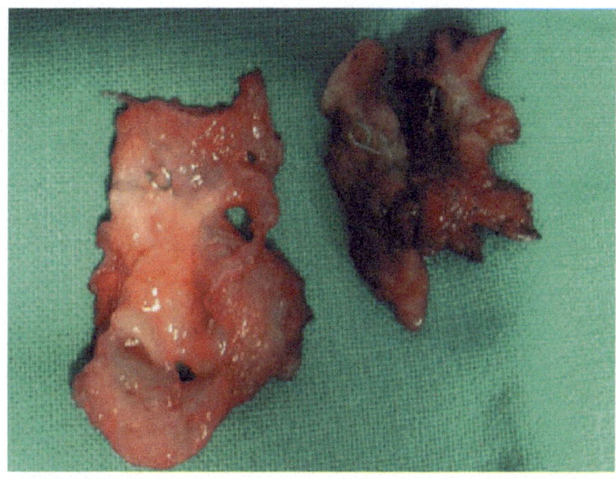

Fig. 2.13 b Polyps are removed

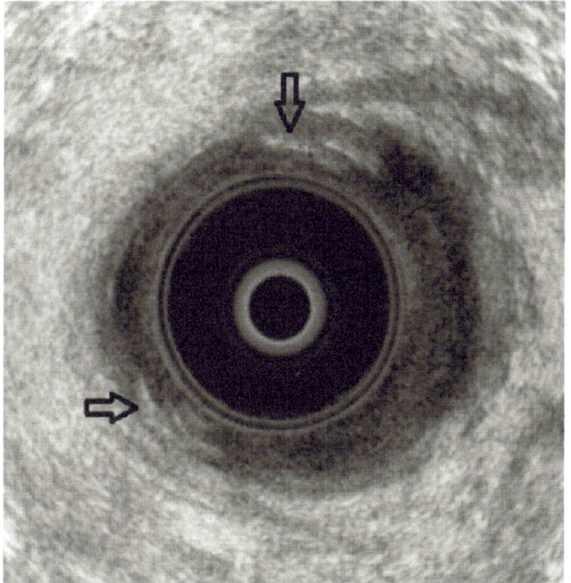

Fig. 2.13 c Transanal ultrasonography with rotating probe of the same patient a month after surgery. Other staples are visible (*arrows*)

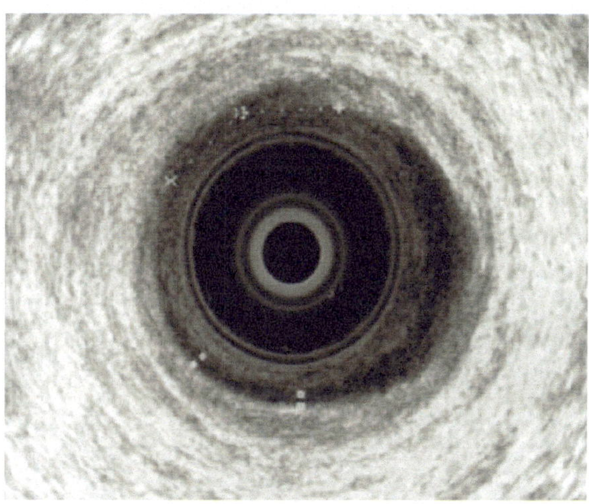

Fig. 2.13 d Endoanal and endorectal wounds have delayed cicatrization because of anal hypertonia, which is treated with calcium-antagonist ointment. *Squares* measure the diameter of the internal sphincter, which is < 2 mm. The *dotted line* shows a postoperative lesion of the internal sphincter

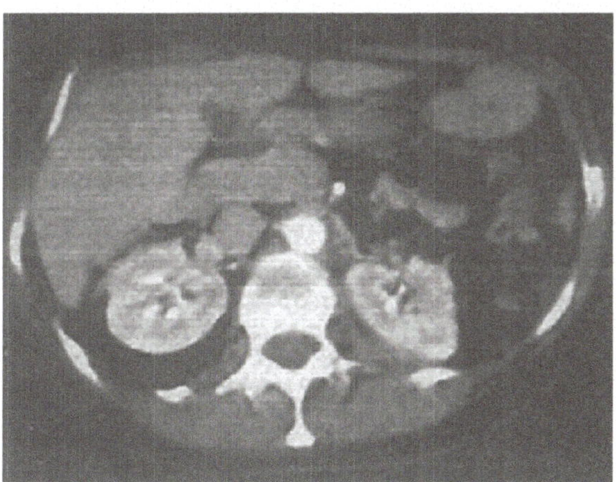

Fig. 2.14 a Retropneumoperitoneum after PPH

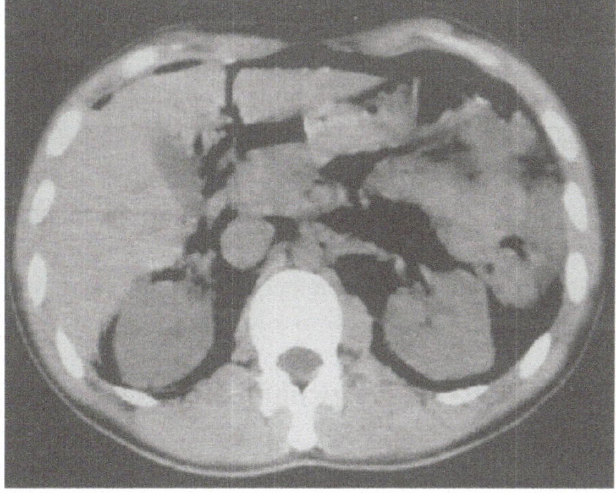

Fig. 2.14 b Pneumoperitoneum after PPH; the bowel loops are separated by air

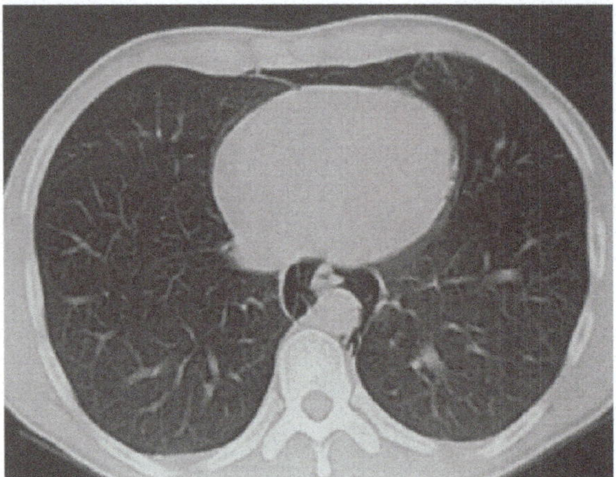

Fig. 2.14 c Pneumomediastinum after stapled hemorrhoidopexy. It is usually treated with conservative therapy

2.4.6 Rectal Inclusion Cysts

This complication was described by Raymond et al. (2008) and by De Nardi et al. (2008) and consists of a palpable, painful and tender perirectal nodule, usually filled with secretions. The suture line remains intact. The nodule must be removed transanally.

2.4.7 Total Obliteration of the Rectal Lumen

Obliteration of the lumen is caused by malpositioning of the purse-string, sometimes of two purse-strings, in a cavity that seems to be the rectal lumen but is actually a false lumen resulting from intussusception (Brown et al., 2007) (Fig. 2.15). This complication has been frequently reported, at least five times between 2005 and 2009, by Cipriani (2002) and Giordano (2008) and others. All patients except one had to undergo a form of rectal resection plus a Delorme mucosectomy. If this complication is suspected, it is important to perform a careful digital rectal examination or rectoscopy to determine whether the lumen is patent

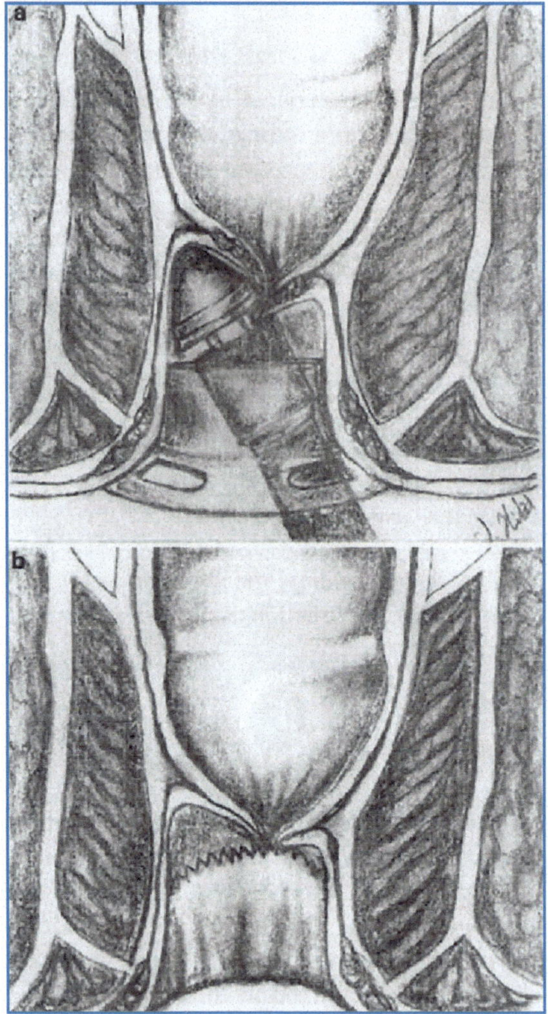

Fig. 2.15 a, b Rectal lumen obliteration after PPH (from Büyükaşik et al., 2009)

2.4.8 Rectal Diverticulum or Rectal Pocket Syndrome

In my experience (a few cases published with colleagues, Pescatori et al., 2007), this complication seems to arise if one or two stitches of the pursesting in the distal rectum are too superficial, so that when the pouch is tightened the suture thread cuts the small portion of mucosa that was included. What remains is a cavity partly isolated from the lumen in which fecoliths and secretions become trapped, dilating the rectal pocket/diverticulum and leading to tenesmus, pain, burning sensation, prostatitis, and sepsis. Treatment consists of laying open the cavity (Fig. 2.16).

The incidence of this complication is around 3%. The most recent cases were described by Serventi et al. (2010) and by Boffi and Podzemny (2011) (Fig. 2.17).

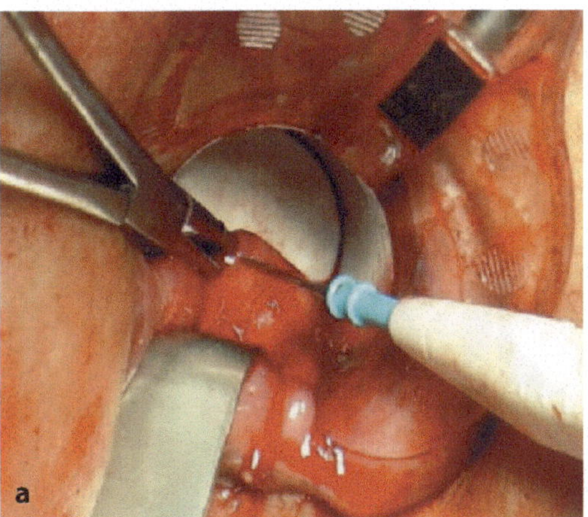

Fig. 2.16 a Operation after PPH carried out to manage a "rectal pocket syndrome", with formation of coproliths and recurrent abscesses causing chronic proctalgia. A Kelly was introduced in the pathological cavity, which is laid open with electrocautery. This syndrome occurs in about 3% of the cases after stapled hemorrhoidopexy

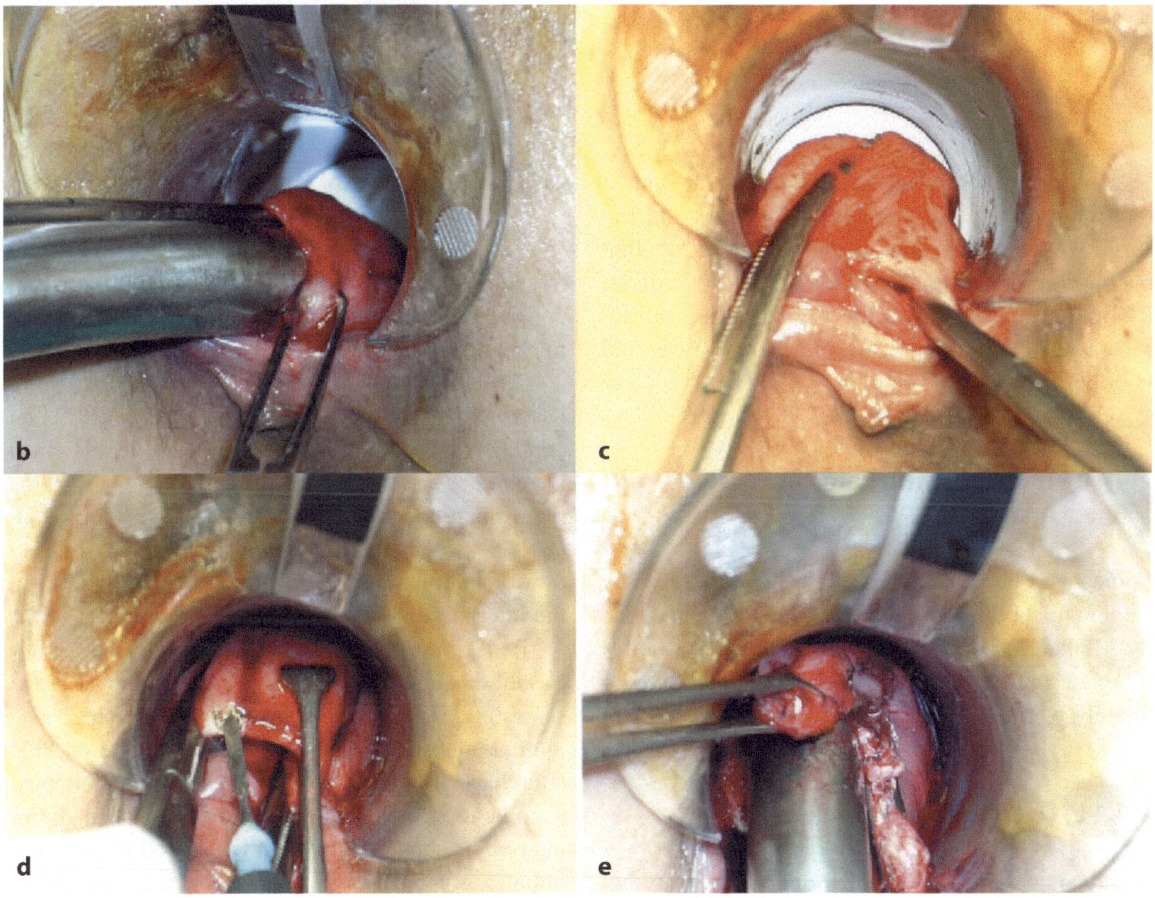

Fig. 2.16 b-e A Hegar is inserted in the pathological cavity, partially laid open. **b** A retained staple is detected at the apex of the pocket

2.4.9 Rectovaginal Fistulae

In a case series of Angelone et al. (2006), which I cited in a review article (2008), the incidence of rectovaginal fistula is only 0.2%. McDonald et al., at St. Mark's Hospital, reported a case in 2004. These fistulas sometimes necessitate reoperation. I once observed a case of an almost asymptomatic fistula that eventually closed spontaneously.

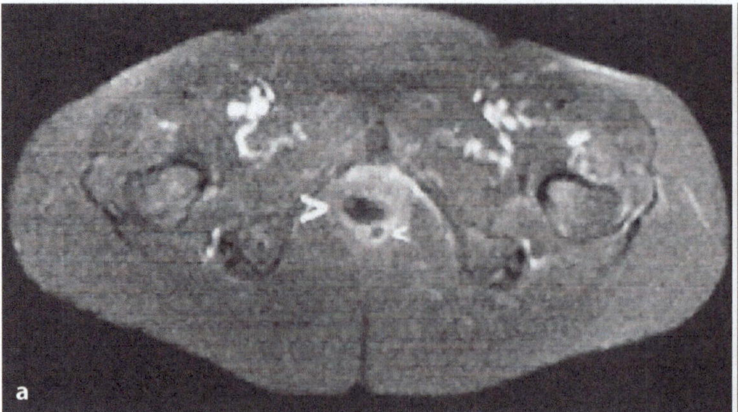

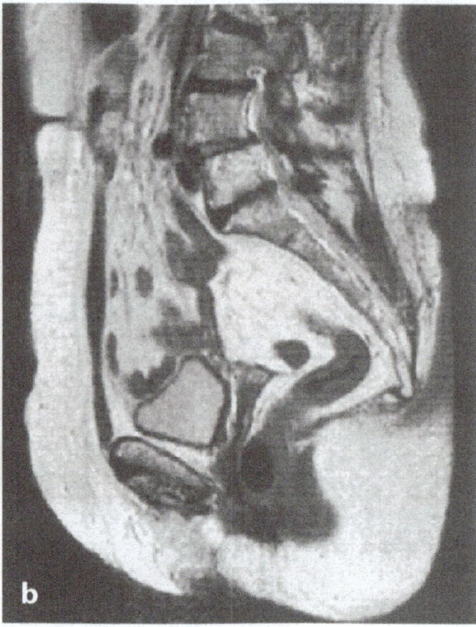

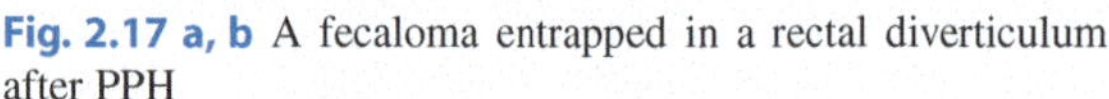
Fig. 2.17 a, b A fecaloma entrapped in a rectal diverticulum after PPH

How does a rectovaginal fistula form? It is most likely not due to a direct lesion that occurs during surgery, but to an area of ischemic tissue that becomes an opening after a few days. Regardless, it is important to protect the vagina with a retractor and to carefully palpate the posterior vaginal wall before firing the stapler.

2.4.10 Trauma to the Penis in Passive Anal Sex

Some cases have been described, including two by Capomagi (1999), one by Kekez (2007), and one by Mlakar (2007). The trauma was due to staples retained in the rectum. Patients should be adequately warned of this potential problem.

2.4.11 Dysplasia and Cancer

Dysplasia or cancer in hemorrhoids is very rare but cases have been described by Brusciano et al. (2004) in articles on re-operations after PPH. Hemorrhoids that may contain neoplastic foci must be removed, not moved up with the PPH. For this reason, I send all removed hemorrhoids to the pathologist. In the patient of Annibali, (Brusciano et al.) the tumor occurred at the level of the mucosal cylinder removed by the stapler.

2.4.12 Retro-rectal Hematoma

In one case of retro-rectal hematoma, described by Vasudevan et al. (2007), the hematoma caused complete obstruction of the rectum and a colostomy was required.

Thirteen cases of retro-rectal hematoma were described in a study conducted by Naldini (2011) on complications after PPH and STARR (46 of which were major complications). A perisigmoid hematoma requiring reoperation was reported by De Santis et al. (2011). If the hematoma cannot be drained, a resection of the rectum or a laparotomy with ligation of the internal iliac arteries may be necessary.

It is interesting to note that, shortly after Vasudevan's article was published, and almost at the same time as the publication of Naldini's, the same journal published a systematic review article on PPH (Burch et al., 2009). In the accompanying "Invited Comment", although the journal has published alarming reports about PPH, Ronan O'Connell wrote, "The initial concerns about potentially severe postoperative complications (after PPH) have been shown to be unfounded."

A few months earlier, the *Corriere della Sera*, a well-known newspaper in Milan, published an interview with Dr. Longo, conducted by Pappagallo, in which PPH was advocated as a "gentle" and "sutureless" procedure. Boffi's commentary on the interview, which emphasized how misleading it was, was published soon thereafter in Techniques in Coloproctology, 2009. His letter gave rise to a series of letters, under the heading "Ethical issues and innovations", by various authors, including presidents and editors of international societies and journals (Seow-Choen, Amato, Gupta, Madoff, Zbar, Kodner). Among their conclusions: 1) there are also companies that are very careful to behave in an ethical manner, 2) around half of the articles in which the authors deny any conflict of interest are actually subsidized by the industry, and 3) to protect patients from misleading information, scientific societies should not allow anyone who gives wrong information to the media to participate in scientific meetings/congresses. In addition, the board of the Italian Society of Colorectal Surgery (Società Italiana di Chirurgia Colo-Rettale SICCR) wrote to the director of the newspaper and reported the debate on "Ethical issues and innovations" on the society's website www.siccr.org.

I mention all this in order to demonstrate that risks and complications may be underestimated by the same people charged with providing accurate information. Patients and surgeons who have not been sufficiently alerted to possible problems associated with operations said to be simple and safe will approach them without enough caution, which in turn can increase the risk of complications. Conclusion: correct information about complications is essential in any attempt to effectively prevent them.

2.4.13 Hemoperitoneum

Fortunately, this is a rare complication. In the patient described by Aumann et al. (2004), the presence of a prolapsed pouch of Douglas and an enterocele facilitated the development of hemoperitoneum, which was then successfully treated with re-operation via abdominal access (Fig. 2.18).

During stapling, to avoid inclusion of the upper part of the vagina, the peritoneum of a prolapsed pouch of Douglas, or, even worse, the ileum or sigmoid colon (thus forming an enterocele), there is a useful trick: Before placing the sutures of the purse-string in the anterior part of the distal rectum, i.e., the at-risk zone, inject physiological solution into the submucosa so that the nearby bowel is distanced from the rectal lumen and the stapler.

2.4.14 Dehiscence of the Rectal Suture and Rectal Lacerations with Hemorrhage and/or Pelvic Sepsis

About 100 cases of dehiscence or rectal laceration, possibly linked to instrument dysfunction, are reported on the website of the United States Food and Drug Administration (FDA); http://www.fda.gov/cdrh/index.html. In general, these complications can be treated by transanal suture placement, but sometimes a defunctioning colostomy is required.

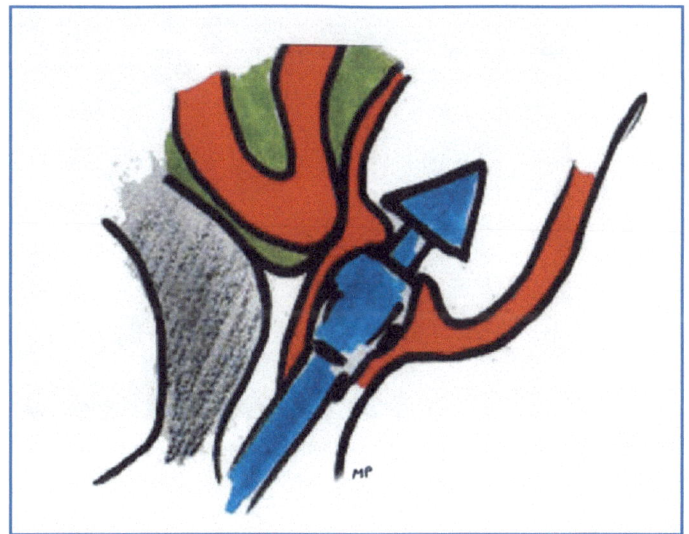

Fig. 2.18 Complications after PPH. In case of enterocele, a bowel loop can be trapped in the stapler, with successive intestinal perforation and/or peritonitis and/or hemoperitoneum

2.4.15 Rectal Perforation and Pelvic Sepsis

The first case was described by Molloy and Kingsmore (2000) and was successfully treated with a Hartmann procedure. The authors recommended antibiotic prophylaxis before PPH. Fu's group, in China, described eight cases (Gao et al., 2010), including five in which the perforation was definitely above the anastomosis, and reviewed those in the literature. Seven patients died (including one of his own) due to this complication and pelviperineal gangrene.

The predisposing factors, according to Gao et al., are: 1) a descent of the anterior wall of the rectum, which is perhaps injured by the pointed cone of the anvil of a stapler inserted too forcefully, in patients who have rectal prolapse or invagination, and 2) ascites that causes the pouch of Douglas to be pushed downwards by the liquid. These conditions thus define a group of high-risk patients. Furthermore, there is clearly a need for staplers with more rounded tips (Fig. 2.19).

According to Ravo et al. (2002), rectal perforation can be demonstrated in one out of every 1,300 cases of PPH. This is why, in their consensus article, Corman et al. (2006) recommended that PPH be performed by colorectal surgeons who are well-informed about the indications and the contraindications (including anal sepsis, high-grade enterocele, pregnancy) as well as the intra- and postoperative complications, and who are able to prevent and treat adverse events.

In 10 years (2000-2010) almost 80 cases of rectal perforation after PPH were reported: 38 on the FDA website (until 2007) and about 40 in various articles. At least half necessitated a colostomy. Seven patients died, as mentioned above. In spite of these striking numbers, at www.comecurarele-morroidi.it, consulted on 12/12/2010, "Longo's operation" was described as a minimally invasive procedure.

A new method of treating pelvic and/or perirectal sepsis after PPH was proposed by Durai and Ng (2009), both working at Lewisham Hospital in

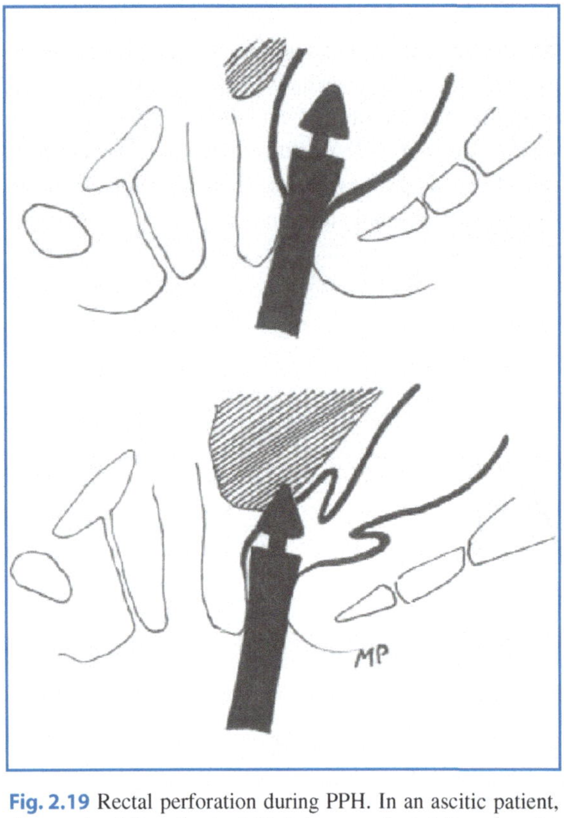

Fig. 2.19 Rectal perforation during PPH. In an ascitic patient, the pouch of Douglas is shifted downwards and it pushes the anterior wall of the distal rectum toward the cone of the stapler "anvil" (from Gao et al., 2010, modified)

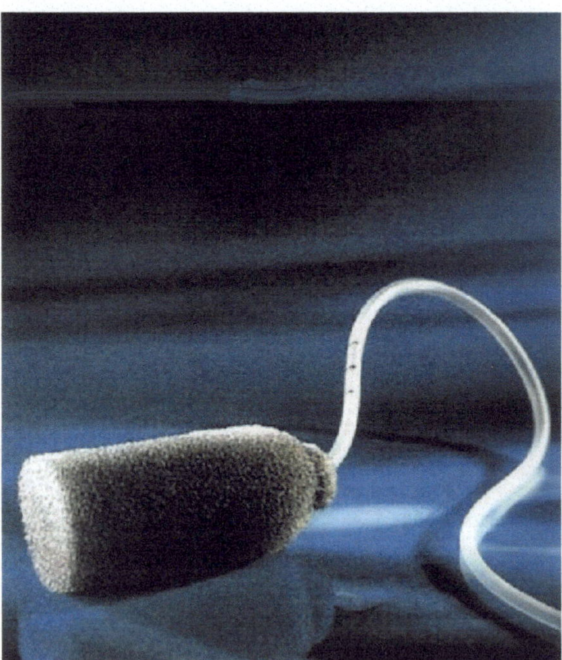

Fig. 2.20 VAC system (vacuum aspiration), with associated Redivac drainage, to treat a postoperative pathological cavity (from Durai and Ng, 2009)

London: VAC system, consisting of vacuum aspiration combined with a Redivac drain (Fig. 2.20). This combined approach also seems to be useful for similar complications after various procedures, such as the sequelae of dehiscence after anterior resection of the rectum. According to the authors, it allowed the successful treatment of a septic presacral cavity that formed in a patient who underwent a Hartmann procedure for pelvic sepsis due to rectal perforation after stapled hemorrhoidopexy.

2.4.16 Thrombosis of the Inferior Vena Cava

One case was described in a report by Nemati Fard in 2006. In this patient, it was necessary to perform a nephrectomy.

2.5 Complications After Other Operations

There are many other operations for hemorrhoids. The following sections describe the complications associated with six operations, five of which I have sometimes performed.

2.5.1 Semi-open or Semi-closed Hemorrhoidectomy

This is mostly used in Japan and Brazil and can be performed in two ways: by removal of the external hemorrhoid and suturing of the internal one (the Reis-Neto technique) or by removing both and marsupializing the surgical wound (the Pescatori technique). Both methods were published, with very clear illustrations, in Techniques in Coloproctology, the first (which is semi-open) in 2002 and the second in 2005.

The advantages of these procedures are good hemostasis and rapid scar formation. In my experience with the semi-open procedure, the complications consisted of only slight bleeding, but a fair amount of pain, with a VAS between 4 and 5 (more than after PPH) 12 hours after surgery. The pain occurred because of a suture in the sensitive epithelium of the anal canal. For this reason I seldom perform this operation. However, it is useful for removing two quadrants although it requires an elastomere with continuous i.v. analgesics.

2.5.2 Farag Suturing of Internal Hemorrhoids

The technique is simple: stitches are used to make the hemorrhoids ischemic. The advantages are that it is quick, easy, and safe. There are no surgical wounds and recovery is uneventful. The only complication, based on the more than 30 of these operations that I performed, was the need to suture a hemorrhagic area in one patient. In addition, stitches that are too deep will cause pain.

2.5.3 Hussein's Manual Hemorrhoidopexy

When this procedure is used at our unit, it is often combined with Ferguson hemorrhoidectomy to treat the third nodule, when it is not external. It is an inexpensive procedure since it does not require the use of sophisticated instruments such as staplers. Hussein who invented it works in Egypt, which may in part explain why the procedure has yet to be more widely adopted.

The original version was described by Hussein in 2010. I presented a modification of it in Techniques in Coloproctology. It is indicated for hemorrhoids that are mainly internal, which are pulled upwards with a U-shaped stitch and then sutured (Farag style). This results in a good anopexy. The advantages of manual hemorrhoidopexy is that there are no surgical wounds in the anal canal, which ensures rapid recovery. Among the potential complications: the hemorrhoids can slide back down unless the sutures are deep, but deep sutures can cause pain.

2.5.4 Whitehead-Rand Hemorrhoidectomy

This operation removes external hemorrhoids, internal hemorrhoids, and associated mucosal prolapse. It is indicated when the lesions are circum-

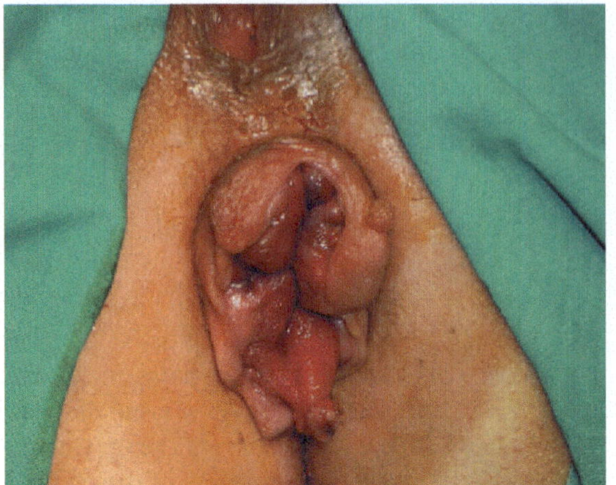

Fig. 2.21 a Circumferential internal and external hemorrhoids with concomitant rectal internal mucosal prolapse; Whitehead-Rand technique. Polypoid internal and external hemorrhoids should be sent for histologic analysis to determine if there is potential dysplasia. Therefore, a stapled hemorrhoidopexy is not indicated in this case. The patient is in the lithotomy position

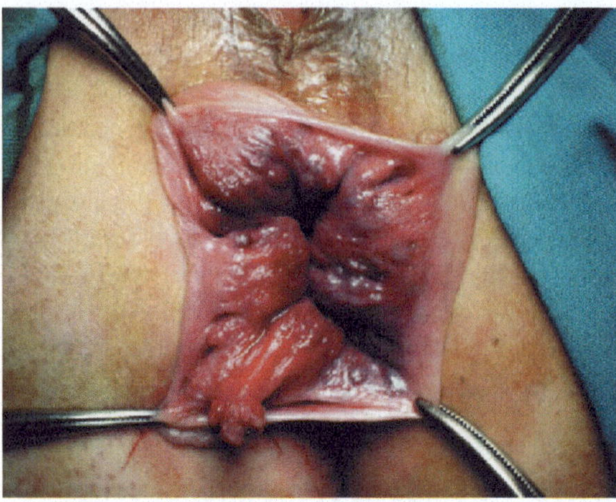

Fig. 2.21 b The piles are stretched. The patient had a recurrence after PPH

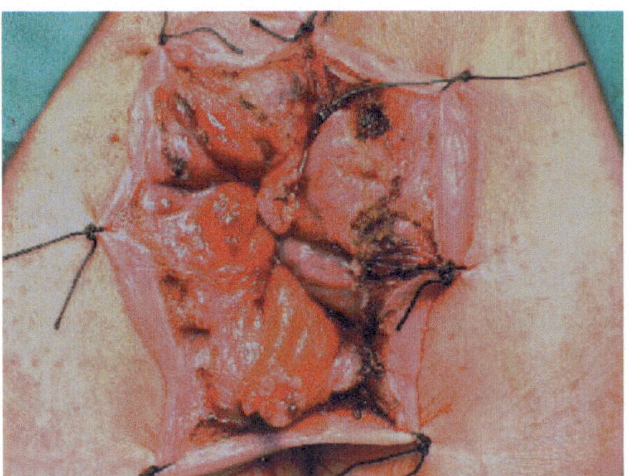

Fig. 2.21 c Cutaneous flaps are fixed to the perianal skin and a circumferential incision is performed immediately above the dentate line

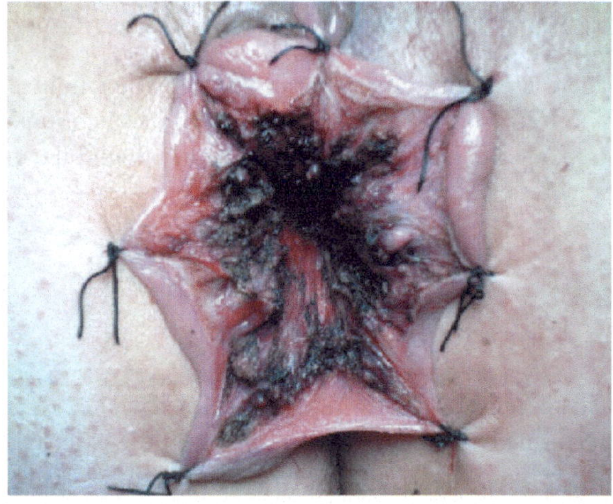

Fig. 2.21 d Diathermic excision of external and internal hemorrhoids and mucosal prolapse. Note the internal sphincter and rectal muscle, which are identified and left intact

ferential (Fig. 2.21). Currently, this is the perfect indication for PPH, possibly not in constipated patients, in order to reduce the risk of recurrence. A modified version of this operation was used by Wolff (1988) at the Mayo Clinic.

The Whitehead-Rand procedure is rather complex and knowledge of plastic surgery is required because of the need to prepare skin flaps. Its advantage is that it is very radical. The complications are not, as perhaps expected, associated with stenosis or incontinence (in contrast to the old Whitehead procedure). I have observed subclinical anal stenosis (treated with dilators) in only one out of 25 patients. However, partial detachment of the skin flap does occur (in 5 cases in my small series) so that a large skin tag forms. In three

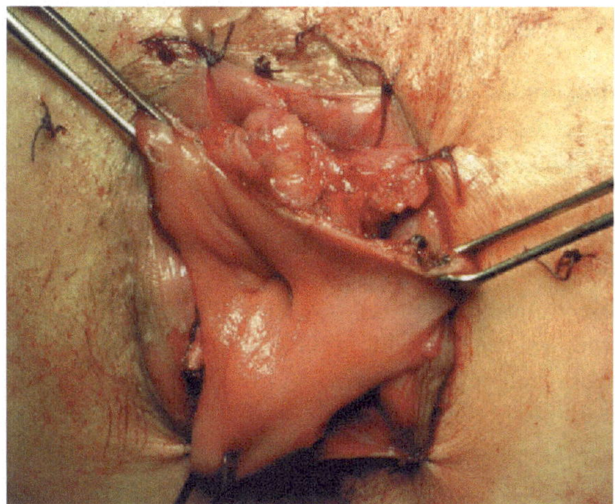

Fig. 2.21 e Mucosal cylinder of the distal rectum before anastomosis with the anal canal

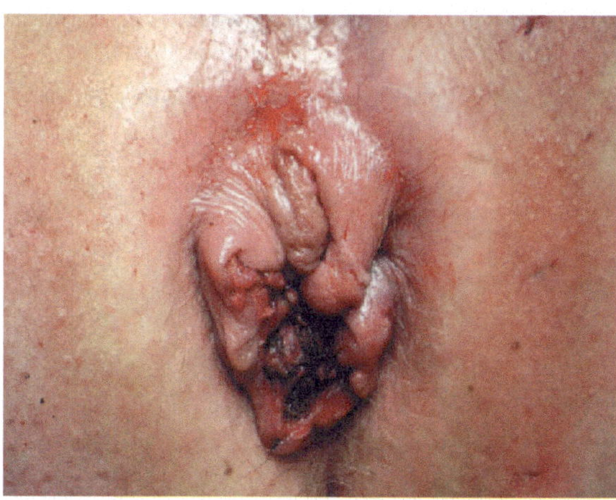

Fig. 2.21 f Cutaneous flaps (i.e., distal anal canal) are preserved

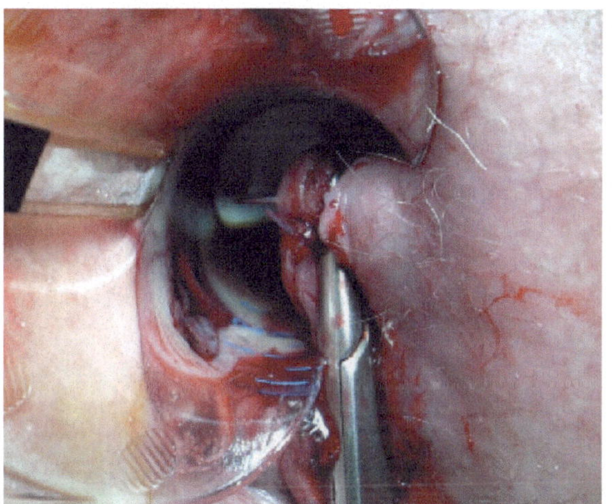

Fig. 2.21 g They are sutured to the distal rectum

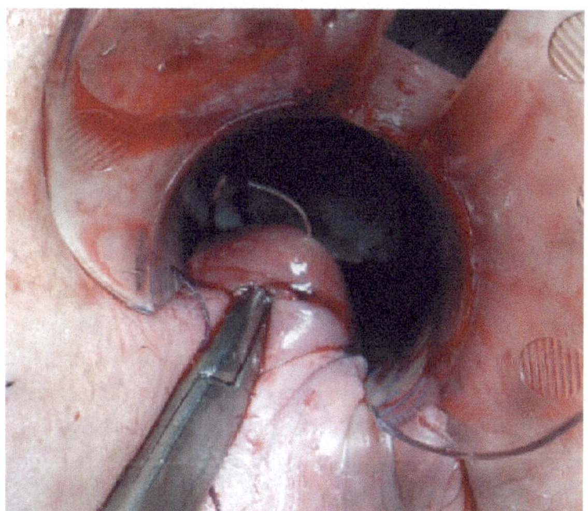

Fig. 2.21 h The suture is completed

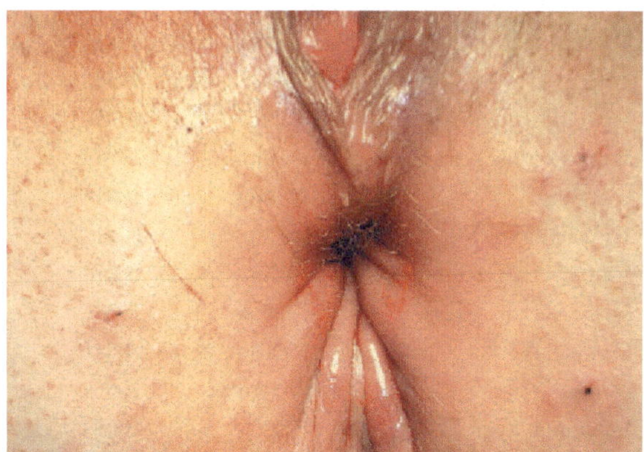

Fig. 2.21 i Final look: cutaneous flaps are pulled upwards by the rectal sutures, with a -pexy effect

cases I had to remove the tag, although always in an outpatient setting with the patient under local anesthesia.

In cases of mucosal ectropion, the Sarafoff procedure (Dodi et al., 1999) can be helpful.

2.5.5 Parks' Submucosal Hemorrhoidectomy

Few surgeons perform this procedure because it is rather long and laborious and always involves intraoperative bleeding. It is the only one of the operations invented by Sir Alan Parks that is now only

Table 2.4 Postoperative complications after 640 cases of Parks' hemorrhoidectomy in 20 years (from Rosa et al., 2005)[a]

Early complications	Number of patients	(%)
Hemorrhage	19	3.0
Intense pain	9	1.4
Fecaloma	3	0.5
Suture dehiscence	2	0.3
Urinary retention	74	11.6
Late complications		
Proctalgia and hypertonia	11	2.9
Recurrence or skin tags	6	1.6
Gas incontinence	3	0.8
Anal fistula	2	0.5
Anal stenosis	1	0.3

[a]Fourth-degree hemorrhoids in 80% of cases; average follow-up of 7.3 years in 374 patients who filled out a mailed questionnaire.

rarely performed at St. Mark's Hospital. While my own experience with this type of hemorrhoidectomy is limited to one patient, Rosa and Milito (2005) used it to treat around 2000 patients, with good results. The advantages are that it allows reconstruction of the entire anal canal and is the only hemorrhoidectomy procedure that preserves the anoderm, which has an important role in the sensory mechanism of continence. As seen in Table 2.4, there are very few complications, which is a recommendation for its use.

While the results are impressive, there is an important bias: almost half of the patients were lost to follow-up. In Milito's case series, among 1315 patients who underwent the procedure, 25% had early postoperative complications, with the most frequent one being urinary retention, and 11.3% had late complications, including 1.6% with anal stenosis and 3.2% with gas incontinence. Follow-up at 65 months after surgery was possible in 88% of the patients.

The results of two prospective randomized trials (Roe et al., 1987 and Hosch et al., 1998) showed that there is less pain, quicker recovery and better anal sensitivity after the Parks procedure than after Milligan-Morgan hemorrhoidectomy.

2.5.6 Coagulation of Hemorrhoids

While I do not use this method, it is perhaps of interest to readers so that the associated complications should be mentioned here. The procedure originated as bipolar coagulation, in the early 1990s. Surgeons in Singapore converted it to monopolar coagulation and, in a prospective randomized trial, compared it with open hemorrhoidectomy performed using diathermy (Quah and Seow-Choen, 2004).

Complications were reported in 5 out of 20 patients (25%), with the development of rectal bleeding that required re-admission to the hospital and, in one patient, a blood transfusion. There were no re-operations. More than half of the patients (11 out of 20, 55%) had residual hemorrhoids or skin tags after the operation. Three patients (15%) developed anal stenosis that required dilatation. None of the patients developed incontinence. The high rate of complications may explain why this method is not widely used.

2.6 Treating the Complications

Not even the best surgeon in the world can avoid complications, so in this section we will look at how they can be treated.

2.6.1 Pain

While not a real complication in the strict sense of the term, it is a frequent occurrence. In an important article, Cheetham and Phillips (2001) proposed various ways to reduce pain. Among their suggestions was the administration of metronidazole, since

Table 2.5 Treatment for postoperative pain after surgery for hemorrhoids

Treatment	Author	Year
Ketorolac	Milito	1996
Metronidazole i.v. & per os	Milito	1996
Metronidazole per os	Phillips	2001
Lactulose	Phillips	2001
Trimebutine	Phillips	2001
Nitroglycerin cream	Phillips	2001
Metronidazole cream	Nicholson	2004
Flavonoids	La Torre	2004
Diltiazem	Silverman	2005
Botulinum toxin A	Patti	2005
Pudendal nerve block	Imbelloni	2008
Opioid cream	Tegon	2009

pain, especially during postoperative days 3-5, can be due to bacterial colonization. Other drugs are used to combat anal hypertonia, for example, trimebutine, nitroglycerin, diltiazem, and Botox. The different treatments are listed Table 2.5.

2.6.2 Urinary Retention

This generally resolves if the patient is given a Foley catheter. In rare cases (as described in "Unforgettable Complications"), more aggressive measures are required; however, these are preventative not curative.

2.6.3 Hemorrhage

Let me begin by mentioning how not to cure hemorrhage. The patient is not immediately returned to the operating room for re-operation. Gauze packs or tampons are not inserted into the patient's anus, since this maneuver causes pain and possibly additional injury to the bleeding wound.

In 37 years, out of almost 900 patients whom I operated on for hemorrhoids, 20 developed severe bleeding, most commonly on postoperative day 4 after a Milligan-Morgan procedure. In 18 of these patients, bleeding resolved when the balloon of a 20-24 French Foley catheter inserted in the rectum was inflated with 20-40 ml of water and pulled until resistance was felt, so that the balloon was compressed between the distal rectum and the anal canal, where the source of bleeding was located. It was then anchored, under traction, to the gluteus muscle and the thigh with a bandage. It is best to irrigate the catheter with cold water, as this helps to obtain hemostasis and to remove the blood from the rectum. It also allows estimation of the extent of blood loss, which is important in preparing patients who are in critical condition for transfusion (I have only had to transfuse 5 patients). The patient should be kept rested and without oral intake. Adrenaline can be administered via irrigation (I occasionally do this) or injected (something I have never done).

After a few hours, the balloon partially deflates and a few hours later it is completely deflated. The catheter should be checked to make sure it is patent, not blocked by blood clots. It can be removed when one is certain that bleeding has stopped (Basso and Pescatori, 1994).

In three cases, the maneuver with the Foley catheter did not work and I had to suture the wound, which was bleeding. One case occurred in the operating room, one on the ward, and one in an outpatient setting. In each of them, I used local anesthesia.

If a perianal hematoma develops (Regadas, already cited), surgical drainage may be necessary.

Late postoperative bleeding can occur after several days, up to the second postoperative week. It is usually due to sepsis and the exposure of a blood vessel beneath the eschar. Late bleeding is rarely severe and rarely requires re-operation, but a collegue of mine had a patient who was over 80 years of age and died at home due to massive rectal bleeding. He went into shock and had a myocardial infarction.

2.6.4 Fecaloma

This is not a severe complication, but it is troublesome for the patient, who will complain of tenesmus and small, painful bowel movements, a sort of paradoxical, mini-diarrhea. The problem usually resolves after the administration of one or two enemas. The patient should be advised to eat less fiber. Only rarely is it necessary to remove the fecaloma under general anesthesia. Warm sitz baths can be helpful. Recently, I had a case of fecaloma formation, whose expulsion and removal by irrigation using a soft catheter caused suture disruption following a Ferguson procedure. It was necessary to reoperate the patient excising tags and marsupializing the wounds (Fig. 2.22).

2.6.5 Thrombosed External Hemorrhoids

This can happen after any type of hemorrhoid surgery but seems to occur most frequently after PPH (5.9%) if the external hemorrhoids are not removed (Boccasanta, 1998), less frequently after THD (Infantino et al. 2010), and almost never after hemorrhoidectomy. The problem can often be successfully treated with medical therapy, either systemic or topical. The latter consists of injections of 0.25% bupivacaine with adrenaline 1:200 000 and

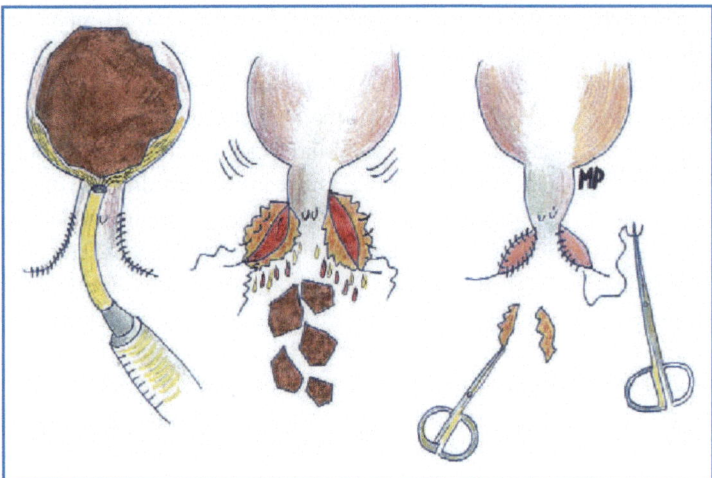

Fig. 2.22 *From left to right*: Fecal impaction following Ferguson hemorrhoidectomy. Excessive straining of the patient, an anxious constipated 43-year-old woman. Irrigation of the rectum with saline and glycerine oil. Complete breakdown of the sutures, bleeding, local sepsis and formation of large skin tags after the fragmentation of the fecaloma. Three weeks later, following a course of antibiotics, the tags have been excised and the wounds marsupialized. The patient is well after three months

hyaluronidase, as suggested by Salvati (1990). Alternatively, an incision or excision can be made in an outpatient setting, with local anesthesia and without suturing of the surgical wound.

Patti et al. (2008) successfully used Botox injections to treat thrombosed hemorrhoids.

What complications can be expected after surgical or conservative treatment of thrombosed hemorrhoids? Allan et al. (2006) carried out a controlled study of 24 patients, 12 of whom had undergone emergency hemorrhoidectomy and 12 conservative treatment. Bleeding occurred in two patients in the surgery group and three patients in the conservative group. Three patients in each group developed anal incontinence.

2.6.6 Anal or Rectal Stenosis

Anal stenosis is seen occasionally after a Milligan-Morgan procedure (1-3% of cases, usually after 3 months). It is very rare after PPH. Chew et al. (2008), from Singapore, described a case of anal stenosis after PPH that was due to keloid formation, which was treated surgically by anoplasty. As previously noted, those surgeons make the tobacco pouch lower than is typically done elsewhere, 2-3 cm above the anal rim. Basically their procedure is a hemorrhoidectomy rather than a hemorrhoidopexy.

In the cases of anal stenosis after hemorrhoidectomy procedures that I or others performed, reviewed in the following paragraphs, the treatment was rarely surgical.

I have treated mild stenosis with Dilatan (the Sapimed dilator, applied by the patient at home) and moderate stenosis with dilatations (using Dilatan, a Hegar dilator, or my fingers) in an outpatient setting, with the patient receiving local anesthesia, Emla cream, or infiltration anesthetics. Severe stenosis is treated in the operating room, with the patient under spinal, local, or general anesthesia, using a Hegar dilator and then digital dilatation; in some cases, radial incisions are made with an electric scalpel. If this is not sufficient, treatment consists of sphincterotomy, or better yet, incision and/or removal of the fibrotic cushions and anoplasty, usually with two lateral sliding V-Y flaps. I prefer the latter and use this method also in patients with mucosal ectropion. In rare cases, a U-, S-, diamond-, or house-shaped flap is necessary.

In 1986, Milsom and Mazier published a maxi-series of 212 patients with postoperative anal stenosis, more than half of whom were treated with one or two sphincterotomies and 40 of whom underwent multiple sphincterotomies.

Caution is warranted in performing "generous" sphincterotomies because they may provoke soiling. They are best avoided in patients who are already at risk of anal incontinence. Gingold (1991) reported his experience with 21 cases of anal stenosis after laser hemorrhoidectomy. Many of the patients who underwent re-operation also had an anal fissure.

In two out of my 40 patients who underwent PPH, a moderate rectal stenosis had to be dilated under anesthesia, followed by local injections of cortisone to maintain the dilatation. It is important to note that in both cases the patient not only had hemorrhoids but also a notable internal mucosal prolapse of the rectum, requiring stapled excision.

Among 85 patients of Regadas et al. (2005), two developed rectal stenosis and were treated with radial incisions using a hot biopsy forceps (endoscopic stricturectomy).

Dilatations must be performed carefully. Kanellos (2004) described a case of stenosis after PPH that was due to suture dehiscence. Immediately after the dilatation, the patient developed retropneumoperitoneum.

2.6.7 Anal Fissure

This complication develops only very rarely after PPH and Ferguson hemorrhoidectomy, but less rarely after Milligan-Morgan procedures if the surgical wound becomes infected and does not heal, in which case it is helpful to close off the edges. Metronidazole cream and flavonoids improve scar formation and reduce pain. Injecting botulinum toxin A into the internal sphincter at the end of the operation serves as a preventive measure (Patti et al., 2005).

It is important to check whether the patient has anal hypertonia in addition to anal fissure. The former should be treated with nitroglycerin (Rectogesic cream, Dermatrans patches, or Antrolin cream, which contains calcium channel blockers). Disinfectants and scarring agents such as Abound, Colostrum gel, Fitostimoline cream/gauze, Cicatrene, or Vulnamin are also effective. If treatment fails, an internal sphincterotomy (with curettage of the fissure) may be necessary, or, in cases of normo/hypotonia, fissure excision and anoplasty.

2.6.8 Abscess or Fistula

There is no difference between the Ferguson and Milligan-Morgan procedures as far as anal sepsis is concerned: it rarely occurs. Sepsis is usually more likely after Ferguson hemorrhoidectomy because there is a suture in a "dirty" area, but if it develops after a closed procedure it usually causes suture dehiscence and as a result drains spontaneously.This is why it is better to use catgut or Vicryl Rapid as the suture material rather than standard vicryl, which is more resistant such that in some cases it is not reabsorbed and must be removed. Patients with sepsis complain of dysuria, pelvic, and/or perineal pain and may have fever and urinary retention.

Sometimes a chronic, occult abscess forms, i.e., subclinical postoperative sepsis develops and the patient then presents with proctalgia, even long after surgery. Endoanal ultrasound examination with a rotating probe may reveal a small intersphincteric mass of mixed echogencity. This happened in four of my patients: in three, I decided to re-operate, but only in one of these patients did I find and remove what was definitely a chronic abscess, with the result that the patient's symptoms resolved.

Anal fistulae rarely develop after hemorrhoid surgery. Most are submucosal and should be laid open, which can even be done in an outpatient setting using local anesthesia.

2.6.9 Skin Tags

According to the meta-analysis of Jayaraman et al. (2007), skin tags are found more frequently after PPH than after excisional hemorrhoidectomy, for the obvious reason that PPH does not remove skin tags. In the meta-analysis performed by Tjandra and Chan (2007), the incidence of skin tags after these two procedures was similar, albeit with a trend in favor of hemorrhoidectomy.

The Swedish surgeon Nyström studied postoperative pain in two groups of patients operated on with stapled hemorrhoidopexy. One group underwent standard PPH, and the other PPH plus skin tag removal. Interestingly, the postoperative VAS evaluation did not show any increase in pain in the second group. It seems therefore that skin tag removal can be combined with PPH without any problems.

Koh and Seow-Choen (2005) proposed an interesting method of ensuring that there are no residual skin tags after PPH. It involves excision of a mucosal flap immediately below the suture, at the level of the residual hemorrhoid. If a small half-moon shaped strip of tissue between the suture and the dentate line is removed and the wound re-sutured with interrupted sutures, the result is a hemorrhoidopexy, with the hemorrhoidal nodule and the skin tag compressed upwards.

Skin tags found after hemorrhoidectomy are usually small and rarely have to be resected; but, if this is indeed necessary, the procedure can be performed in an outpatient setting using local anesthesia. This was the case in three of my patients, after I had performed 25 hemorrhoidectomies using the Whitehead-Rand procedure, which is indicated in cases of circumferential hemorrhoids associated with internal mucosal prolapse of the rectum.

Even after THD-mucopexy, especially if performed for fourth-degree hemorrhoids (Ratto et al., 2011), there can be residual skin tags. These can be removed during the procedure if they are medium- or large-sized.

2.6.10 Anal Incontinence

I refer to "anal" not "fecal" because stool incontinence after hemorrhoidectomy is rare. More often, there is mucus soiling or gas incontinence due to a small lesion of the internal sphincter.

Antidiarrheal drugs, a diet rich in fiber, the use of enemas, and physiokinesis therapy (exercises favoring anal contractions) are usually effective. Biofeedback and electrostimulation (transanal or pudendal nerve stimulation, Fig. 2.23) are less commonly required but should be used when retained staples in the rectum put the patient at risk of burns or laceration if an electric probe or other type of probe is inserted. There is rarely a need to inject bulking agents into the lacuna of the internal sphincter once it has been identified with transanal or perineal ultrasound. Sphincteroplasty is very rarely performed. It was used by Brusciano et al. (2004) to treat incontinence after PPH. They reported a 20% incidence of continence problems after re-operation because of recurrence or complications after stapled hemorrhoidopexy.

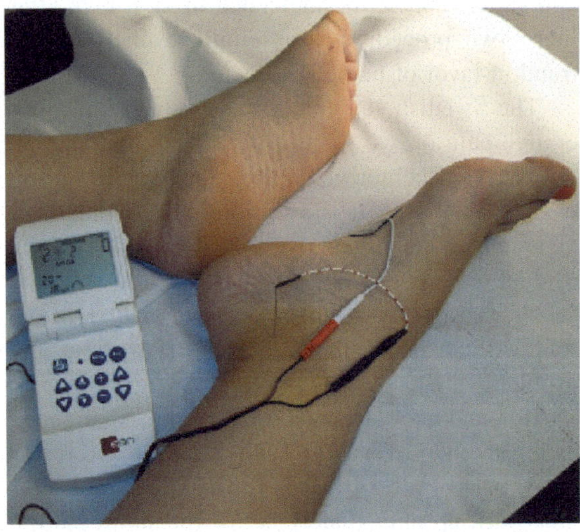

Fig. 2.23 Posterior tibial nerve electrostimulation in postoperative anal incontinence after hemorrhoidopexy or hemorrhoidectomy. It is preferred over transanal electrostimulation when there are endoanal painful scars or "floating" staples in the rectal lumen which may cause burning

2.6.11 Severe Anal Sepsis

Table 2.6 lists several of these cases and briefly notes the results.

In a review article, McCloud et al. (2006) described cases of severe anal sepsis after hemorrhoidectomy that required aggressive medical therapy or re-operation. The latter was usually surgical drainage of the perianal abscess or area of perineal necrosis after manual hemorrhoidectomy, and laparotomy plus defunctioning colostomy after stapled hemorrhoidopexy. Sadly, some patients died.

As shown in the table, in 15 years, there have been eight cases of severe sepsis after hemorrhoidectomy, four re-operations with a colostomy, and two deaths. For PPH, the numbers are seven cases in 4 years, six re-operations, all with a colostomy, and one death. Thus, severe sepsis occurred more frequently after PPH. The need for re-operation and the creation of a defunctioning stoma was greater after stapled hemorrhoidopexy. Among the five patients who required perineal necrosectomy, sepsis was clearly developing into Fournier's gangrene, after both PPH and stapled hemorrhoidopexy. The patient who underwent PPH died in spite of the necrosectomy. The two patients who died due to severe sepsis after hemorrhoidectomy did not have defunctioning stomas. One of them (not included in the table) had a liver abscess.

Table 2.6 Severe anal sepsis after surgical treatment of hemorrhoids (in general, one case per author)

Author	Year	Re-operation	Defunctioning colostomy	Death
Post-hemorroidectomy				
Timerbulatov	1988	drainage	no	no
Kriss	1990	no	no	no
Parikh (2 cases)	1994	no	no	no
Mohammedi	1996	drainage	no	YES
Basoglu	1997	necrosectomy	YES	no
Cihan	1999	necrosectomy	YES	no
Ibanez	2003	no	no	YES
Post-PPH				
Molloy	2000	Hartmann	YES	no
Roos	2000	necrosectomy	YES	no
Bonner	2001	necrosectomy	YES	YES
Giebel	2002	necrosectomy	YES	no
Ripetti	2002	laparotomy	YES	no
Maw	2002	no	no	no
Wong	2003	Hartmann	YES	no

2.6.12 Fournier's Gangrene

In 2004, Lehnhardt et al. described a case of Fournier's gangrene that developed 2 days after a Milligan-Morgan hemorrhoidectomy in an elderly, obese patient. Since necrosectomy with creation of a defunctioning stoma was not sufficient, because the entire rectum was necrotic, an abdominoperineal resection was performed. The authors referred to two other cases of Fournier's gangrene after hemorrhoidectomy, reported by Başoğlu et al. in 1997 and 1999. One case involved drug-induced agranulocytosis.

This complication, which in the case reported by Lehnhardt et al. occurred in spite of the use of rubber band ligation and dilatation of the anal stenosis, always requires extensive necrosectomy and very often the construction of a defunctioning colostomy.

Estrada et al. (2009) described two cases in which fecal contamination of the necrotic areas was avoided by inserting a large tube into the anus (Flexi-Seal Fecal Management System). They called this potentially very useful method "fecal diversion without colostomy."

In 1991, Heppel and Bernard wrote an excellent review article on the treatment of Fournier's gangrene. The authors listed the four key treatment steps (Table 2.7).

Table 2.7 Treatment of Fournier's gangrene

Re-animation	Analgesia, IV liquids, Blood transfusion, Control of diabetes
Monitoring	Central venous pressure, Diuresis, Arterial blood gases, Arterial line, Pulmonary arteriovenous pressure
Surgery	Extended necrosectomy, Second look after 24 hours, Defunctioning stoma if necessary, Total parenteral nutrition
Laboratory tests	Coagulation, Bilirubin, Creatinine

Patients with Fournier's gangrene have perineal pain, sepsis, edema of the scrotum (if male) and perineum followed by formation of watery pus with a fetid odor and necrosis, and subcutaneous emphysema with crepitus. They are hypotensive, disoriented, febrile, and tachypneic. They are also at high risk for septic shock and death unless immediately given appropriate therapy, which consists of wide and aggressive excision of all necrotic skin, fascia, and muscle. This is the only treatment that in many cases allows patients to improve quickly. Simple incision and drainage are not sufficient. It should also be noted that any maneuver, even application of a simple dressing, is very painful, so it is best to administer morphine.

What happens to the perineal wound once the patient recovers? Four out of five times the skin and underlying tissues spontaneously form scar tissue, although usually only after a long time. If not, a skin graft is necessary and sometimes even more extensive measures, for instance graciloplasty.

2.6.13 Unusual Complications after PPH

These were described earlier, often with comments on their treatment. However, worthy of mention is a trick for the complete (or almost complete) obliteration of the distal rectum.

Gently insert a small (2-3 mm) Hegar dilator to find the lumen and dilate the stenotic segment. After the segment has been enlarged with the dilator, introduce a very thin (10-12 mm) Foley catheter, inflate the balloon, and pull. This will draw the critical point towards you, thus allowing the most opportune maneuvers to be comfortably performed. The first of these maneuvers is cutting the knot of the purse-string in order to "open" the lumen.

In cases of rectovaginal fistula, watch and wait. The fistula may resolve spontaneously. If it does not, surgery is needed; for example, excision and levatorplasty.

Retropneumoperitoneum (sometimes with pneumomediastinum and cervical emphysema) can almost always be treated conservatively. This will be discussed elsewhere.

For rectal pocket/diverticulum, if it is small, then laying open is adequate treatment. If it is large, resection of the diverticulum after introflexion may be necessary.

A bleeding granulomatous polyp can simply be removed.

The third most frequent (20%) re-operation after PPH (Brusciano et al., 2004) is the removal of retained staples. If this is the case, and, as certainly or very likely, the staples are causing intense pain, one can consider an en bloc removal with a strip of rectal tissue (mucosa, submucosa, and part or all of the muscle layer) followed by manual re-anastomosis. This is not a simple operation if a large segment has to be removed, and its effectiveness cannot be guaranteed. In fact, a fibrotic area will probably be left behind (or recur after the procedure), resulting in chronic stimulation of the pudendal nerve endings.

There is not much information on this subject in the literature. Wunderlich (from Vienna, where there is a center dedicated to transanal stapling and therefore such complications are frequent) reported encouraging results. The Israeli colorectal surgeon Rabau told me about a few cases of his that went fairly well. However there is little to induce one to try this procedure.

Recently, Petersen et al. (2011) reviewed the literature on what they call "agrapphectomy" and conclude that the procedure may be more helpful for bleeding than for chronic pain.

We now consider rectal perforations and their treatment. If pelvic sepsis has developed, a Hartmann procedure can be performed. Since a patient with hemorrhoids is usually not very old and usually does not have comorbidities, the stoma can almost always be closed. More than half of the rectal perforations that occur after PPH, as described in the literature or on the FDA website, especially supra-anastomotic perforations, necessitate the creation of a diverting stoma.

In cases of re-operation for recurrent hemorrhoids after PPH, there is a greater risk of postoperative hemorrhage (Brusciano et al., 2004) and postoperative pain (White et al., 2011).

2.7 Tricks of the Trade

1. One trick was already mentioned in Sect. 2.2: coagulating on forceps rather than directly on the tissue when excising a hemorrhoidal nodule, as there will be less bleeding, and then performing the excision by pressing on the forceps and slowly moving the tip along the tissue.
2. This maneuver can be used to obtain hemostasis and to avoid the need for an anal tampon, which might cause pain if, at the end of a Ferguson procedure, the sutured wound is leaking blood or if, after a Milligan-Morgan procedure, large amounts of blood ooze from the wound that has been left open. In such cases, coagulation should not be continued since this may cause burns and necrosis as well as postoperative pain; nor should the wound margins be re-sutured (after a Ferguson procedure) because of the risk of lacerations in the anal canal followed by stenosis. Instead, anchor a small piece of Tabbotamp (hemostatic gauze) to the bleeding

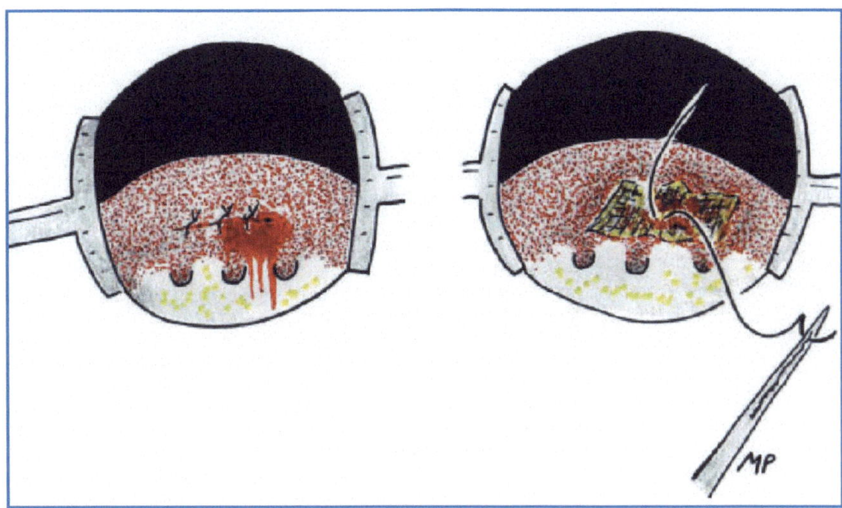

Fig. 2.24 In case the wound is open inside the rectum and hemorrhage persists despite diathermy, a hemostatic gauze of Tabbotamp can be sutured to the bleeding site

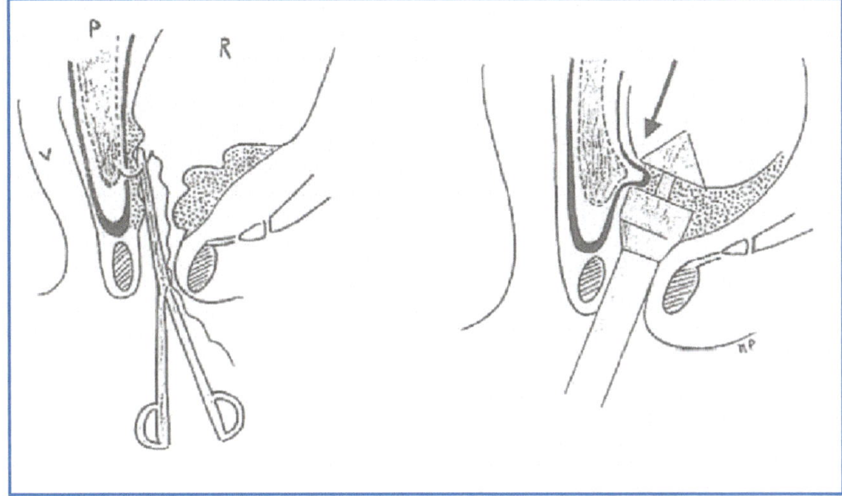

Fig. 2.25 Circular stapled hemorrhoidopexy: "Purse-string" suture in the distal rectum. In an enterocele, a stitch can approximate the peritoneum and bowel with the rectal lumen, with the risk that they are caught in the stapler and injured

tissue with a couple of stitches (Fig. 2.24). This trick can be used for any bleeding endoanal wound, for instance, after surgery for fistulas or villous adenomas.

3. The following trick is useful when performing a PPH on an elderly woman, with a descending perineum, a prolapsed pouch of Douglas, and possibly an enterocele: Before stitching the purse-string to the anterior wall of the distal rectum, infiltrate the area with saline solution in order to distance the submucosa from the rectum and nearby organs. This will reduce the risk of passing the stitches of the purse-string or staples through them and thus provoking ischemia, lesions, or perforations followed by peritonitis or hemoperitoneum (Fig. 2.25 and 2.26). The trick was described in a previously published article (Pescatori and Quondamcarlo, 1999).
4. This is another trick to use when performing a PPH, in order to prevent rectal pocket syndrome, i.e., the formation of a rectal diverticulum/rectal inclusion cyst. When constructing the purse-string, be careful not to make any of the stitches too superficial. If you suspect that this is indeed so, pull hard on the stitch. A small laceration during surgery is better than complications afterwards.
5. In a Milligan-Morgan procedure, if there are residual accessory nodules on the mucocuta-

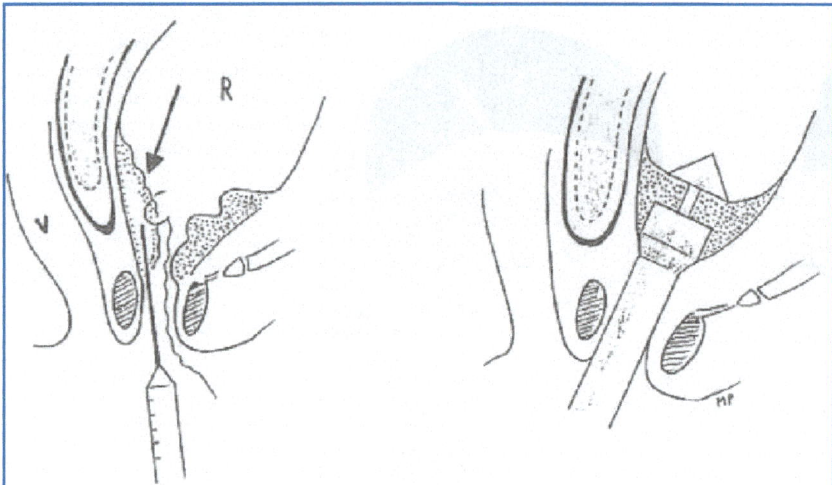

Fig. 2.26 This complication can be prevented with saline injection in the anterior submucosal plane of the distal rectum before the procedure (from Pescatori and Quondamcarlo, 1999)

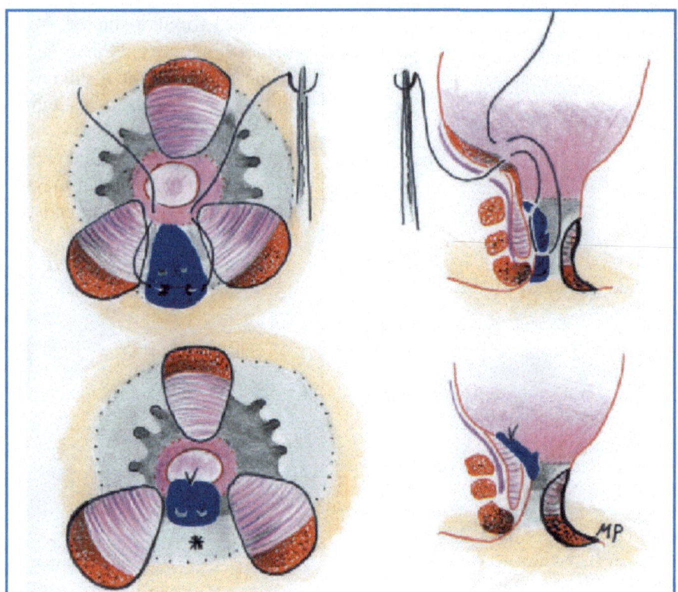

Fig. 2.27 Technique for the treatment of a secondary hemorrhoid (*blue*) in a residual mucocutaneous bridge after Milligan-Morgan hemorrhoidectomy. Three surgical wounds are visible. An ischemizing pexy is performed by means of a U-shaped stitch that is fixed to the muscularis of the distal rectum without dissecting bridge epithelium in the anal canal (*asterisk*). This technique is used to prevent anal stenosis. In the last image, the hemorrhoid is sutured to the anorectal ring

neous bridges after the three main nodules have been excised, U-shaped sutures can be placed (as Parks used to do): one suture per bridge. The first passage of the needle is vertical, into the distal rectum immediately above the anorectal ring, and deep into the tissue, to grab the muscularis layer. The second and third passages are low down and horizontal, penetrating the hemorrhoidal nodule on the mucocutaneous bridge, immediately above the dentate line, thereby avoiding the highly innervated zone of the anal canal epithelium. The fourth passage is vertical, to close the U, and slightly lateral to the first (Fig. 2.27).

An adroit move: before placing stitches, make two "strips" using diathermy coagulation on the two segments of tissue, one in the distal rectum and the other in the anal canal. These strips will be pulled together once the suture knots are tied, thus ensuring greater adhesion because the epithelium on the tissue has been destroyed by electrocautery. Use the flat part of the electric scalpel so that these two strips do not bleed. Just barely coagulating the epithelium is sufficient since obviously there is no need to cut. The last step is tightening the suture knot; this results in a -pexy effect and ischemia of the residual nodule while preserving the integrity of the "bridge," which is a guarantee against stenosis of the anal canal.

6. To perform a Ferguson procedure without (or almost without) intraoperative bleeding following removal of the hemorrhoid, prior to exeresis, place two stitches at the base of the nodule, a superficial stitch and then, pulling on the thread, a stitch further down, at the base of the nodule, where the hemorrhoidal pedicle is located. Even if the pedicle is not always there, the trick often works.
7. How can the problem of "dog ears" at the distal end of the suture line in a Ferguson hemorrhoidectomy be avoided? Those raised parts of the skin not only become unaesthetic skin tags, they also cause edema and postoperative pain. If they have formed because you have not cut off enough skin when starting the excision of the nodule, making a pointed "V," leave out the last stitch on the perianal skin when you finish suturing, make a knot, and go back 2-3 cm towards the anal border with the same thread. Then make a knot either at the anal border or at the level of the former dentate line. This maneuver results in a sort of - pexy and should prevent the formation of "dog ears." It usually works.
8. Another trick for the Ferguson procedure was taught to me by Nivatvongs of the Mayo Clinic, and was already mentioned in this chapter. Use Vicryl Rapid (or catgut if available) to suture the surgical wound. This way, if an infection develops and a small abscess starts to form, it will drain spontaneously when the suture thread is reabsorbed (Fig. 2.28). Additional advice, perhaps not very original, is: if infection develops, in other words pus, edema, and pain, cut the knot that you made at the distal end of the suture line to facilitate drainage.
9. Now for a trick that can be used not to prevent a complication, anal stenosis, but to treat it. I have used this trick in a couple of cases of stenosis after PPH. Following dilatation with a Hegar dilator, either in the operating room or in an outpatient setting, inject cortisone into the area of the former stenosis. This will

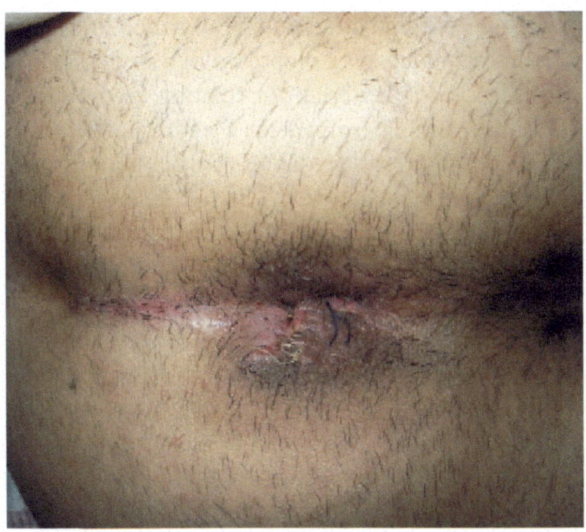

Fig. 2.28 After Ferguson hemorrhoidectomy, early suture release allows spontaneous drainage of a local sepsis. Drainage is facilitated by using Vicryl Rapid or catgut, as recommended by Nivatvongs of the Mayo Clinic)

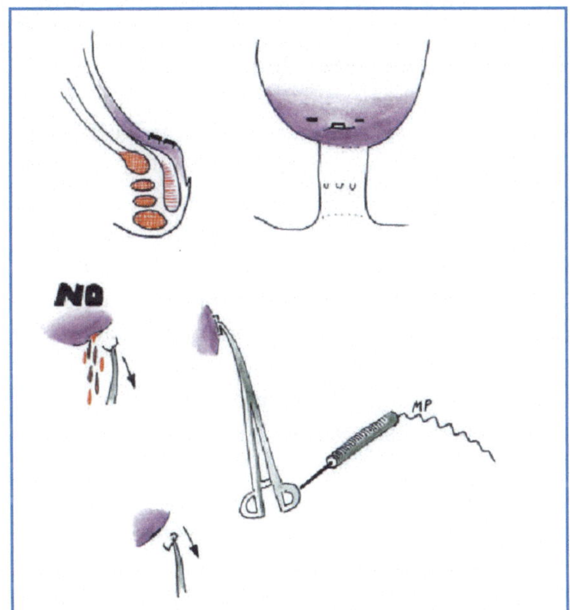

Fig. 2.29 A simple, but useful "trick" to remove retained staples, a possible cause of bleeding or proctalgia after PPH (or STARR). Instead of grabbing the stitch with a Kelly, pulling it and tearing the rectal mucosa causing bleeding, diathermy is performed on the Kelly. The stitch is easily removed, coagulating the mucosa and leaving a small eschar

"stabilize" the dilatation. I described this trick in Techniques in Coloproctology in 2002.

10. Here is another trick for treating a complication, in this case pain or bleeding after PPH caused by retained staples. This commonplace but useful maneuver, which I learned from Sandro Palazzi, my colleague. Once you have identified the staple, refrain from doing what is usually done, i.e., grabbing it with a Kelly and pulling it out of the tissue. This will definitely cause laceration and bleeding. Instead, after grabbing it with the Kelly, coagulate on the Kelly itself. The heat is transmitted to the staple, which in turn coagulates just a few millimeters of tissue around it. The staple will then come out without any damage to the tissue (Fig. 2.29).

2.8 Two Unforgettable Complications

2.8.1 Case Number One

One morning, years ago, while I was working in the clinic, which was located on a hill among the pine trees of the "Roma Nord" district of Rome, the head nurse of the general surgery ward came into my office. She told me that a patient had been admitted to the Urology unit as an emergency case (a rare occurrence) and the urologists had asked me to see her because she had a history of recent hemorrhoid surgery. I entered the examination room, where I saw before me a small shrunken form lying on the bed. It was a young woman (35 years old), suffering greatly, confused, very thin and sharp-featured, dyspneic, and with a large distended abdomen only half covered by the sheet. Her abdomen looked like that of a pregnant woman. Seeing that she was so worn out I thought, "she has a tumor," but then I recalled "a recent history of hemorrhoidectomy." I was puzzled. The blood test results arrived from the laboratory. Her blood urea level was 70 mg/100 ml.

So what do you think this patient had?

In my presence, they catheterized her bladder. One bag filled with urine, then another, and another. And there was still urine coming out—a total of 4 liters. Her abdomen slowly became smaller. The patient continued to touch her perineum and grimace with pain.

The urologists organized hemodialysis for her. There was no time to be lost. With such a high urea reading she was at risk of cardiac arrest due to hyperkalemia.

A few hours later, having in the meantime looked through the patient's chart from the small country hospital from which she had been transferred, and when things had calmed down, I was able to talk to the patient. She recounted that she began to have urinary retention after a Milligan-Morgan hemorrhoidectomy with internal sphincterotomy (she had also had a fissure). She had been suffering excruciating pain at home and had been unable to urinate. Undecided as to what to do, she finally returned to the hospital. The doctor on call immediately notified the clinic in Rome as it was the closest one with a Urology unit.

This case demonstrates that urinary retention is not always a trivial complication, but can sometimes be life-threatening. In this patient, retention did not occur immediately and it seemed to be related to the intense postoperative pain.

Once the critical phase had passed and after more than one session of hemodialysis, there was still anal stenosis, which did not resolve after dilatation and therefore necessitated anoplasty. The case was described in Techniques in Coloproctology (Basso et al., 2001).

2.8.2 Case Number Two

The complication was severe chronic proctalgia after PPH and the saddest thing about this case is that the patient L., underwent 10 operations in 3 years but at presentation felt even worse. She was a strong woman, almost 40 years old, and had tried to remain active even though she suffered from severe chronic pain. Every now and then she sends me an e-mail and still hopes for the best.

A gynecologist performed the first of the series of operations: a colpo-perineoplasty for rectocele. It is unclear whether the operation was essential. The patient was rather young and nulliparous. I suspect that from the start she was a victim of excessive "surgical intent." Her case serves as a reminder to surgeons (myself included) that sometimes it is important to wait rather than to operate.

After the gynecological operation, L. was well for a year. Then she went to see a surgeon because she suffered from hemorrhoids. The surgeon found two second-degree piles and suggested PPH. She told me later that the operation was described to her as "painless" and cure was promised (no doubt in good faith). She was reassured and decided to undergo surgery.

Some readers will perhaps think, as I do, that PPH is excessive for second-degree hemorrhoids. In the SICCR guidelines (Altomare et al., 2006), PPH is indicated for third-degree hemorrhoids. It is, however, worthy of note that surgeons at the University of Aberdeen (Shanmugan et al. 2010) reported a case series of PPH for second-degree hemorrhoids. In my patient, a few weeks later the gradually intensifying proctalgia, which the patient has suffered from ever since, began.

We cannot know for certain whether the surgical wound from the gynecological operation (or other factors that will be mentioned) were partly responsible for the proctalgia. It is, however, a fact that re-operation increases a patient's risk of developing complications. Pain is one of these. The branches of the pudendal nerves extend into the perineum and the levator ani muscles and the formation of a second scar is certainly not beneficial.

A pause for thought. Imagine a young nulliparous woman with severe proctalgia after PPH. What would you have done at this point to treat her?

For the sake of brevity, I will omit most of what happened in the following two years. I shall only say that L. underwent seven other operations: staple's removal, internal prolapsectomy with the Delorme technique, transgluteal neurolysis of the pudendal nerve, removal of endometriotic nodules from the pouch of Douglas, removal of a granuloma from the rectovaginal septum, and positioning of a provisional electrode for sacral neuromodulation plus laying open of an anal fistula.

"But she could have had conservative therapy!" you might say. She did! Biofeedback, total parenteral nutrition, psychotherapy, acupuncture, treatment of pain with Lyrica and other agents, hypnosis, local infiltration anesthesia, and cortisone injections into the levator ani muscles. All failed to help.

Fortunately severe chronic proctalgia after PPH is relatively rare. In Ravo's multicenter study (2002), 2% of 1300 patients were affected, and in other studies (Cheetham et al., 2003) up to 16%. The majority of authors reported an incidence of severe chronic proctalgia under 5%. However, when it does occur it is difficult to treat.

There is definite evidence that L. had some psychological problems; for example, after decades she still had not accepted the death of her mother, which had occurred when she was still a little girl. Her separation from her husband had been very traumatic. She suffered because she had no children. All this may have had some connection to her problems with chronic pain. Yet regarding the implacable persistence of the pain it is clear that the determining factors were the excessive number of operations and the large amount of scar tissue in a highly innervated area. I think an even more important factor was that instead of having rubber band ligation she underwent PPH.

Summary

There are many complications that can occur after an operation for hemorrhoids. The majority of them can be prevented by correct surgical maneuvers.

Both Milligan-Morgan hemorrhoidectomy and stapled hemorrhoidopexy are sometimes followed by severe hemorrhage, but the incidence is under 5%. The incidence of rectal bleeding after the Ferguson procedure is often under 1%. There is rarely a need for re-operation if rectal tamponade with a Foley catheter is used in the procedure.

Stool incontinence is rare and may be caused by a lesion of the internal sphincter. It can be treated conservatively with bulking agents.

If there is anal stenosis, it is usually after the Milligan-Morgan procedure, but it almost never requires anoplasty and often resolves after dilatation. After Ferguson hemorrhoidectomy there can be suture dehiscence (25% of patients). Chronic anal fissure occurs more frequently after Milligan-Morgan hemorrhoidectomy.

Unusual complications may occur after PPH, for instance, obliteration of the rectum, retropneumoperitoneum, or rectovaginal fistula, all of which are very rare. Fecal urgency and tenesmus are more common and often temporary.

Rectal intussusception and perforations of the rectum, more likely if the pouch of Douglas is prolapsed, have been described. Pelvic sepsis often makes colostomy necessary. In three out of 100 cases, a rectal pocket forms.

Severe proctalgia after PPH is hard to treat and has a negative effect on the quality of life.

The least invasive operation is THD-mucopexy. The incidence of complications (which are usually minor), such as hemorrhoidal thrombosis, is under 10%.

Urinary retention is associated more commonly with the type of anesthesia used, and the age and sex of the patient. It can occur after any surgical treatment of hemorrhoids.

Suggested Readings

Aigner F, Bonatti H, Peer S et al (2010) Vascular considerations for stapled haemorrhoidopexy. Colorectal Dis 12:452-458

Allan A, Samad AJ, Mellon A et al (2006) Prospective randomised study of urgent haemorrhoidectomy compared with non-operative treatment in the management of prolapsed thrombosed internal haemorrhoids. Colorectal Dis 8:41-45

Altomare D, Infantino A, Bottini C et al (2010) Prospective randomized multicenter study comparing stapled hemorrhoidopexy (SH) with Doppler-guided transanal hemorrhoid dearterialization (THD) for III degree hemorrhoids. Dis Colon Rectum 53:580

Altomare DF, Milito G, Andreoli R et al (2008) Ligasure Precise vs. conventional diathermy for Milligan-Morgan hemorrhoidectomy: a prospective, randomized, multicenter trial. Dis Colon Rectum 51:514-519

Altomare DF, Roveran A, Pecorella G et al (2006) The treatment of hemorrhoids: guidelines of the Italian Society of Colorectal Surgery. Tech Coloproctol 10:181-186

Amato A, Seow-Choen F (2009) Ethical issues and innovation in colorectal surgery. Tech Coloproctol 13:83-85

Amoli HA, Notash AY, Shahandashti FJ et al (2011) A randomized, prospective, double-blind, placebo-controlled trial of the effect of topical diltiazem on posthaemorrhoidectomy pain. Colorectal Dis 13:328-332

Andrews BT, Layer GT, Jackson BT et al (1993) Randomized trial comparing diathermy hemorrhoidectomy with the scissor dissection Milligan-Morgan operation. Dis Colon Rectum 36:580-583

Angelone G, Giardiello C, Prota C (2006) Bleeding after stapled haemorhoidopexy using PPH 03 instrument. ANZ J Surg 76:672-673

Angelone G, Giardiello C, Prota C (2006) Stapled hemorrhoidopexy. Complications and 2-year follow-up. Chir Ital 58:753-760

Angelone G, Giardiello C, Prota C (2007) Bleeding after stapled haemorrhoidopexy using the PPH 03 stapler device. Experience and results in 100 consecutive patients. Chir Ital 59:225-229

Arbman G, Krook H, Haapaniemi S (2000) Closed vs. open hemorrhoidectomy-is there any difference? Dis Colon Rectum 43:31-34

Arroyo A, Pérez F, Miranda E et al (2004) Open versus closed day-case haemorrhoidectomy: is there any difference? Results of a prospective randomised study. Int J Colorectal Dis 19:370-373

Arroyo A, Pérez-Vicente F, Serrano P et al (2006) Proctitis complicating stapled hemorrhoidectomy: report of a case. Int J Colorectal Dis 21:197-198

Augustin G, Smud D, Kinda E et al (2009) Intra-abdominal bleeding from a seromuscular tear of an ascending rectosigmoid intramural hematoma after stapled hemorrhoidopexy. Can J Surg 52:14-15

Aumann G, Petersen S, Pollack T et al (2004) Severe intra-abdominal bleeding following stapled mucosectomy due to enterocele: report of a case. Tech Coloproctol 8:41-43

Baraza W, Shorthouse A, Brown S (2009) Obliteration of the rectal lumen after stapled hemorrhoidopexy: report of a case. Dis Colon Rectum 52:1524-1525

Başoğlu M, Gül O, Yildirgan I et al (1997) Fournier's gangrene: review of fifteen cases. Am Surg 63:1019-1021

Basso L, Bernardi C, Ayabaca S et al (2001) Life-threatening urinary retention after haemorrhoidectomy and internal sphincterotomy. Tech Coloproctol 5:109-111

Basso L, Pescatori M (1994) Outcome of delayed hemorrhage following surgical hemorrhoidectomy. Dis Colon Rectum 36:743-746

Basso L, Pescatori M (2003) Subcutaneous emphysema after associated colonoscopy and transanal excision of rectal adenoma. Surg Endosc 17:1677

Beer-Gabel M, Carter D, Venturero M et al (2010) Ultrasonographic assessment of patients referred with chronic anal pain to a tertiary referral centre. Tech Coloproctol 14:107-112

Behboo R, Zanella S, Ruffolo C et al (2011) Stapled haemorrhoidopexy: extent of tissue excsion and clinical implications in the early postoperative period. Colorect Dis 13:697-702

Berstock JR, Bunni J, Torrie AP (2010) The squelching hip: a sign of life-threatening sepsis following haemorrhoidectomy. Ann R Coll Surg Engl 92:39-41

Bessa SS (2008) Ligasure vs. conventional diathermy in excisional hemorrhoidectomy: a prospective, randomized study. Dis Colon Rectum 51:940-944

Beuke AC, Pedersen ME, Qvist N (2008) Rectal perforation and faecal peritonitis after stapled operation for grade IV haemorrhoids. Ugeskr Laeger 170:460

Bittorf B, Ringler R, Forster C et al (2006) Cerebral representation of the anorectum using functional magnetic resonance imaging. Br J Surg 93:1251-1257

Blouhos K, Vasiliadis K, Tsalis K et al (2007) Uncontrollable intra-abdominal bleeding necessitating low anterior resection of the rectum after stapled hemorrhoidopexy: report of a case. Surg Today 37:254-257

Boccasanta P, Venture M, Orio A et al (1998) Circular hemorrhoidectomy in advanced hemorrhoidal disease. Hepato-gastroenterology 45:962-969

Boccasanta P, Venturi M, Roviaro GC (2007) Stapled Transanal Rectal Resection versus stapled anopexy in the cure of hemorroids with rectal prolapse. A randomized controlled trial. Int J Colorectal Dis 22:245-251

Boffi F (2008) Retained staples causing rectal bleeding and severe proctalgia after the STARR procedure. Tech Coloproctol 12:135-136

Boffi F (2008) Sutureless PPH and STARR. Tech Coloproctol 12:352

Boffi F, Podzemny V (2011) Obstructed defecation, rectocele, recurrent hemorrhoids and rectal diverticulum following the procedure for prolapsed hemorrhoids. Tech Coloproctol 15:255-256

Bondurri A, Zbar AP, Tapia H et al (2011) The relationship between etiology, symptom severity and indications for surgery in cases of anal incontinence: a 25-year analysis of 1046 patients at a tertiary coloproctology practice. Tech Coloproctol 15:159-164

Bozdag AD, Nazli O, Tansug T et al (2008) Videoanoscope-assisted stapled haemorrhoidopexy: analysis of 18 patients. Tech Coloproctol. 12:123-126

Brown S, Baraza W, Shorthouse A (2007) Total rectal lumen obliteration after stapled haemorrhoidopexy: a cautionary tale. Tech Coloproctol 11:357-358

Brown SR, Shanmugan P, Dobbs P (2006) Stapled haemorrhoidopexy for prolapsing haemorrhoids. Colorectal Dis 8:525-526

Brusciano L, Ayabaca SM, Pescatori M et al (2004) Reinterventions after complicated or failed stapled hemorrhoidopexy. Dis Colon Rectum 47:1846-1851

Bufo A, Galasse S, Amoroso M (2006) Recurrent severe postoperative bleeding after stapled hemorrhoidopexy requiring emergency laparotomy. Tech Coloproctol 10:62-63

Burch J, Epstein D, Sari AB et al (2009) Stapled haemorrhoidopexy for the treatment of haemorrhoids: a systematic review. Colorectal Dis 11:233-243

Büyükaşik O, Hasdemir OA, Cöl C (2009) Rectal lumen obliteration from stapled hemorrhoidopexy: can it be prevented? Tech Coloproctol 13:333-335

Capomagi A, Mannetta V, Balestrieri A et al (1999) Circular haemorrhoidectomy using stapler is the "gold standard" for the treatment of hemorrhoids? Preliminary data regarding 206 consecutive patients. Ital J Coloproctol 2:782–785

Carapeti EA, Kamm MA, McDonald PJ et al (1998) Double-blind randomised controlled trial of effect of metronidazole on pain after day-case haemorrhoidectomy. Lancet 351:169-172

Carapeti EA, Kamm MA, McDonald PJ et al (1999) Randomized trial of open versus closed day-case haemorrhoidectomy. Br J Surg 86:612-613

Carriero A, Dal Borgo P, Pucciani F (2001) Stapled mucosal prolapsectomy for haemorrhoidal prolapse with Lone Star Retractor System. Tech Coloproctol 5:41-46

Cheetham MJ, Cohen CR, Kamm MA et al (2003) A randomized, controlled trial of diathermy hemorrhoidectomy vs. stapled hemorrhoidectomy in an intended day-care setting with longer-term follow-up. Dis Colon Rectum 46:491-497

Cheetham MJ, Mortensen NJ, Nystrom PO et al (2000) Persistent pain and faecal urgency after stapled haemorrhoidectomy. Lancet 356:730-733

Cheetham MJ, Phillips RK (2001) Evidence-based practice in haemorrhoidectomy. Colorectal Dis 3:126-134

Chen JG, Yang XD, Quian Q et al (2010) Rectal perforation after procedure for prolapse and hemorrhoids. Dis Colon Rectum 52:1439-1445

Chew MH, Chiow A, Tang CL (2008) Keloid formation after stapled haemorrhoidectomy causing anal stenosis: a rare complication. Tech Coloproctol 12:351-352

Chik B, Law WL, Choi HK (2006) Urinary retention after haemorrhoidectomy: impact of stapled haemorrhoidectomy. Asian J Surg 29:233-237

Chung YC, Wu HJ (2003) Clinical experience of sutureless closed hemorrhoidectomy with LigaSure. Dis Colon Rectum 46:87-92

Cihan A, Menteş BB, Sucak G et al (1999) Fournier's gangrene after hemorrhoidectomy: association with drug-induced agranulocytosis. Report of a case. Dis Colon Rectum 42:1644-1648

Cipriani S, Pescatori M (2002) Acute rectal obstruction after PPH stapled haemorrhoidectomy. Colorectal Dis 4:367-370

Cirocco WC (1996) Local epinephrine injection for delayed hemorrhage after hemorrhoidectomy. Tech Coloproctol 4:147-149

Cirocco WC (2008) Life threatening sepsis and mortality following stapled hemorrhoidopexy. Surgery 143:824-829

Corman ML, Carriero A, Hager T et al (2006) Consensus conference on the stapled transanal rectal resection (STARR). Colorect Dis 8:98-101

Cotton MH (2005) Pelvic sepsis after stapled hemorrhoidectomy. J Am Coll Surg 200:983

Dal Monte PP, Tagariello C, Sarago M et al (2007) Transanal haemorrhoidal dearterialisation: nonexcisional surgery for the treatment of haemorrhoidal disease. Tech Coloproctol 11:333-338

Daniel F, Sultan S, de Parades V et al (2006) Anal fissure and minor anorectal sepsis after stapled hemorrhoidectomy. Dis Colon Rectum 49:693-694

De Nardi P, Corsetti M, Passaretti S et al (2008) Evaluation of sensory and motor rectal response after hemorrhoidopexy with electronic barostat. Dis Colon Rectum 51:1255-1260

De Santis G, Gola P, Lancione L et al (2011) Sigmoid intramural hematoma and hemoperitoneum: an early severe complication after stapled hemorrhoidopexy. Tech Coloproctol [Epub ahead of print]

Dodi G, Cavallari F, Ventura S et al (1999) Sarafoff's anoplasty for incontinence following Whitehead's hemorrhoidectomy. Tech Coloproctol 3:63-66

Drummond R, Wright DM (2007) Continued rectal bleeding following stapled haemorrhoidectomy. Colorectal Dis 9:669-670

Durai R, Ng PC (2009) Perirectal abscess following procedure for prolapsed haemorrhoids successfully managed with a combination of VAC sponge and Redivac systems. Tech Coloproctol 13:307-309

Ertem M, Karatas A, Gök H, Yilmaz S (2009) Rare complication following Longo operation: giant rectal haematoma. Case report. ANZ J Surg 79:956-957

Estrada O, Martinez I, Del Bas M, Salvans S, Hidalgo LA (2009) Rectal diversion without colostomy in Fournier's gangrene. Tech Coloproctol 13:157-159

Eu KW, Teoh TA, Seow-Choen F, Goh HS (1995) Anal stricture following haemorrhoidectomy: early diagnosis and treatment. Aust N Z J Surg 65:101-103

Farag AE (1978) Pile suture: a new technique for the treatment of haemorrhoids. Br J Surg 65:293-295

Fareed M, El-Awady S, Abd-El monaem H, Aly A (2009) Randomized trial comparing LigaSure to closed Ferguson hemorrhoidectomy. Tech Coloproctol 13:243-246

Farouk R, Lieske B, Conaghan P (2010) Doppler guided hemorrhoid artery ligation and rectoanal repair for grade 2 and 3 hemorrhoids: outcomes after surgery. Dis Colon Rectum 53:580

Faucheron JL, Poncet G, Voirin D et al (2011) Doppler-guided hemorrhoidal artery ligation and rectoanal repair (HAL-RAR) for the treatment of grade IV hemorrhoids: long-term results in 100 consecutive patients. Dis Colon Rectum 54:226-231

Festen S, van Hoogstraten MJ, van Geloven AA, Gerhards MF (2009) Treatment of grade III and IV haemorrhoidal disease with PPH or THD. A randomized trial on postoperative complications and short-term results. Int J Colorectal Dis 24:1401-1405

Filingeri V, Gravante G (2005) Pneumoretroperitoneum, pneumomediastinum and subcutaneous emphysema of the neck after stapled hemorrhoidopexy. Tech Coloproctol 9:86

Filingeri V, Gravante G (2006) Stapled hemorrhoidopexy followed by fecal urgency and tenesmus: methodological complication or surgeon's mistake? Tech Coloproctol 10:149

Folgado Alberto S, Oro I, Sánchez P et al (2009) Rectal ulcer as a complication of the Longo circular hemorrhoidopexy. Rev Esp Enferm Dig 101:733-735

Fondran JC, Porter JA, Slezak FA (2006) Inflammatory polyps: a cause of late bleeding in stapled hemorrhoidectomy. Dis Colon Rectum 49:1910-1913

Forrest NP, Mullerat J, Evans C, Middleton SB (2010) Doppler-guided haemorrhoidal artery ligation with recto anal repair: a new technique for the treatment of symptomatic haemorrhoids. Int J Colorectal Dis 25:1251-1256

Gaj F, Trecca A (2005) Hemorrhoids and rectal internal mucosal prolapse: one or two conditions? A national survey. Tech Coloproctol 9:163-165

Ganio E, Altomare DF, Gabrielli F, Milito G, Canuti S (2001) Prospective randomized multicentre trial comparing stapled with open haemorrhoidectomy. Br J Surg 88:669-674

Gao XH, Wang HT, Chen JG, Yang XD, Qian Q, Fu CG (2010) Rectal perforation after procedure for prolapse and hemorrhoids: possible causes. Dis Colon Rectum 53:1439-1445

Garg P, Sidhu G, Nair S et al (2011) The fate and significance of retained staples after stapled hemorrhoidopexy. Colorect Dis 13:572-575

Giamundo P, Cecchetti W, Esercizio L et al (2010) Doppler-guided hemorrhoidal laser procedure for the treatment of symptomatic hemorrhoids: experimental background and short-term clinical results of a new mini-invasive treatment. Surg Endosc 25:1369-1375

Gingold BS (1991) Complications of anorectal laser therapy. Persp Colon rect Surg 4:305-312

Giordano A, della Corte M (2008) Non-operative management of a rectovaginal fistula complicating stapled haemorrhoidectomy. Int J Colorectal Dis 23:727-728

Giordano P, Bradley BM, Peiris L (2008) Obliteration of the rectal lumen after stapled hemorrhoidopexy: report of a case. Dis Colon Rectum 51:1574-1576

Giordano P, Gravante G, Sorge R et al (2009) Long-term outcomes of stapled hemorrhoidopexy vs conventional hemorrhoidectomy: a meta-analysis of randomized controlled trials. Arch Surg 144:266-272

Gravante G, Venditti D (2007) Pos anal stenoses with Ligasure hemorrhoidectomy. World J Surg 31:245

Gravié JF, Lehur PA, Huten N et al (2005) Stapled hemorrhoidopexy versus milligan-morgan hemorrhoidectomy: a prospective, randomized, multicenter trial with 2-year postoperative follow up. Ann Surg 242:29-35

Guenin MO, Rosenthal R, Kern B et al (2005) Ferguson hemorrhoidectomy: long-term results and patient satisfaction. Dis Colon Rectum 48:1523-1527

Gupta PJ (2004) A comparative study between radiofrequency ablation with plication and Milligan-Morgan hemorrhoidectomy for grade III hemorrhoids. Tech Coloproctol 8:163-168

Gupta PJ (2009) Ethical issues on newer technologies in colorectal practice. Tech Coloproctol 13:329-330

Guy RJ, Seow-Choen F (2003) Septic complications after treatment of haemorrhoids. Br J Surg 90:147-156

Halberg M, Raahave D (2006) Perirectal, retroperitoneal, intraperitoneal and mediastinal gas after stapled haemorrhoidopexy. Ugeskr Laeger 168:3139-3140

Hall NR, Goldberg SM (2003) Reoperative surgery for persistent hemorrhoidal disease and complications of surgical hemorrhoidectomy. In: Longo WE, Northover JMA (eds) Reoperative colon and rectal surgery. London, Martin Dunitz

Heppel J, Benard F (1991) Life-threatening perineal sepsis. Persp Colon Rect Surg 4:1-16

Ho KS, Ho YH (2006) Prospective randomized trial comparing stapled hemorrhoidopexy versus closed Ferguson hemorrhoidectomy. Tech Coloproctol 10:193-197

Ho YH, Foo CL, Seow-Choen F, Goh HS (1995) Prospective randomized controlled trial of a micronized flavonidic fraction to reduce bleeding after haemorrhoidectomy. Br J Surg 82:1034-1035

Ho YH, Seow-Choen F, Tsang C, Eu KW (2001) Randomized trial assessing anal sphincter injuries after stapled haemorrhoidectomy. Br J Surg 88:1449-1455

Holzheimer RG (2004) Hemorrhoidectomy: indications and risks. Eur J Med Res 9:18-36

Hosch SB, Knoefel WT, Pichlmeier U et al (1998) Surgical treatment of piles: prospective, randomized study of Parks vs. Milligan-Morgan hemorrhoidectomy. Dis Colon Rectum 41:159-164

Huang WS, Chin CC, Yeh CH et al (2007) Randomized comparison between stapled hemorrhoidectomy and Ferguson hemorrhoidectomy for grade III hemorrhoids in Taiwan: a prospective study. Int J Colorectal Dis 22:955-961

Hussein AM (2001) Ligation-anopexy for treatment of advanced hemorrhoidal disease. Dis Colon Rectum 44:1887-1890

Hwang DY, Yoon SG, Kim HS, Lee JK, Kim KY (2003) Effect of 0.2 percent glyceryl trinitrate ointment on wound healing after a hemorrhoidectomy: results of a randomized, prospective, double-blind, placebo-controlled trial. Dis Colon Rectum 46:950-954

Ibrahim S, Tsang C, Lee YL, Eu KW, Seow-Choen F (1998) Prospective, randomized trial comparing pain and complications between diathermy and scissors for closed hemorrhoidectomy. Dis Colon Rectum 41:1418-1420

Imbelloni LE, Gouveia MA, Vieira EM, Cordeiro JA (2008) Selective sensory spinal anaesthesia with hypobaric lidocaine for anorectal surgery. Acta Anaesthesiol Scand 52:1327-1330

Infantino A, Bellomo R, Dal Monte PP et al (2010) Transanal haemorrhoidal artery echodoppler ligation and anopexy (THD) is effective for II and III degree haemorrhoids: a prospective multicentric study. Colorectal Dis 12:804-809

Jayaraman S, Colquhoun PH, Malthaner RA (2007) Stapled hemorrhoidopexy is associated with a higher long-term recurrence rate of internal hemorrhoids compared with conventional excisional hemorrhoid surgery. Dis Colon Rectum 50:1297-1305

Jayaraman S, Colquhoun PHD, Malthaner RA (2006) Stapled versus conventional surgery for hemorrhoids. Cochrane Database of Systematic Reviews Issue 4 Art. No: CD005393

Jensen C, Jørgensen H (2001) Late, life-threatening bleeding after hemorrhoidectomy. Ugeskr Laeger 163:41-42

Jóhannsson HO, Påhlman L, Graf W (2006) Randomized clinical trial of the effects on anal function of Milligan-Morgan versus Ferguson haemorrhoidectomy. Br J Surg 93:1208-1214

Kam MH, Lim JF, Ho KS, Ooi BS, Eu KW (2009) Short-term results of DST EEA 33 stapler and neu@ anoscope for stapled haemorrhoidectomy: a prospective study of 1,118 patients from a single centre. Tech Coloproctol 13:273-277

Kanellos I, Blouhos K, Demetriades H, Pramateftakis MG, Betsis D (2004) Pneumomediastinum after dilatation of anal stricture following stapled hemorrhoidopexy. Tech Coloproctol 8:185-187

Karanlik H, Akturk R, Camlica H, Asoglu O (2009) The effect of glyceryl trinitrate ointment on posthemorrhoidectomy pain and wound healing: results of a randomized, double-blind, placebo-controlled study. Dis Colon Rectum 52:280-285

Keighley MR, Williams NS (1993) Surgery of the anus, rectum and colon. Sounders Elsevier, Philadelphia

Kekez T, Bulic K, Smudj D, Majerovic M (2007) Is stapled hemorrhoidopexy safe for the male homosexual patient? Report of a case. Surg Today 37:335–337

Khubchandani I (2002) Internal sphincterotomy with hemorrhoidectomy does not relieve pain: a prospective, randomized study. Dis Colon Rectum 45:1452-1457

Khubchandani I (2005) Open vs. closed hemorrhoidectomy. Tech Coloproctol 9:256

Khubchandani I, Fealk MH, Reed JF 3rd (2009) Is there a post-PPH syndrome? Tech Coloproctol 13:141-144

Knight JS, Senapati A, Lamparelli MJ (2008) National UK audit of procedure for prolapsing haemorrhoids on behalf of the Association of Coloproctology of Great Britain and Ireland. Colorectal Dis 10:440-445

Kodner IJ (2009) Innovations in colorectal surgery. Tech Coloproctol 13:167-168

Koh PK, Seow-Choen F (2005) Mucosal flap excision for treatment of remnant prolapsed hemorrhoids or skin tags after stapled hemorrhoidopexy. Dis Colon Rectum 48:1660-1662

Kosorok P, Mlakar B (2005) Haemorrhoidectomy as a one-day surgical procedure: modified Ferguson technique. Tech Coloproctol 9:57-59

Kraemer M, Parulava T, Roblick M et al (2005) Prospective, randomized study: proximate PPH stapler vs. LigaSure for hemorrhoidal surgery. Dis Colon Rectum 48:1517-1522

Kriss BD, Porter JA, Slezak FA (1990) Retroperitoneal air after routine hemorrhoidectomy. Report of a case. Dis Colon Rectum 33:971-973

La Torre F, Nicolai AP (2004) Clinical use of micronized purified flavonoid fraction for treatment of symptoms after hemorrhoidectomy: results of a randomized, controlled, clinical trial. Dis Colon Rectum 47:704-710

Lacerda-Filho A, Assunção GM, de Oliveira TA (2009) Neuropathic pain after stapled hemorrhoidopexy. Tech Coloproctol 13:255-256

Laughlan K, Jayne DG, Jackson D, Rupprecht F, Ribaric G (2009) Stapled haemorrhoidopexy compared to Milligan-Morgan and Ferguson haemorrhoidectomy: a systematic review. Int J Colorectal Dis 24:335-344

Lehnhardt M, Steinstraesser L, Druecke D, Muehlberger T, Steinau HU, Homann HH (2004) Fournier's gangrene after Milligan-Morgan hemorrhoidectomy requiring subsequent abdominoperineal resection of the rectum: report of a case. Dis Colon Rectum 47:1729-1733

Lim YK, Eu KW, Ho KS, Ooi BS, Tang CL (2006) PPH03 stapled hemorrhoidopexy: our experience. Tech Coloproctol 10:43-46

Lin YH, Liu KW, Chen HP (2010) Haemorrhoidectomy: prevalence and risk factors of urine retention among post recipients. J Clin Nurs 19:2771-2776

Lindsey I, Jones OM, Smilgin-Humphreys MM, Cunningham C, Mortensen NJ (2004) Patterns of fecal incontinence after anal surgery. Dis Colon Rectum 47:1643-1649

Lo O, Ong K, Kam M, Eu K (2010) Transanal hemorrhoidal dearterialization a short-term prospective case series in a single institution. Dis Colon Rectum 53:581

Longo WE, Northover J (2003) Reoperative colon and rectal surgery. Martin Dunitz - Medical

Luo CH, Zang CB, Zhang GK, Liu HY (2010) Haemorrhoidectomy by vessel sealing system under local anaesthesia in an outpatient setting: preliminary experience. Colorectal Dis 12:236-240

Marino F (2009) Gabapentin therapy for chronic proctalgia following stapled haemorrhoidopexy. Colorectal Dis 11:788

Martellucci J, Papi F, Tanzini G (2009) Double rectal perforation after stapled haemorrhoidectomy. Int J Colorectal Dis 24:1113-1114

Martínez-Serrano MA, Parés D, Pera M et al (2009) Management of lower gastrointestinal bleeding after colorectal resection and stapled anastomosis. Tech Coloproctol 13:49-53

Mattana C, Coco C, Manno A et al (2007) Stapled hemorrhoidopexy and Milligan-Morgan hemorrhoidectomy in the cure of fourth-degree hemorrhoids: long-term evaluation and clinical results. Dis Colon Rectum 50:1170-1175

Maw A, Eu KW, Seow-Choen F (2002) Retroperitoneal sepsis complicating stapled hemorrhoidectomy: report of a case and review of the literature. Dis Colon Rectum 45:826-828

McCloud JM, Doucas H, Scott AD, Jameson JS (2007) Delayed presentation of life-threatening perineal sepsis following stapled haemorrhoidectomy: a case report. Ann R Coll Surg Engl 89:301-302

McCloud JM, Jameson JS, Scott AN (2006) Life-threatening

sepsis following treatment for haemorrhoids: a systematic review. Colorectal Dis 8:748-755

McDonald PJ, Bona R, Cohen CR (2004) Rectovaginal fistula after stapled haemorrhoidopexy. Colorectal Dis 6:64-65; Comment on: Colorectal Dis 2003; 5:304-310

Meyer P, Stieger R (2004) Retroperitoneal hematoma due to seam insufficiency after stapled hemorrhoidectomy. Chirurg 75:1125-1127

Milito G, Cadeddu F, Muzi MG, Nigro C, Farinon AM (2010) Haemorrhoidectomy with LigaSure vs conventional excisional techniques: meta-analysis of randomized controlled trials. Colorectal Dis 12:85-93

Milito G, Cortese F, Brancaleone C, Casciani CU (1997) Submucosal haemorrhoidectomy: surgical results and complications in 1,315 patients. Tech Coloproctol 1:128-132

Milito G, Gargiani M, Cortese F (2002) Randomised trial comparing LigaSure haemorrhoidectomy with the diathermy dissection operation. Tech Coloproctol 6:171-175

Milsom JW, Mazier WP (1986) Classification and management of postsurgical anal stenosis. Surg Gynecol Obstet 163:60-64

Mlakar B (2007) Should we avoid stapled hemorrhoidopexy in males and females who practice receptive anal sex? Dis Colon Rectum 50:1727

Molloy RG, Kingsmore D (2000) Life threatening pelvic sepsis after stapled haemorrhoidectomy. Lancet 355:810

Mongardini M, Custureri F, Schillaci F et al (2005) Rectal stenosis after stapler hemorrhoidopexy. G Chir 26:275-277

Muzi MG, Milito G, Nigro C et al (2007) Randomized clinical trial of LigaSure and conventional diathermy haemorrhoidectomy. Br J Surg 94:937-942

Naldini G (2011) Serious unconventional complications of surgery with stapler for haemorrhoidal prolapse and obstructed defaecation because of rectocoele and rectal intussusception. Colorectal Dis 13:323-327

Naldini G, Martellucci J, Moraldi L et al (2009) Is simple mucosal resection really possible? Considerations about histological findings after stapled hemorrhoidopexy. Int J Colorectal Dis 24:537-541

Nemati Fard M (2006) Sardinian congress of the Italian society of colorectal surgery. Tech Coloproctol 10:383-384

Ng KH, Ho KS, Ooi BS et al (2006) Experience of 3,711 stapled haemorrhoidectomy operations. Br J Surg 93:226-230

Ng KH, Ho KS, Ooi BS et al (2007) Pudendal block with bupivacaine for postoperative pain relief. Dis Colon Rectum 50:1656-1661

Nicholson TJ, Armstrong D (2004) Topical metronidazole (10 percent) decreases posthemorrhoidectomy pain and improves healing. Dis Colon Rectum 47:711-716

Nienhuijs SW, de Hingh IH (2010) Pain after conventional versus LigaSure haemorrhoidectomy. A meta-analysis. Int J Surg 8:269-273

Nisar PJ, Acheson AG, Neal KR et al (2004) Stapled hemorrhoidopexy compared with conventional hemorrhoidectomy: systematic review of randomized, controlled trials. Dis Colon Rectum 47:1837-1845

Nyström PO, Qvist N, Raahave D et al (2010) Randomized clinical trial of symptom control after stapled anopexy or diathermy excision for hemorrhoid prolapse. Brit J Surg 97:167-176

Occelli G, Bruni T (2006) The Italian Society of Colo-Rectal Surgery (SICCR) Annual Report of the Coloproctology Units (UCP Club)

Ommer A, Wenger FA, Rolfs T, Walz MK (2008) Continence disorders after anal surgery – a relevant problem? Int J Colorectal Dis 23:1023-1031

Ong K, Kam M, Eu K (2010) Pain scores after stapled hemorrhoidopexy vs transanal hemorrhoidal dearterialization: a prospective study of 70 consecutive patients. Dis Colon Rectum 53:578

Ortiz H, Marzo J, Armendáriz P et al (2005) Stapled hemorrhoidopexy vs. diathermy excision for fourth-degree hemorrhoids: a randomized, clinical trial and review of the literature. Dis Colon Rectum 48:809-815

Oughriss M, Yver R, Faucheron JL (2005) Complications of stapled hemorrhoidectomy: a French multicentric study. Gastroenterol Clin Biol 29:429-433

Palazzo FF, Francis DL, Clifton MA (2002) Randomized clinical trial of Ligasure versus open haemorrhoidectomy. Br J Surg 89:154-157

Patti R, Almasio PL, Arcara M et al (2006) Botulinum toxin vs. topical glyceryl trinitrate ointment for pain control in patients undergoing hemorrhoidectomy: a randomized trial. Dis Colon Rectum 49:1741-1748

Patti R, Almasio PL, Muggeo VM et al (2005) Improvement of wound healing after hemorrhoidectomy: a double-blind, randomized study of botulinum toxin injection. Dis Colon Rectum 48:2173-2179

Patti R, Arcara M, Bonventre S et al (2008) Randomized clinical trial of botulinum toxin injection for pain relief in patients with thrombosed external haemorrhoids. Br J Surg 95:1339-1343

Pescatori M (1995) Closed hemorrhoidectomy. Ann Ital Chir 66:787-790

Pescatori M (2002) Management of post-anopexy rectal stricture. Tech Coloproctol 6:125-126

Pescatori M (2002) Prospective randomized multicentre trial comparing stapled with open haemorrhoidectomy. Br J Surg 89:122

Pescatori M (2002) Two-quadrant semiclosed hemorrhoidectomy. A preliminary report. Tech Coloproctol 6:105-108

Pescatori M (2006) Chronic anorectal pain after stapled hemorrhoidopexy. The use and abuse of surgery. Osp It Chir 12:259-265

Pescatori M, Ayabaca S, Caputo D (2004) Can anal manometry predict anal incontinence after fistulectomy in males? Colorectal Dis 6:97-102

Pescatori M, Favetta U, Amato A (2000) Anorectal function and clinical outcome after open and closed haemorrhoidectomy, with and without internal sphincterotomy. A prospective study. Tech Coloproctol 4:17-23

Pescatori M, Favetta U, Dedola S, Orsini S (1997) Transanal stapled excision of rectal mucosal prolapse. Tech Coloproctol 1:96-98

Pescatori M, Favetta U, Navarra L (1998) Anal pressures after hemorrhoidectomy. Int J Colorectal Dis 13:149

Pescatori M, Gagliardi G (2008) Postoperative complications after procedure for prolapsed hemorrhoids (PPH) and stapled transanal rectal resection (STARR) procedures. Tech Coloproctol 12:7-19

Pescatori M, Quondamcarlo C (1999) Prevention of intraoperative complications during stapled excision of rectal mucosal prolapse. Tech Coloproctol 3:103-104

Pescatori M, Spyrou M, Cobellis L et al (2006) The rectal pocket syndrome after stapled mucosectomy. Colorectal Dis 8:808-811

Pescatori M, Spyrou M, Pulvirenti d'Urso A (2007) A prospective evaluation of occult disorders in obstructed defecation using the 'iceberg diagram'. Colorectal Dis 9:452-456

Petersen S, Hellmich G, Schumann D et al (2004) Early rectal stenosis following stapled rectal mucosectomy for hemorrhoids. BMC Surg 21:6

Petersen S, Jongen J, Scwenck W (2011) Agraffectomy after low rectal stapling procedures for hemorrhoids and rectocele. Tech Coloproctol [Epub ahead of print]

Phillips RKS (2009) Stapled obliteration of rectal lumen after PPH. Dis Colon Rectum 52:1525

Pigot F, Dao-Quang M, Castinel A et al (2006) Low hemorrhoidopexy staple line does not improve results and increases risk for incontinence. Tech Coloproctol 10:329-333

Quah HM, Seow-Choen F (2004) Prospective, randomized trial comparing diathermy excision and diathermy coagulation for symptomatic, prolapsed hemorrhoids. Dis Colon Rectum 47:367-370

Ramcharan KS, Hunt TM (2005) Anal stenosis after LigaSure hemorrhoidectomy. Dis Colon Rectum 48:1670-1671

Rand AA (1969) Skin-flap graft operation for hemorrhoids, a modification of the Whitehead. Dis Colon Rectum 265-276

Rasmussen OO, Larsen KG, Naver L et al (1991) Emergency haemorrhoidectomy compared with incision and banding for the treatment of acute strangulated haemorrhoids. A prospective randomised study. Eur J Surg 157:613-614

Ratto C, Giordano P, Donisi L et al (2010a) Transanal hemorrhoidal dearterialization for IV degree hemorrhoids. Dis Colon Rectum 53:578

Ratto C, Giordano P, Donisi L et al (2011) Transanal haemorrhoidal dearterialization (THD) for selected fourth-degree haemorrhoids. Tech Coloproctol 15:191-197

Ratto C, Parello A, Zaccone G et al (2010b) Assessment of hemorrhoidal arteries location within the rectum using endorectal ultrasound and echo-color doppler. Dis Colon Rectum 53:578

Ravo B, Amato A, Bianco V et al (2002) Complications after stapled hemorrhoidectomy: can they be prevented? Tech Coloproctol 6:83-88

Raymond TM, Raman SR, Basnyat PS (2008) First case of rectal inclusion cyst after stapled haemorrhoidopexy (PPH). Colorectal Dis 10:733-734

Regadas FS, Regadas SM, Rodrigues LV et al (2005) Transanal repair of rectocele and full rectal mucosectomy with one circular stapler: a novel surgical technique. Tech Coloproctol 9:63-66

Reis Neto JA, Reis JA Jr, Kagohara O et al (2005) Semi-open hemorrhoidectomy. Tech Coloproctol. 9:159-161

Roe AM, Bartolo DC, Vellacott KD et al (1987) Submucosal versus ligation excision haemorrhoidectomy: a comparison of anal sensation, anal sphincter manometry and postoperative pain and function. Br J Surg 74:948-951

Rosa G, Lolli P, Piccinelli D, Vicenzi L et al (2005) Submucosal reconstructive hemorrhoidectomy (Parks' operation): a 20-year experience. Tech Coloproctol 9:209-214

Sakr MF (2010) LigaSure versus Milligan-Morgan hemorrhoidectomy: a prospective randomized clinical trial. Tech Coloproctol 14:13-17

Sakr MF, Moussa MM (2010) LigaSure hemorrhoidectomy versus stapled Hemorrhoidopexy: a prospective, randomized clinical trial. Dis Colon Rectum 53:1161-1167

Salvati EP (1990) Management of acute hemorrhoidal disease. Persp Colon Rect Surg 3:309-314

Schmidt J, Dogan N, Langenbach R et al (2009) Fecal urge incontinence after stapled anopexia for prolapse and hemorrhoids: a prospective, observational study. World J Surg 33:355-364

Senagore AJ, Singer M, Abcarian J et al (2004) A prospective, randomized, controlled, multicenter trial comparing stapled hemorrhoidopexy and Ferguson hemorrhoidectomy: perioperative and one-year results. Dis Colon Rectum 47:1824-1836

Serventi A, Rassu PC, Giaminardi E et al (2010) Fecaloma in an iatrogenic diverticulum: an unusual complication of the procedure for prolapsed hemorrhoids (PPH). Tech Coloproctol 14:371-372

Shanmugam V, Muthukumarasamy G, Cook JA et al (2010) Randomized controlled trial comparing rubber band ligation with stapled haemorrhoidopexy for Grade II circumferential haemorrhoids: long-term results. Colorectal Dis 12:579-586

Shanmugam V, Thaha MA, Rabindranath KS et al (2005) Systematic review of randomized trials comparing rubber band ligation with excisional haemorrhoidectomy. Br J Surg 92:1481-1487

Siddiqui MRS, Abraham-Igwe C, Shangumanandan A et al (2011) A literature review on the role of chemical sphincterotomy after Milligan–Morgan hemorrhoidectomy. Int J Colorectal Dis 26: 685-682

Sileri P, Stolfi VM, Franceschilli L et al (2008) Reinterventions for specific technique-related complications of stapled haemorrhoidopexy (SH): a critical appraisal. J Gastrointest Surg 12:1866-1872

Silverman R, Bendick PJ, Wasvary HJ (2005) A randomized, prospective, double-blind, placebo-controlled trial of the effect of a calcium channel blocker ointment on pain after hemorrhoidectomy. Dis Colon Rectum 48:1913-1916

Slawik S, Kenefick N, Greenslade GL et al (2007) A prospective evaluation of stapled haemorrhoidopexy/rectal mucosectomy in the management of 3rd and 4th degree haemorrhoids. Colorectal Dis 9:352-356

Smellie GD (1965) Control of post-haemorrhoidectomy bleeding with a Foley catheter and a pack. J R Coll Surg Edinb 11:328

Soudan D, Castinel A, Suduca J et al (2010) One-year outcome of hemorrhoidectomy: a prospective, multicenter French study. Dis Colon Rectum 53:581

Spyrou M, De Nardi P (2005) The last images. Fecal incontinence after stapled transanal rectotomy managed with Durasphere injection. Tech Coloproctol 9:87

Sultan S, Rabahi N, Etienney I et al (2010) Stapled haemorrhoidopexy: 6 years' experience of a referral centre. Colorectal Dis 12:921-926

Szmulowicz U, Gurland B, Garofalo T et al (2010) Hemorrhoidal arterial ligation: the experience of a single institution. Dis Colon Rectum 53:579

Tegon G, Pulzato L, Passarella L et al (2009) Randomized placebo-controlled trial on local applications of opioids after hemorrhoidectomy. Tech Coloproctol 13:219-224

Tenschert G, Freitas A, Langmayr J et al (2006) Reinterventions after stapled hemorrhoidopexy. Proktologia, Supplement, 2006 (abstract)

Teo JY, Kam MH, Eu KW (2010) Letter to the editor on the article "Treatment of grade III and IV haemorrhoidal disease with PPH or THD. A randomized trial on postoperative complications and short-term results". Int J Colorectal Dis 25:1385

Thaha MA, Irvine LA, Steel RJ, Campbell KL (2005) Postdefecation pain syndrome after circular stapled anopexy is abolished by oral nifedipine. Br J Surg 92:208–210

Theodoropoulos GE, Sevrisarianos N, Papaconstantinou J et al (2010) Doppler-guided haemorrhoidal artery ligation, rectoanal repair, sutured haemorrhoidopexy and minimal mucocutaneous excision for grades III-IV haemorrhoids: a multicenter prospective study of safety and efficacy. Colorectal Dis 12:125-134

Tjandra JJ, Chan MK (2007) Systematic review on the procedure for prolapse and hemorrhoids (stapled hemorrhoidopexy). Dis Colon Rectum 50:878-892

Toyonaga T, Matsushima M, Sogawa N et al (2006) Postoperative urinary retention after surgery for benign anorectal disease: potential risk factors and strategy for prevention. Int J Colorectal 21:676-682

van Wensen RJ, van Leuken MH, Bosscha K (2008) Pelvic sepsis after stapled hemorrhoidopexy. World J Gastroenterol 14:5924-5926

Vasudevan SP, Mustafa el A, Gadhvi VM, Jhaldiyal P, Saharay M (2007) Acute intestinal obstruction following stapled haemorrhoidopexy. Colorectal Dis 9:668-669

Vindal A, Lal P, Chander J, Ramteke VK (2008) Rectal perforation after injection sclerotherapy for hemorrhoids: case report. Indian J Gastroenterol 27:84-85

Wang JY, Lu CY, Tsai HL et al (2006) Randomized controlled trial of LigaSure with submucosal dissection versus Ferguson hemorrhoidectomy for prolapsed hemorrhoids. World J Surg 30:462-466

Wasvary HJ, Hain J, Mosed-Vogel M, Bendick P, Barkel DC, Klein SN (2001) Randomized, prospective, double-blind, placebo-controlled trial of effect of nitroglycerin ointment on pain after hemorrhoidectomy. Dis Colon Rectum 44:1069-1073

Watson AJ, McLaren CM, Chapman AD, Binnie NR, Loudon MA (2003) Further cautionary tales from histopathology of stapled haemorrhoidopexy specimens. Colorectal Dis 5:271-272

Wexner SD (2001) Persistent pain and faecal urgency after stapled haemorrhoidectomy. Tech Coloproctol 5:56-57

Wilkerson PM, Strbac M, Reece-Smith H, Middleton SB (2009) Doppler-guided haemorrhoidal artery ligation: long-term outcome and patient satisfaction. Colorectal Dis 11:394-400

Wolff BG, Culp CE (1988) The Whitehead hemorrhoidectomy. An unjustly maligned procedure. Dis Colon Rectum 31:587-590

Wong LY, Jiang JK, Chang SC, Lin JK (2003) Rectal perforation: a life-threatening complication of stapled hemorrhoidectomy: report of a case. Dis Colon Rectum 46:116-117

Yao L, Zhong Y, Xu J, Xu M, Zhou P (2006) Rectal stenosis after procedures for prolapse and hemorrhoids (PPH)—a report from China. World J Surg 30:1311-1315

You SY, Kim SH, Chung CS, Lee DK (2005) Open vs. closed hemorrhoidectomy. Dis Colon Rectum 48:108-113

Zacharakis E, Kanellos D, Pramateftakis MG et al (2007) Long-term results after stapled haemorrhoidopexy for fourth-degree haemorrhoids: a prospective study with median follow-up of 6 years. Tech Coloproctol 11:144-147

Zbar AP (2008) Postoperative complications after procedure for prolapsing haemorrhoids (PPH) and stapled transanal rectal resection (STARR). Tech Coloproctol 12:136-137 (correspondence)

Zbar AP (2009) Innovations in coloproctology. Tech Coloproctol 13:331-332

3 Anal Abscesses and Fistulae

3.1 Introduction

A patient with anal fissures and hemorrhoids may be operated on by a general surgeon, but a patient with anal fistula needs to be managed by a specialist. Professor Goligher, in his book which for decades has been the bible of large-bowel surgery, wrote that it is more difficult to successfully operate on a patient with a complex recurrent anal fistula than on a patient with rectal cancer.

More than the risk of a recurrence, what concerns the patient with anal fistula prior to surgery is postoperative fecal incontinence (Ellis, 2010). Clearly, the colorectal surgeon understands, better than the general surgeon, the anatomy and function of the anal sphincter as well as the other factors responsible for anal continence. Therefore, this chapter will mainly deal with postoperative incontinence, which, as Professor Phillips wrote in his book (Chapman & Hall, 1996), sometimes is "the price to pay" for cure.

However, this chapter begins with a description of other complications.

3.2 Postoperative Bleeding

Severe hemorrhage may occur following surgery for anal fistula, albeit less frequently than after a procedure for hemorrhoids. Over a period of nearly 40 years, with over 800 operations for anal fistula, only three of my patients have had severe postoperative bleedings. While none of them needed a blood transfusion, in one case an emergency re-intervention was necessary. The first bleeding incident occurred about 20 years ago, following the lay-open of a high intersphincteric tract. At that time, I did not routinely marsupialize the surgical wound. During the night, this male patient bled from the wound at the level of the submucosal plexus, just above the anorectal ring, such that I had to position and inflate a Foley catheter in the rectum to stop the hemorrhage. The second episode occurred about a year ago. This female patient had a large chronic ischiorectal abscess with a trans-sphincteric fistula, and acutely bled into the wound one hour after surgery, from the inferior aspect of the levator muscles. Despite vigorous compression of the ischiorectal cavity with a wad of gauze, the bleeding did not stop and the patient developed tachycardia and hypotension. She was therefore given intravenous fluids returned to the operating theatre, and placed under general anesthesia, in order to suture the bleeding site. Some muscular fibers had been injured during excision of the abscess. While re-exploring the ischiorectal space, it became clear that a careful and effective hemostasis had not been carried out, because at the end of the first operation I had relied upon compression of the gauze introduced inside the ischiorectal cavity. Fortunately, the patient had no further troublesome consequences. The third and last bleeding incident occurred a few months ago and involved a young male who had undergone a lay-open of a low posterior intersphincteric fistula. He also had first-degree internal hemorrhoids, which slightly bled during fistulotomy but were cauterized using diathermy (Fig. 3.1). Five days later, probably when the eschar sloughed off, a delayed hemorrhage occurred and the patient was taken to the Emergency Department of the nearest hospital, where local compression using gauzes soaked with a pro-coagulant drug was used to stop the bleeding. By that time, I had been marsupializing the surgical wounds in such procedures, but in

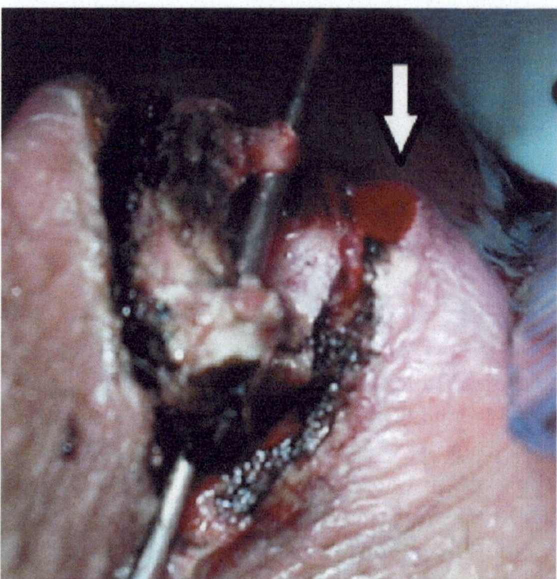

Fig. 3.1 Lay-open of a low posterior intersphinteric fistula. The patient was placed in the lithotomy position. Mild intraoperative bleeding was observed, coming from a submucosal venous plexus. A few days after surgery, severe rectal bleeding required urgent tamponade with gauze soaked in coagulant. Surgical wound marsupialization at the end of operation might have prevented the complication

that particular patient I thought that this was unnecessary, as the fistulotomy wound was rather small and prevalently external. In retrospect, I should have marsupialized the wound.

If we look at the literature, it is clear that I have been rather lucky, as a bleeding rate of 20% after fistulotomy and after seton, and of 10% following fistulectomy and rectal flap advancement have been reported (Ho and Ho, 2005).

To prevent or at least minimize the risk of postoperative bleeding, it is better:

1. Not to rely upon the gauze filling the residual cavities, also because excessive compression, which is likely to cause postoperative pain, should be avoided; instead, a careful hemostasis should be carried out, if necessary using Surgicel or Tabbotamp.
2. To marsupialize even small wounds, especially if they are associated with internal piles, which might bleed afterwards; marsupialization significantly decreases the wound size (Fig. 3.2), thus shortening the convalescence, and reduces the risk of bleeding without increasing postoperative pain (Pescatori et al., 2006; Malik and Nelson, 2008).

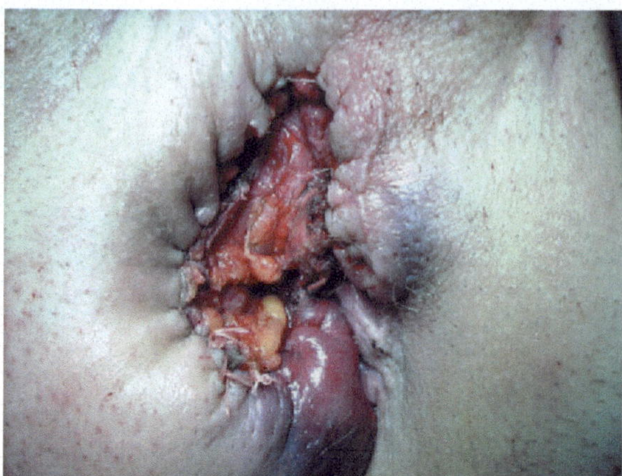

Fig. 3.2 Surgical wound marsupialization after fistulotomy (from Pescatori, 2011)

3. To carefully inspect the surgical wound once the patient has returned to the ward; if the gauze has become bloodied, it is advisable to take it out and to control any active bleeding.

3.3 Iatrogenic Fistula

This condition may be caused by excessive intraoperative probing. In patients with a trans-sphincteric fistula, once a probe has been inserted through the external orifice, we should bear in mind that, after a few centimeters, the tract direction is likely to change: rather than proceed cranially, towards the anorectum, it will cross the external sphincter. By continuing to push the probe upwards, a false tract is created, i.e., an extra-sphincteric iatrogenic fistula, across the levator ani muscle to the supralevator space, which thereafter will communicate with the external orifice at the level of the perianal skin.

3.4 Persisting or Early Recurrent Local Sepsis

After the operation, when seeing the patient in the ward, there is nothing worse than hearing: "Doctor, listen, I feel a painful induration here, close to the anus," or "Look, there is some pus coming out here in the groin…" or "….here on the tip of the coccyx, I feel discomfort, is there anything wrong?". Upon examination, we may unfortunately find residual sepsis, an undiscovered abscess, or a neglected tract. This happened to me twice early in my career, in a female patient with Crohn's disease who had septic extension to the inguinal region and in a male patient who had a concomitant anal fistula and pilonidal sinus. Since then, I routinely prepare a wide operative field in patients in whom sepsis extends far from the perianal region, in order to be able to evaluate the extent by adequate inspection, palpation, and probing. It should be noted that an inguinal sepsis is likely to be neglected if the patient is examined only in the Sims position.

What happens if there is either residual abscess or a fistula tract? How did I manage the two above-mentioned patients? The small groin abscess of the patient with Crohn's disease (who was maintained on antibiotics) was successfully curetted in the office after ten days, at the first postoperative visit. The male with the pilonidal sinus was successfully managed with a simple lay-open, carried out in the office after a week under local anesthesia.

Horse-shoe fistulae, by definition, have retro-anal and/or retro-rectal, deep and/or superficial extensions. Therefore, the posterior spaces need to be adequately drained, with a retro-anal incision if necessary; otherwise, a closed space will be at risk of persistent or recurrent sepsis due to the growth of anaerobic germs. Two lateral incisions might not be sufficient to achieve adequate drainage. Khoeler et al. (2004) reported that satisfactory results can be obtained by means of two incisions, provided that the posterior spaces are adequately drained with silicon setons or drains and the internal orifice is either sutured or covered with a rectal advancement flap. In case residual sepsis persists, due to insufficient surgical drainage and/or inadequate dressing, the patient needs to be re-operated on, as shown in Figs. 3.3 and 3.4. When fibrin glue is used or stem cells are injected, an early sepsis may occur, as reported by Garcia-Olmo et al. (2009) in 12 of their 49 patients. However, according to these authors, in only half of the cases was the abscess due to the procedure itself, namely to the fibrin glue, the use of which is declining compared with other methods.

An early anal abscess requiring drainage occurred postoperatively in three out of eight patients following a combined operation consisting of placement of a plug and rectal mucosal flap advancement (Mitalas et al., 2010). Due to this complication, the authors had to interrupt a pilot study.

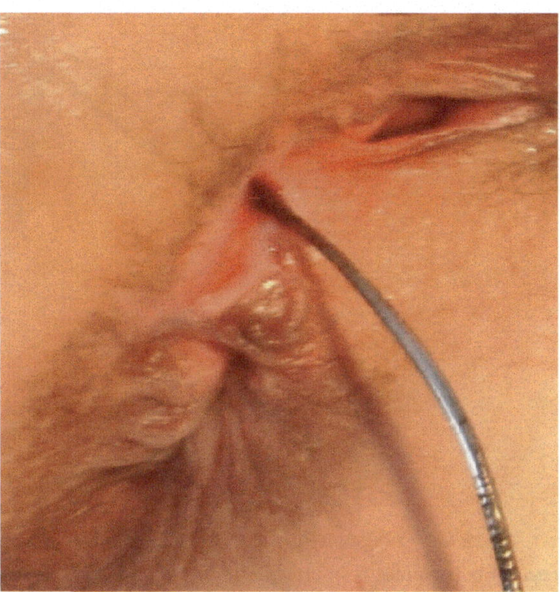

Fig. 3.3 Fistulectomy and a rectal advancement flap were performed in a woman with an anal fistula caused by a suppurative Bartholin's cyst. Postoperatively, the surgical wound did not heal due to persisting sepsis. Antibiotic therapy was preferred to re-operation, but the sinus created a trans-sphincteric fistula that required a new operation. The patient is in the Sims position and a probe has been inserted into the tract

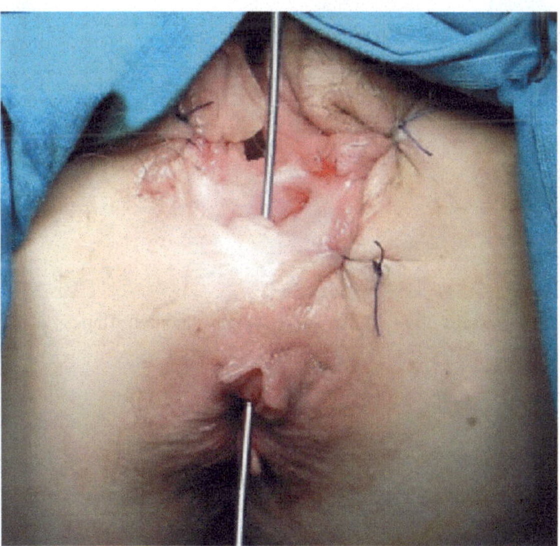

Fig. 3.4 a Patient in the lithotomy position. The high anterior fistula was located above the external sphincter. The patient was 50 years old and had previously undergone two anal operations. The second, a fistulotomy, was followed by anal incontinence. The decision was made to perform a re-do flap, that is, to make a new rectal flap after curettage of the septic tissue of the fistula

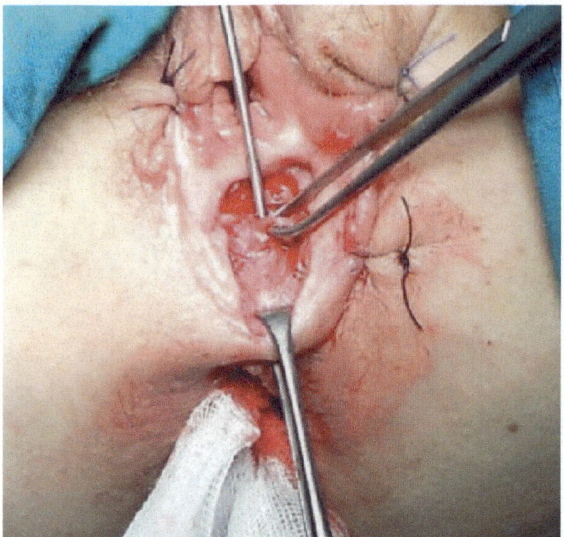

Fig. 3.4 b The probe is inserted in the fistula, which included the entire external sphincter

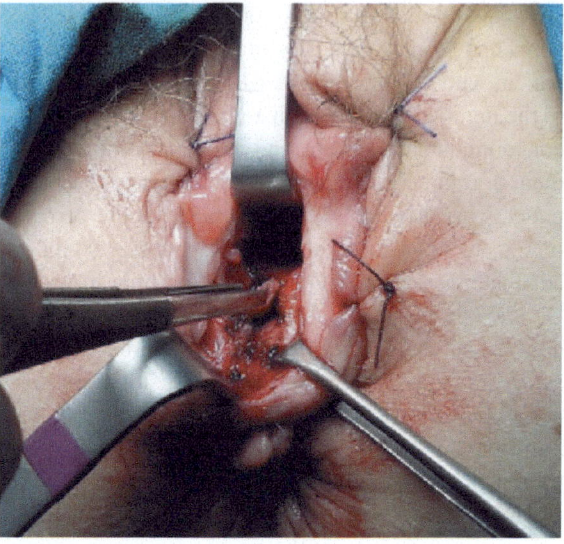

Fig. 3.4 c The fistula tract is removed

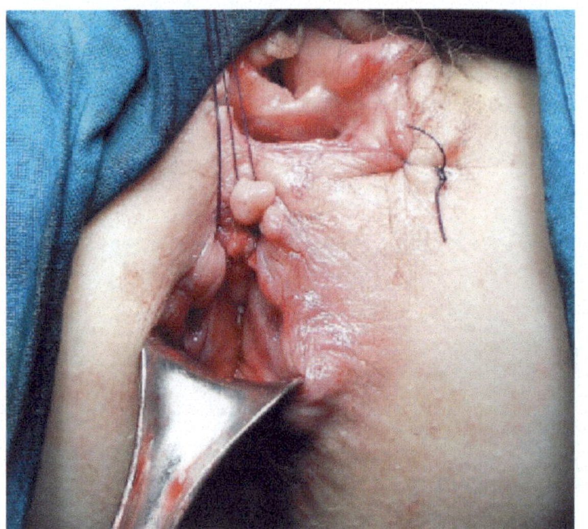

Fig. 3.4 d Re-do of a mucosal rectal advancement flap

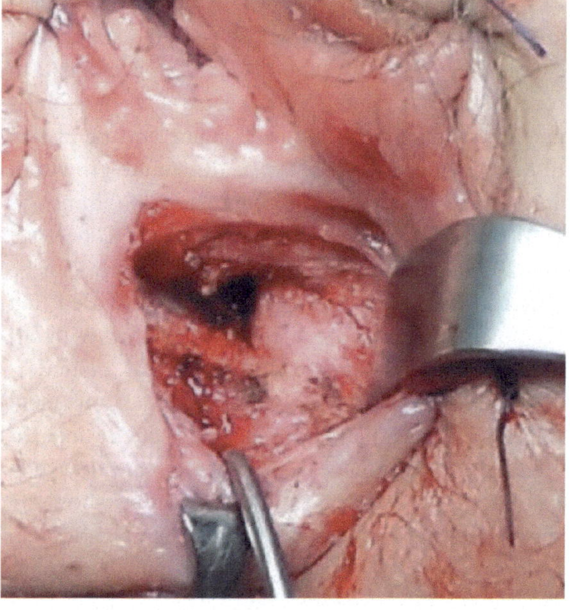

Fig. 3.4 e Anterior levatorplasty to create another diaphragm between the anal canal and perineum with vital tissue not previously used. The lateral left branch of the puborectalis muscle is shown

3.5 Suture Dehiscence and Non-healing Wounds

The following patients are at greater risk of suture dehiscence and/or a non-healing wound: a) those with diabetes, obesity, Crohn's disease, or immunosuppression (HIV and AIDS); b) those with anal hypertonicity and an endoanal wound; c) those who do not appropriately care for the wound or carry out adequate perineal hygiene by means of hip baths; and d) those who are highly sensitive to

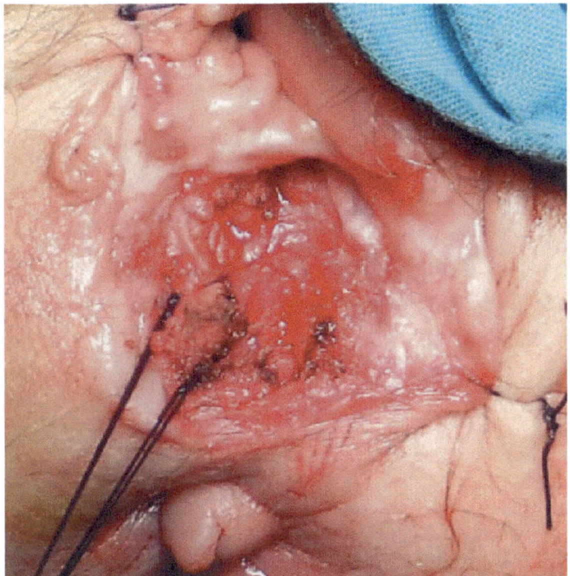

Fig. 3.4 f Both puborectalis branches are sutured one to the other during anterior levatorplasty

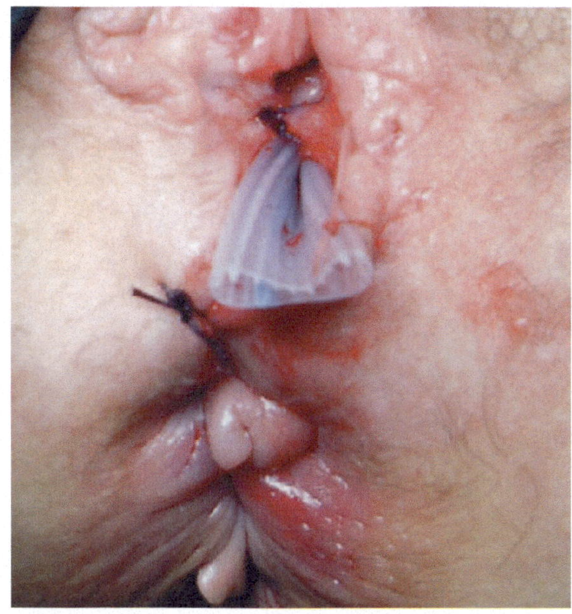

Fig. 3.4 g Aspect of the operating field at the end of the operation

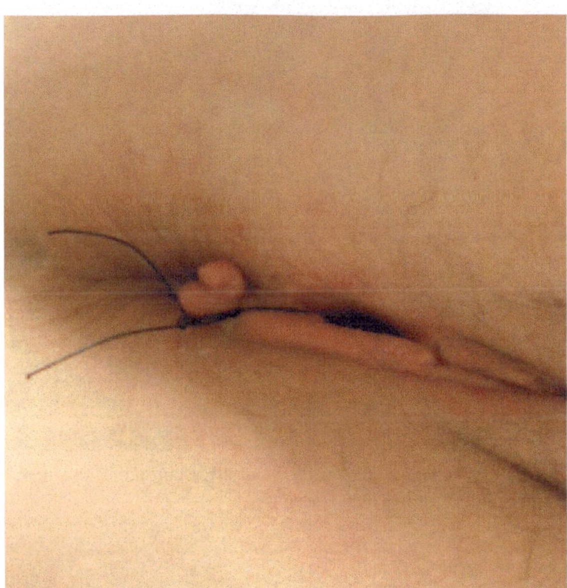

Fig. 3.4 h Complication 10 days postoperatively, when the patient, after a week of peripheral parenteral nutrition and Loperamide, had the first bowel movement. The small dehiscence of the rectal flap was treated by positioning a draining seton, to prevent sepsis. This seton was eventually converted to a cutting one

pain, as they will not tolerate a proper dressing and an effective postoperative curettage of the wound, due to excessive gluteal contraction. In these cases, in which painful maneuvers are necessary, the patients should be sedated. Curettage of the wound should be performed during an office visit by the surgeon, using a Volkmann spoon. It might be also suggested to the patient to clean the wound at home with a toothbrush or gauze. If subclinical chronic sepsis occurs, it is likely to affect wound healing, in which case re-intervention might be indicated: the chronic ulcer with its hardened margins excised and the defect covered with an advancement anoplasty (Fig. 3.5). If the residual wound is wide, a VAC (vacuum-assisted closure) procedure may be successfully used as it favors rapid healing by means of negative pressure, as reported by the group of Professor Ronan O'Connell in 2010. Further details on the use of the VAC system in coloproctology were provided in an interesting review published by Bemelman in 2009. More rarely, the wound becomes chronic and fibrotic and leads to perianal retraction, preventing anal closure and causing incontinence. In this case, anal-perineoplasty might be needed, as reported in 12 patients who underwent re-operation on our unit (Bernardi and Pescatori, 2001). A full-thickness skin graft was successfully used by Binda and Trizi (2007).

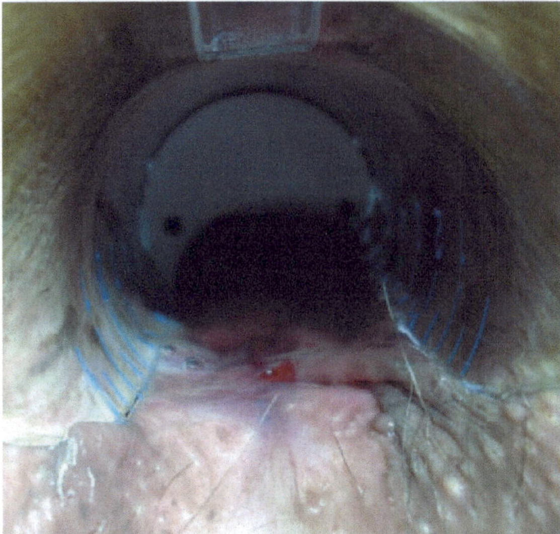

Fig. 3.5 a Non-healing endoanal wound that developed into a chronic ulcer in a heavy smoker, who underwent re-operation due to the recurrence of an intersphincteric posterior anal fistula. Preoperative transanal ultrasound showed a small posterior chronic abscess below the surgical wound. The patient was placed in the lithotomy position in the operating theatre for a surgical revision

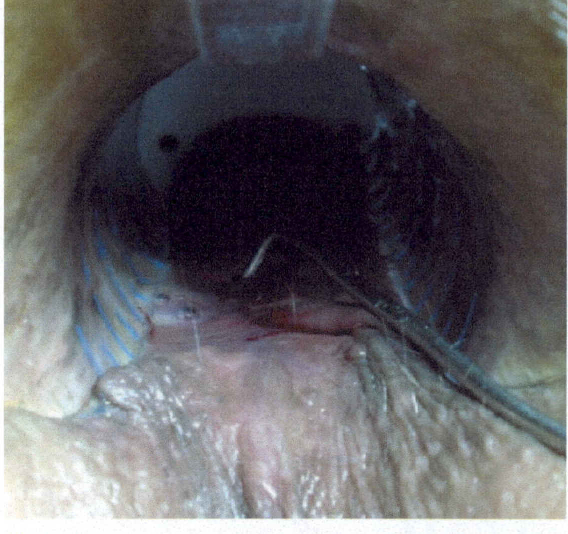

Fig. 3.5 b A probe was inserted in the ulcer but a fistula orifice was not found

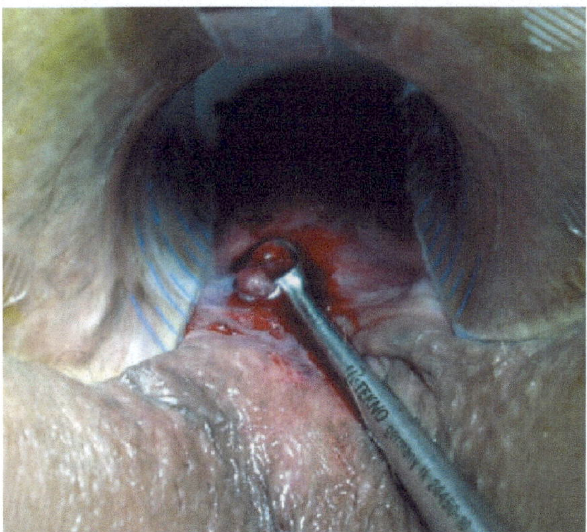

Fig. 3.5 c Curettage of the small chronic abscess

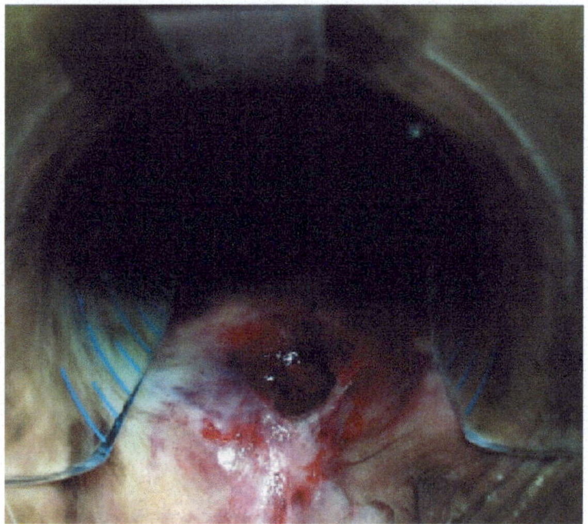

Fig. 3.5 d Endoanal surgical wound after curettage and trimmings of the fibrotic ulcer margins

The presence of parasites in the stool or the persistence of a foreign body might also prevent wound healing, as happened in two patients on our unit. One was an elderly woman whose wound did not heal for years after a fistula operation performed elsewhere. Following a course of perianal electrostimulated acupuncture, a procedure which enhances tissue trophism, a retained surgical gauze was surprisingly expelled through the underskin below the wound, which then healed. The other patient was a young female who had undergone fistulectomy and a rectal advancement flap procedure. The flap suture healed properly in due time, but the perianal wound was still open and became

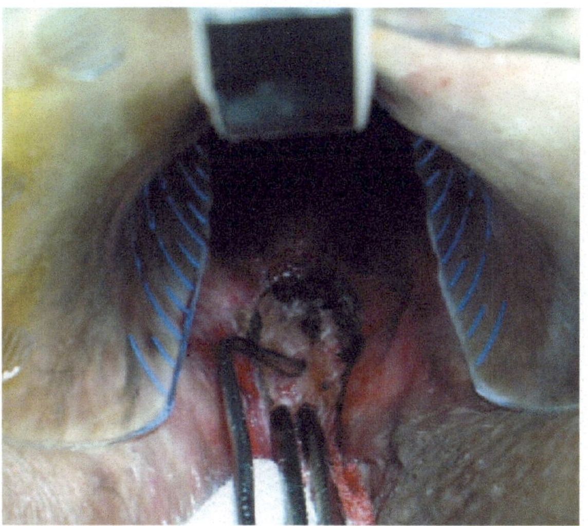

Fig. 3.5 e The whitish fibers of the internal sphincter can be seen at the base of the wound

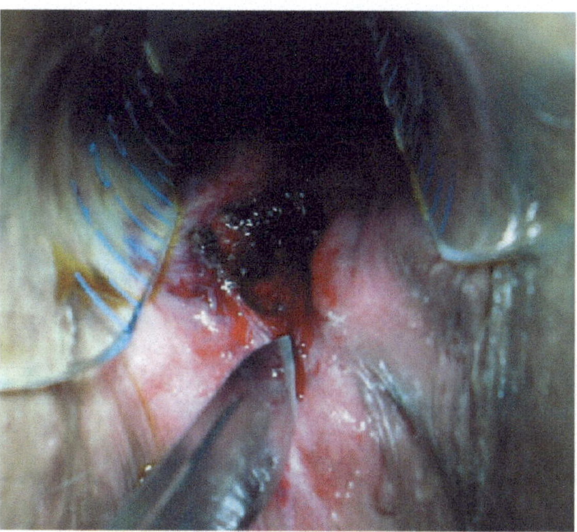

Fig. 3.5 f A 0.5-cm section of the internal sphincter, in its middle portion, was performed to carry out a lay-open

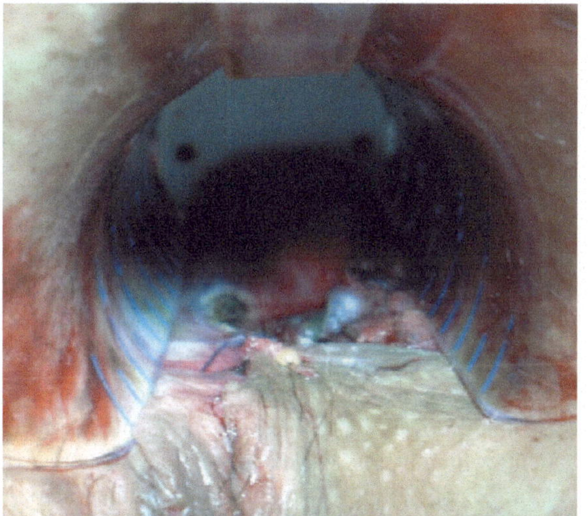

Fig. 3.5 g In the posterior anal canal, there is fibrosis and ischemia, both of which delay healing. The decision was made to perform an anoplasty, with a cutaneous flap to cover the wound

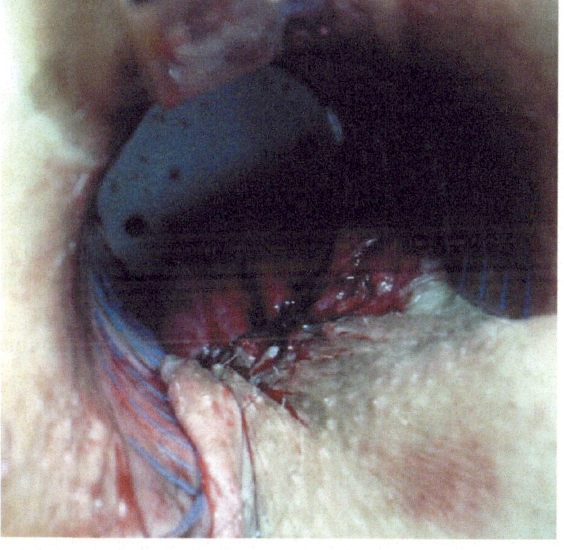

Fig. 3.5 h The anoplasty has been completed and a well-vascularized cutaneous flap sutured to the anal canal

infected after a month, until we found that she had an oxyuriasis and gave her proper treatment. The wound fully healed in a couple of weeks. Since then, we routinely carry out a parasitological exam prior to performing anal fistula surgery.

Careful local disinfection together with the use of cicatrizing agents, both local and systemic, also promotes healing of the wound. Van Koperen et al. (2010) stressed the importance of excising the granulomatous tissue, i.e., the pathological epithelium, at the posterior aspect of the fistula when performing a lay-open. This maneuver encourages wound healing. The completeness of diseased tissue excision may be appreciated by palpating the deep part of the surgical wound, which should be soft. If it is hard, the residual fibrotic tissue is like-

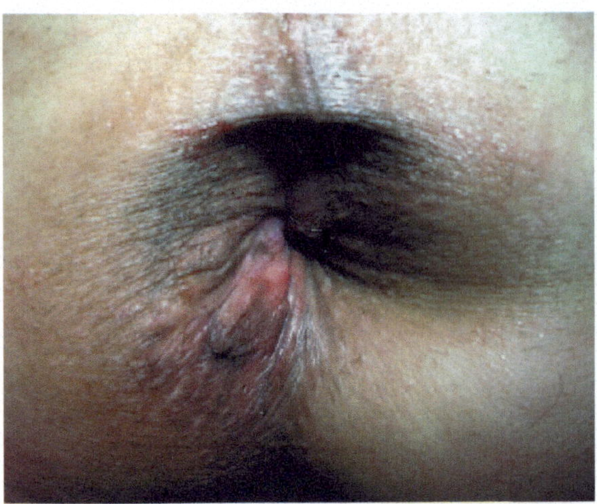

Fig. 3.5 i At the end of the operation, the anus was closed. The patient received nil by mouth and was kept constipated with Loperamide, receiving intravenous fluids and antibiotic therapy for 5 days. The patient is continent and without recurrence after six months

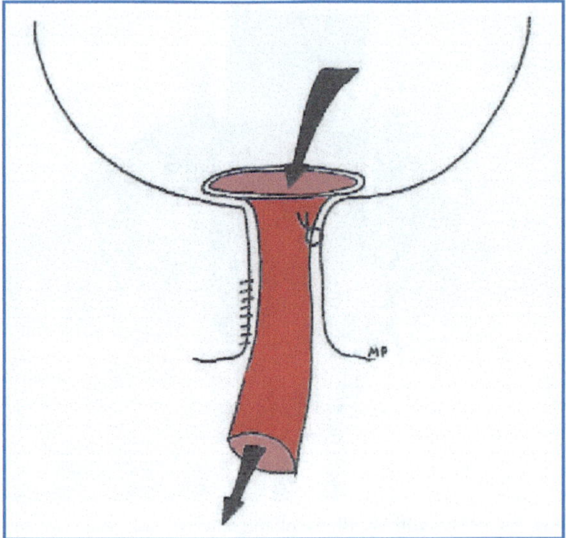

Fig. 3.6 Kosorok tube to preserve endoanal surgical wounds from fecal contamination

ly to prevent healing and necessitates removal using either a Volkmann spoon or scissors.

A "technological" alternative to conventional curettage consists of destruction of the diseased tissue by means of a laser probe (Biolitec), carried out by introducing the probe in the fistula tract through the external orifice. This approach was used by Wilhelm (2011), who reported no postoperative complications in a series of 11 patients apart from one case of soiling.

A brief mention is needed on the management of suture dehiscence, i.e., the breakdown of a rectal advancement flap—usually constructed to cover the endoanal defect—following the excision of a trans-sphincteric or high intersphincteric fistula. The risk of dehiscence is greater in the presence of proctitis or pus, in patients with Crohn's diease, and in heavy smokers (Zimmerman et al., 2003). If fibrin glue is used, the shorter the tract, the greater the risk of dehiscence. The association of a rectal flap with the use of fibrin glue is unlikely to ensure better healing and increases the risk of suture breakdown, as reported by Van Koperen et al. (2008) and Alexander et al. (2008). A soft rubber tube with a proximal rigid end, aimed at keeping the tube in place above the anorectal ring, i.e., the Kosorok device, may also be used to successfully protect the endoanal suture of a rectal flap (Pescatori, 1997) (Fig. 3.6).

3.6 The Prevention of Postoperative Anal Incontinence

In patients who clearly require treatment for an anal fistula, even prior to the examination it may become apparent that he/she is at risk of postoperative incontinence, simply based on an inquiry about bowel habits and on the obstetric and clinical history. Patients of advanced age, a short woman who has had more than one vaginal delivery with heavy babies, patients with associated inflammatory bowel disease or irritable bowel syndrome with frequent diarrhea, patients with a history of anal surgery and hysterectomy, or, of course, those with episodes of fecal incontinence need special care to preserve the integrity of the anal sphincter, the length of the anal canal, and its sensitive epithelium. With the patient in the Sims position, merely by looking at the perineum and the anus we may be able to predict the risk of incontinence. Perineal descent, gaping or deformed anus, perianal scars, and mucosal prolapse protruding through the anus are all signs of a weak sphincter and short anal canal. Using a few simple maneuvers—such as asking the patient to squeeze while the perianal skin is gently touched with a needle and the reflex contraction of the external sphincter, i.e., the anal reflex, is evaluated—gross signs of pudendal neuropathy potentially can be determined. Based on this finding, and if the patient is constipated, a reduced rectal sensation can be suspected. This can be measured by simply inflating a latex balloon in the rectum to assess the onset of feeling (around 20 ml of air), the urge to pass stool (60 ml), and the maximal urgency (120). If these responses are altered, they may predict postoperative incontinence, even in male patients with intact anal sphincters (Pescatori et al., 2004). Patients should be questioned repeatedly, as almost none is happy to admit fecal incontinence. If the patient is simply asked: "Do you lose stool?" the answer is likely to be: "No, I don't." But if we ask: "In cases in which you have had diarrhea but there was no toilet nearby, did the stool ever leak?" the answer is likely to be: "Yes, it did, sometimes." Therefore, it is important to spend some time talking with the patient, alone, without relatives in the room.

If a patient has indeed had episodes of incontinence, we need to know why, i.e., the altered component of the continence mechanism must be identified. It may be anatomical, e.g., localized sphincter injury related to previous fistula surgery, or simply a functional disorder, such as deficient innervation causing a weak squeeze or a lack of rectal sensitivity. Regardless, the patient should undergo further examination by anal-vaginal or dynamic perineal ultrasound (US), defecography, anal manometry and manovolumetry, or, in some cases, magnetic resonance imaging, which may well evidence obstetric injuries and asymmetries of the upper pelvic floor muscles. In selected cases in which voluntary contraction is found to be of short duration and the anal reflex is deficient, it may be useful to measure PNTML (pudendal nerve terminal motor latency) to confirm the suspicion of pudendal neuropathy. If this alteration is present, pelvic floor rehabilitation, especially aimed at improving rectal sensation by means of transanal electrostimulation, might be indicated prior to (or after) fistula surgery in order to minimize the risk of postoperative incontinence. A fibrotic internal sphincter, poor voluntary contraction, and perineal scars are negative predictors of outcome following biofeedback training in these incontinent patients (Terra et al., 2006).

Ellis (2010), interviewing 78 patients who were candidates for fistula surgery, determined that for the majority of them the main goal was, rather than cure and the avoidance of anal sepsis recurrence, not to become incontinent after the operation. This markedly increased the number of operations carried out by colorectal surgeons that were aimed at preserving anal continence, i.e., sphincter-sparing procedures. In fact, these procedures accounted for 50% of anal continence procedures in the 1990s but more recently increased to 80%, according to a report by Abcarian's group in Chicago (Blumetti et al., 2010). Nevertheless, a recent paper from St. Marks Hospital (Atkin et al., 2011) concluded that, when dealing with high fistulae, the lay-open is still the best option, as the British authors did not report a significant incontinence rate using this more aggressive policy, which is more radical but is associated with a very low number of recurrences.

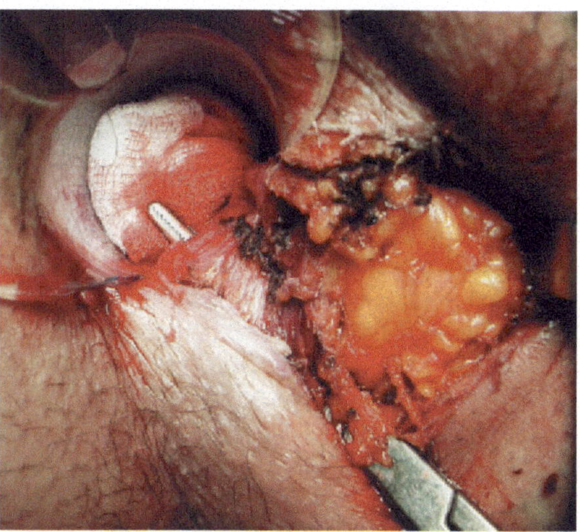

Fig. 3.7 Trans-sphincteric anal fistula. A lay-open is likely to cause fecal incontinence, because the three portions of the external sphincter (subcutaneous, superficial, and deep) were below the fistula. Patient in the lithotomy position

My personal policy is to carry out a sphincter saving procedure in all high trans-sphincteric fistulae (Fig. 3.7).

De Stefano, a colorectal surgeon from Orbassano, recounted a story told at a Congress by Bruno Roche, in which a patient with a recurrent anal fistula preferred to permanently keep a seton rather than undergo a lay-open of the fistula tract, which might have rendered him incontinent.

As far as the risk of incontinence, it was noted above that bowel habit, clinical history, rectal sensation, and the integrity of the anal sphincters are important factors. But what is even more important is the type of fistula to be managed, as this strongly influences the choice of the operation:

- Lay-open (fistulotomy) or fistulectomy, described by many authors.
- Fistulectomy alone, with seton (Hanley and many other investigators) or with internal sphincteromy (Parks).
- The Mann and Clifton re-routing procedure (Mann and Clifton, 1985), with the technical variation reported by Zbar and Pescatori (2004).
- Rectal advancement flap (Aguilar et al., 1999).
- Cutaneous flap (Nelson et al., 2000).
- Primary suture of the internal orifice (Athanasiadis et al., 2004).
- Fibrin glue (Buchanan et al., 2003) or Permacol, i.e., porcine collagen (Hammond et al., 2011) injection.
- Plug insertion (Christoforidis et al., 2009; Lenisa et al., 2010).
- The not novel but revisited LIFT (ligation of the intersphincteric fistula tract) procedure originally proposed by Phillips (Rojanasakul, 2009; Bleier et al., 2010).
- The novel bio-lift (Ellis, 2010).
- Stem cells injection (Garcia-Olmo et al., 2009).
- Video-assisted ablation of the fistula tract (VAAFT), the "triumph" of modern technology (Meinero and Mori, 2011).

Of the above mentioned techniques, all but one (fistulotomy) are aimed at sparing the anatomy and function of the anal sphincter and decreasing the risk of postoperative incontinence, especially in case of high and trans-sphincteric tracts. Interestingly, St. Mark's Hospital's policy is still fistulotomy-oriented, even in case of high fistulae. At our unit, 40% of the cases are still treated with a lay-open, compared with 50% in Chicago (Abcarian, in Blumetti et al., 2010) and 80% at St. Mark's Hospital (Phillips, in Atkin et al., 2011).

As far as the risk of postoperative incontinence is concerned, according to personal experience and as reported in the literature, the surgeon's policy should be based on the following principles: First, a low posterior intersphinteric fistula in a young continent male who does not suffer from diarrhea and has never had anal surgery may be laid-open with minimal risk of complications. Second, a high anterior trans-sphincteric fistula of an elderly multiparous (vaginal) female with diarrhea, weak sphincters, and perineal descent, rectal hyposensation, and previous anal surgery cannot be laid-open as there is a risk of postoperative incontinence. Instead, the patient will need a fistulectomy with a sphincter-saving technique, possibly without seton, as anteriorly the external sphincter is thin and there is no puborectalis muscle (Fig. 3.8). Therefore, in the operating theatre, prior to "cutting" we need to carefully inspect, palpate, gently probe, and visualize (by injecting methylene blue, peroxide water, or milk).

However, it also should be noted that between the two above-described possibilities there is a wide range of intermediate conditions, which renders our subspecialty more difficult but also more appealing and allows us to better appreciate why a patient with anal fistula and abscess should be dealt with by an experienced colorectal surgeon, as stated at the beginning of this chapter.

In the following, we consider the various options, i.e., the dos and don'ts when dealing with different anatomical and physiological patterns, while always bearing in mind the final goals: to prevent or minimize postoperative incontinence and to achieve permanent eradication of the sepsis. If the tract is either high or anterior, it is better not to perform a fistulotomy. If it is trans-sphincteric and the sphincters are weak, it is likewise better to avoid a lay-open. In these two cases, fistulectomy is the preferred option.

Following fistulectomy, what is the best way to preserve anal function? It does not involve a seton, which is expected to cause some degree of muscle fibrosis and likely to leave an anal deformity, which might favor soiling. Instead, a plug, fibrin glue, and rectal mucosal flap advancement (less costly) are advantageous strategies, as they do not affect the sphincters and keep most of the sensitive epithelium intact.

The literature findings are as follows: fibrin glue was reported to cause local sepsis, pruritus, and pain in 47% of the patients in one series (Zmora et al., 2005), whereas in other reports there were no significant postoperative complication when fibrin glue was mixed with Permacol (Hammond et al., 2011).

O'Connor et al. (2006) did not observe any adverse events in their patients treated by the insertion of a Surgisis plug, made of porcine lyophilized intestinal submucosa, into the curetted fistula tract. Among these patients, 80% were

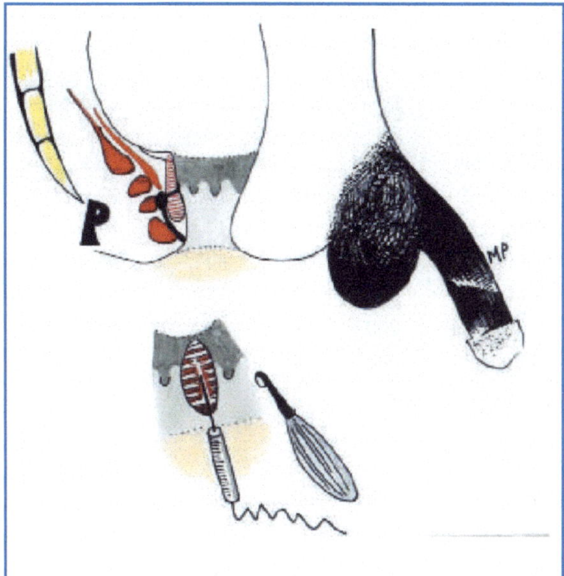

Fig. 3.8 a In a male patient, a posterior low intersphincteric fistula (P) can be usually laid-open without continence problems. The puborectalis muscle is in the posterior aspect. After fistulotomy, curettage is performed with a Volkman's spoon to prevent residual sepsis

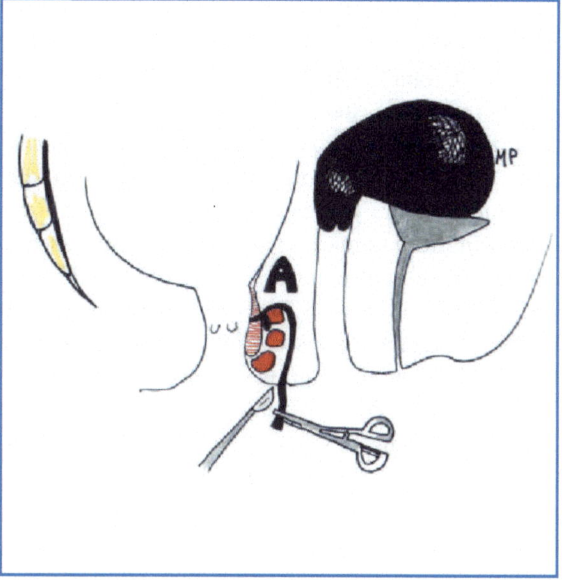

Fig. 3.8 b In a female, a laid-open high anterior trans-sphincteric (or intersphincteric) fistula would almost always be followed by incontinence. Fistulectomy is more often preferred. Anteriorly, there is no puborectalis muscle

cured, with no case of new-onset anal incontinence, as no sphincter division was carried out. It should be said, however, that O'Connor is a consultant of the company manufacturing the plug, as noted by the author at the end of the article. American authors are requested by law to disclose any potential conflict of interest. In a prospective study, European (Italian and Spanish) authors, with no conflicts of interest, reported just three complications (pain and edema) out of 60 patients surgically treated with a plug; there was no case of anal incontinence (Lenisa et al., 2010). Similar findings, i.e., the absence of incontinence, were reported in 49 patients operated upon at the University of Minnesota by Christoforidis et al. (2008). Unfortunately, incidental protrusion of the plug occurred in 14 patients. The same complication occurred in 22% of the 43 patients who also had the plug procedure, carried out by Thekkinkattil et al. (2009). However, recurrence rates of 80% with the plug vs. 13% using a rectal advancement flap (Ortiz et al., 2009) and 69% (including persisting fistulae) with fibrin glue Loungarath et al. (2004) have been reported. Therefore, due to the high complication and failure rates, neither the plug nor the glue has become popular. By contrast, a trial comparing seton with fibrin glue showed superiority of the seton in terms of recurrence (Altomare et al., 2011).

Three prospective studies, by Shukla et al. (1991), Ho et al. (2001), and Zbar et al. (2003), reported a low incontinence rate (5, 8, and 5%, respectively) with respect to flatus and liquid stool following fistulectomy and seton. Similarly, the rate of incontinence in our patients after the same procedure was 5% (Pescatori et al., 1995). Overall, no case of incontinence to solid stool was reported in about 700 patients in the above quoted studies. Ritchie et al. (2009) reviewed 37 studies in which a cutting seton was used and reported a higher incontinence rate (12%), but many series were retrospective and also included patients with Crohn's diseases, who are more prone to continence problems due to the liquid stool. In 63 patients treated for complex fistulae with a Silastic or Penrose seton, Abarca et al. (2010) reported recurrence in just 6% and incontinence, mostly to flatus, in 10%. Finally, Sung et al. (2010) had no case of postoperative incontinence among their patients who received a seton following fistulectomy performed for trans-sphincteric tracts, and none of the patients of Thornton et al. (2005) who were treated with long-standing seton and Depezzer tube complained of anal incontinence after surgery for complex Crohn's fistulae.

Therefore, as stated by Abarca et al. (2010) regarding the low recurrence and incontinence rate, "The cutting seton still has a place in the armamentarium of the colorectal surgeon." According to Altomare et al. (2011), based on the results of a multicentric study of the Italian Society of Colo-Rectal Surgery, partly supported by the manufacturer (as declared by the authors), fibrin glue is the first option in incontinent patients with trans-sphincteric fistulae.

The following describes the surgical approach that I use when dealing with a middle-high trans-sphincteric fistula, in patients in whom the lay-open is likely to cause postoperative incontinence. Due to the high costs and the high failure rate, I do not use a plug or glue; instead, I perform a fistulectomy, i.e., hollowing out of the tract, followed by a seton or a rectal mucosal advancement flap (I just carried out one LIFT procedure). I prefer the first option when the patient does not have weak sphincters, and the second when the rectum is not inflamed and there is no acute abscess. After the skin has been incised, I use a cutting seton with 0 or 2/0 suture, loosely knotted around the muscle to avoid causing pain. Two-thirds of surgeons prefer to use Silicone, Silastic, or Prolene (Ritchie et al., 2009). I use silk, as it is likely to induce a greater degree of fibrosis, which is the aim of the procedure, during the slow section of the sphincter. Usually, I divide the inferior portion of the internal sphincter to achieve effective drainage of the intersphincteric plane, which is often the site of the primary sepsis. This maneuver was taught to me by Sir Alan Parks, in the 1980s, but it is unnecessary if there is no sign of either acute or chronic sepsis at the level of the anal glands (which may be located in the external sphincter) and it is contraindicated in patients who suffer from anal incontinence prior to surgery. The Parks maneuver is thought to minimize the risk of recurrence. However, according to a systematic review by Vial et al. (2010), based on 18 studies and 448 patients, when division of the internal sphincter is associated with a seton procedure, the postoperative incontinence rate is 25.2%, whereas without dividing the sphincter it is much lower (5.6%). The recurrence rate is similar with or without sphincterotomy (3 and 5%, respectively). In my experience, carrying out the Parks maneuver when using the seton, the incontinence rate is likewise only around 5%. But, again, I do not divide the internal sphincter routinely. Therefore, with a tailored approach (avoiding sphincterotomy in the presence of weak sphincters) this maneuver can still be useful.

Table 3.1 Anal continence following rectal-mucosa and skin-flap advancement procedures for trans-sphincteric and high intersphincteric anal fistulae

Author	Year	Cases (*n*)	Follow-up (months)	Continence defects (%)
Rectal flap				
Schouten	1999	99	12	35[a]
Ortiz	2000	103	12	8
Mizrahi	2002	66	40	9[b]
Koehler	2004	52[c]	48	32
Van der Haagen	2007	41	72	51[d]
Jarrar	2010	44	38	3
Anocutaneous flap				
Zimmerman	2001	23	NR	30
Amin	2003	18	19	0
Sungurtekin	2004	65	32	0
Ho	2005	20	4	1.3[e]
Hossack	2005	13	NR	30[c]

[a]Probably due to the prolonged use of the Parks anal retractor.
[b]Continence disorders in patients who previously had sphincter reconstruction.
[c]33 cases with rectal flap, 9 with anocutaneous flap, and 11 with primary suture.
[d]After more than one attempt with a rectal flap.
[e]Mean Wexner incontinence score.

Regarding the flap, a skin flap may be used and in heavy smokers is thought to be at less risk of dehiscence than a rectal flap. Both types of flap have been used to cover the internal orifice of the excised fistula, and the outcome achieved with each one has been reported in several studies, as shown in Table 3.1. The rectal flap is preferred by most surgeons and is more often performed at our unit, where a large base flap consisting of mucosa, submucosa, and part of the rectal muscle is harvested using a cold knife rather than with diathermy, to avoid ischemia and to minimize the risk of dehiscence. The flap is then sutured without tension to the subcutaneous part of the external sphincter.

A more complex, but apparently effective and safe procedure is the one recently carried out by Baeten's group, in Maastricht (Van Der Hagen et al., 2011). These authors positioned a seton to keep the

Table 3.2 Fistulectomy and suture of the internal orifice in 90 patients operated on by Athanasiadis et al. (2004)

Complication	No. of cases	%
Suture dehiscence	15	14
Male:female ratio	12.3	17.1
Postoperative day of dehiscence (median)	4-10	8.1
Dehiscence with persisting fistula	12	13
Dehiscence with spontaneous healing	3	3.3
Post-wound-healing recurrent fistula	7	6.6
Re-interventions due to fistulae	19	18
Re-interventions due to abscesses	5	4.5

Table 3.3 Anal continence following fistulotomy for trans-sphincteric tracts

Author	Year	Patients (%)	Follow-up (months)	Incontinence (% of patients)
Van Tets	1994	312	12	24
Garcia-Aguilar	1996	375	29	54
Mylonakis	2001	74	3	21
Cavanaugh	2002	110	24-60	64
Westerterp	2003	60	12-48	50
Atkin	2011	58	>1	35[a]

[a]Only 9% needed to use pads due to anal incontinence.

fistula drained for 3 months and then constructed a rectal flap that was reinforced with a high platelet concentration plasma injection following curettage, through the external perianal orifice, aimed at decreasing the risk of flap dehiscence. They operated on 10 patients with high trans-, supra-, and extra-sphincteric fistulae, reporting no postoperative complication and just one recurrence at one year.

An unusual but interesting option following the excision of a trans-sphincteric tract is primary suture of the internal orifice without a flap. The outcome is detailed in Table 3.2.

The results of fistulectomy and primary suture are satisfactory compared with those obtained with flap construction, which has a 20% failure rate (30% in Crohn's fistulae) and a recurrence rate of less than 10% in specialists' hands, as reported by Phillips and Lunniss in their book cited above. Koehler et al. (2004), in a study carried out in patients with horseshoe fistulae, showed that primary suture may be safely performed if the anal canal is smooth and elastic, not fibrotic. However, the re-intervention rate following primary suture is not negligible, and this procedure has not gained popularity. Recently, a novel video-assisted anal fistula technique (VAAFT) was proposed by Meinero. It is similar to the Athanasiadis technique in that primary closure of the internal orifice is achieved using a linear stapler. Meinero and Mori (2011) reported one case of postoperative local sepsis, two of scrotal edema, and two of urinary retention. Out of 103 surgically treated patients, most with complex fistulae, 87 were followed up and 22% of them had a persisting fistula wound after 3 months. The procedure is rather costly, as a fistuloscope, stapler, and cyanoacrylate injections are needed, but it has the advantage that it may be performed on an outpatient basis. In their Abstract, presented at the last Congress of the ECTA (Eurasian Colorectal Technology Association), the authors did not report cases of postoperative incontinence, but more detailed data are needed before sound conclusions can be made.

The rectal advancement flap may also be associated with "re-routing" of the fistula tract (Zbar and Pescatori 2004), a technique that offers a greater chance of postoperative anal continence, as the internal sphincter is left intact, unlike in Parks' partial sphincterotomy or sphincterectomy, performed to drain the intersphincteric plane.

In a patient with a high intersphincteric fistula, lay-open of the whole tract is likely to cause postoperative incontinence. If carried out using radiofrequency therapy, there is less pain and bleeding (Gupta 2003; Malik and Nelson 2008). However, as stated by Phillips and Lunnis, some degree of incontinence may be "the price to be paid" to eliminate the disease. By doing so, Nicholls reported in an early study that while one-third of the patients had continence disorders almost none suffered a recurrence (lecture at the Congress of the Italian Society of Surgery in Rome, 1983). More recently, avoidance of the lay-open in patients with high fistulae resulted in only a few cases of incontinence but two out of ten patients will have a recurrence. Recently, in a study at St. Mark's Hospital, Atkin et al. (2011) reported a high cure rate with acceptable functional results, concluding that "lay-open of high fistulae is still a good option."

The functional results achieved by carrying out a lay-open in patients with trans-sphincteric fistulae are described in Table 3.3.

Table 3.4 Anal incontinence rate following surgery for the various types of anal fistulae (from Jordàn et al., 2010)

Type of fistula	Postoperative incontinence (% of patients)
Suprasphincteric	42.3
Extrasphincteric	40.0
Trans-sphincteric	17.5
Intersphincteric	5.9
Complex	17.6
Simple	8.1
Recurrent	24.6
Primary	8.7

The fact that there have been very few such reports over the last decade is due to the trend towards sphincter-sparing procedures, also because, prior to surgery, patients' main concern is postoperative incontinence. In fact, the "fistulotomy rate" of Blumetti et al., from Chicago (2010), has markedly decreased, from 80% to 50%, in the last decade.

Among the other sphincter-saving procedures, one has the merit to be costless, i.e. the LIFT or Ligation of Intersphincteric Fistula Tract, followed by simple curettage of the external tract. Professor Rojanasakul from Thailand is the one who popularized this technique, modified from the operation described by the group of Professor Phillips at St Mark's Hospital (Matos et al., 1993), which consisted of a fistula tract ligation plus fistulectomy and suture. In a prospective multicentric study, Buier, Moloo and Goldberg reported a good outcome on 39 patients with trans- and suprasphincteric fistulae after 20 weeks. No case of anal incontinence occurred, and successful closure of the fistula tract was achieved in 57% of the cases (2010).

In August 2011, Professor Goldberg reported good clinical and functional outcome on a larger series of 120 patients (unpublished data, personal communication).

Table 3.5 lists the main LIFT series recently published, with the infrequent and minor postoperative complications that occurred.

My experience is just initial (but encouraging), therefore the review is based on the recent literature. The surgical steps, as recently described by Arun Rojanasakul in the "How I do it" section of Techniques in Coloproctology (2009), are reported in Figure 3.9.

What about the risk of postoperative incontinence in a patient with an acute abscess that has been drained? The systematic review by Malik and Nelson (2007) cited five studies: Hebjorn et al. (1987), Schouten et al. (1991), Tang et al. (1996), Ho et al. (1997), and Oliver et al. (2003). The most impressive finding was that, if surgery is limited to draining the abscess, the anal incontinence rate is around zero whereas it increases up to 39% if the concomitant fistula is also operated on. Only in one series were both the abscess and the fistula treated without postoperative incontinence (Tang et al., 1996). By contrast, Ohana et al. (2004) reported the occurrence of epidural abscess following drainage of a perianal sepsis. The patient had lumbar pain and fever and needed neurosurgical decompression. When dealing with an acute anal abscess, it is advisable to drain and then, as a precaution, leave a loose seton. A second operation, possibly carried out by a specialist, will be aimed at managing the underlying fistula, once the acute sepsis has subsided.

Patients with both high and recurrent fistulae, especially if suprasphincteric, are at greater risk of postoperative continence disorders (Table 3.4).

In intersphincteric fistulae, the most frequent type, Toyonaga et al. (2007) reported that the neg-

Table 3.5 Postoperative complications following the sphincter-preserving LIFT procedure, carried out for both inter-, supra-, and trans-sphincteric fistulae

Author	Year	No. of pts	Complications	%
Royanasakul	2007	15	delayed wound healing anal incontinence	6.5 0
Shanwani	2010	45	delayed wound healing anal incontinence	17.8 0
Buier	2010	39	anal fissure persistent pain anal incontinence	1 1 0
Aboulian	2010	22	failed wound healing anal incontinence	23 23

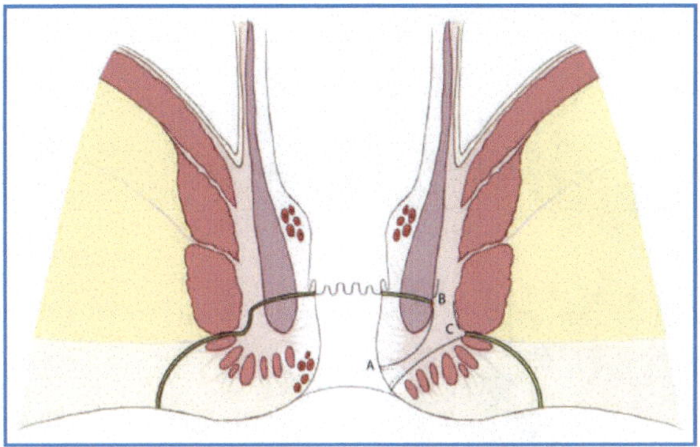

Fig. 3.9 a Illustration showing the basic concept of the LIFT technique. *A*, Approach via intersphincteric groove; *B*, suture ligation of tract to close the internal opening; *C*, suture ligation of defect in the external anal sphincter after removal of all infected granulation tissue

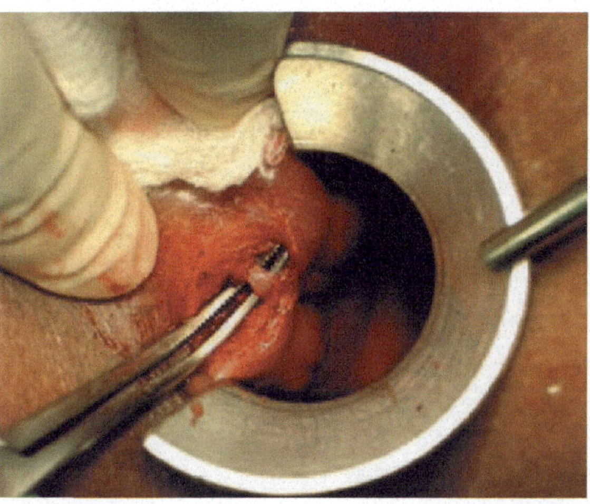

Fig. 3.9 b Intersphincteric fistulous tract hooked up with a Mixter forceps

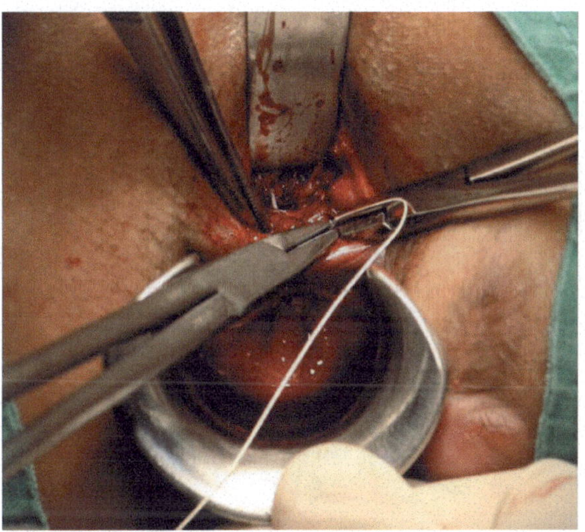

Fig. 3.9 c Sutured ligation of intersphincteric tract to close the internal opening in the internal anal sphincter

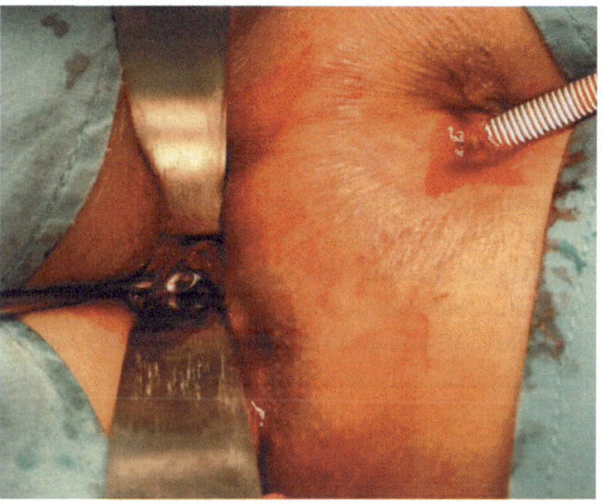

Fig. 3.9 d Curetting the fistulous tract (from Rojanasakul, 2009)

ative predictors of postoperative incontinence are previous abscess drainage and a low squeeze pressure at anal manometry.

In trans-sphincteric fistulae, which are known to be difficult to treat, no postoperative continence disorders after the LIFT procedure have been reported. Bleier et al., already cited, had just two complications among 39 patients who were operated on: an anal fissure and a case of severe pain for which the patient required a re-operation.

3.7 The Management of Postoperative Anal Incontinence

In case of minor incontinence, the patient may benefit from pelvic floor rehabilitation, consisting of sphincter-strengthening exercises, biofeedback, and transanal electrostimulation. According to a multicentric Dutch trial by Terra et al. (2006), internal sphincter deficiency, reduced voluntary contraction,

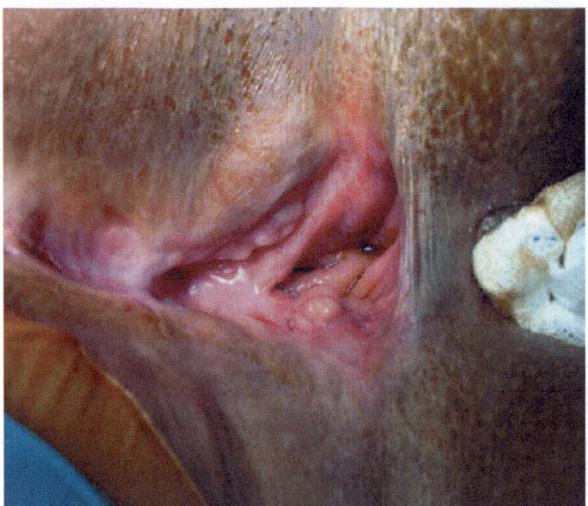

Fig. 3.10 a This patient (female, 34 years old, nulliparous), shown in the prone position, needed sphincter reconstruction because of a small and fibrotic external sphincter, following several surgeries for posterior trans-sphincteric anal fistula. She underwent a diverting sigmoidostomy. The sacrococcygeal area is shown on *the left side*, and the vagina with a gauze inserted on *the right*. The image shows the gaping anus, shortened anal canal, rectal mucosa, and postoperative cavity with a fibrosis area at its back side

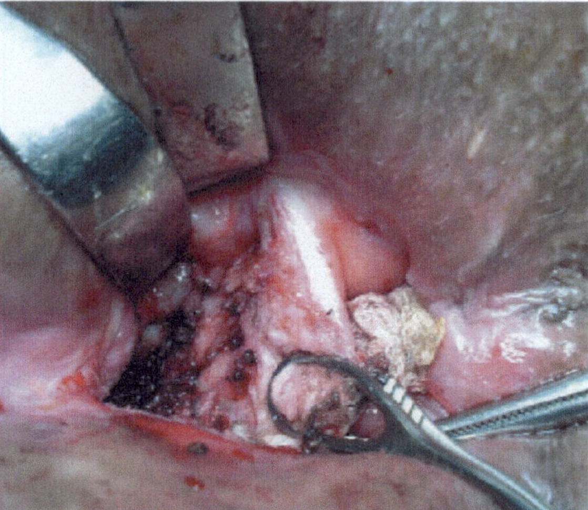

Fig. 3.10 b Curvilinear post-anal incision with anterior concavity. The intersphincteric space was identified, leaving in front the partially fibrotic internal sphincter and the posterior portion of the anal canal. On the posterior side, there was an area of scarring in which the ends of the external sphincter, retracted and fibrotic, were identified

and perineal scars may predict a poor outcome after pelvic floor rehabilitation. Better results were reported by Lacima et al. (2010). Alternatively, transcutaneous electrostimulation of the posterior tibial nerve (Eleouet, 2010) may be effective. Sacral neuromodulation is another option (Altomare et al., 2010; Matzel, 2011), but a relatively high re-intervention rate (25%) has been reported following this procedure (Faucheron et al., 2010).

If the injury is limited to the internal sphincter, the injection of a bulking agent is indicated; the method is costly but safe. There are several different substances that may be used, e.g., PTQ implants or Silicon microspherules, Coaptite, and Durasphere (Tjandra, 2004; Trompetto, 2008; Altomare, 2008). However, according to Altomare et al., in a multicentric prospective trial among the coloproctology units of the Italian Society of Colorectal Surgery (SICCR), Durasphere improves anal continence without improving the quality of life. A costless method, used by our unit prior to the introduction of Durasphere, is the injection of centrifuged autologous fat, harvested from the thigh (Bernardi et al., 1998). Unfortunately, the fat is likely to dislocate far from the injection site and thus lose its efficacy.

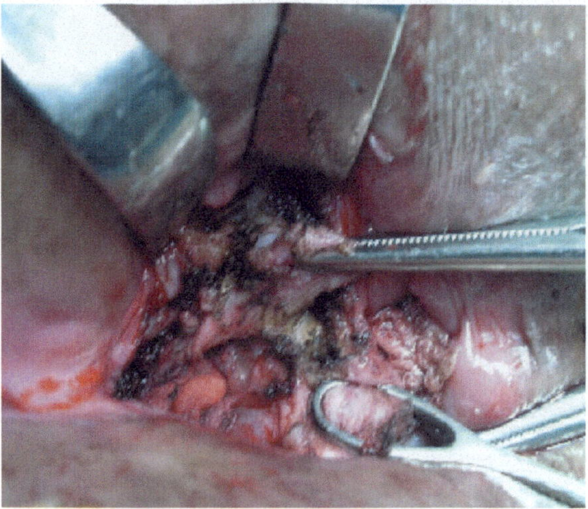

Fig. 3.10 c A ring clamp was positioned on the whitish fibers of the internal sphincter, thus raising the posterior part of the anal canal. *Left*, the external sphincter was isolated for no more than 2 cm to avoid devascularization

When the external sphincter has been injured during fistula surgery, sphincter reconstruction may improve anal continence (Fig. 3.10). However, the association of irritable bowel syndrome and rectal hyposensation are negative predictors of outcome (Chaudary et al., 2010; Nordestam et al., 2010). Both conditions may be easily diagnosed based on the clinical history and by simply inflating a rubber balloon in

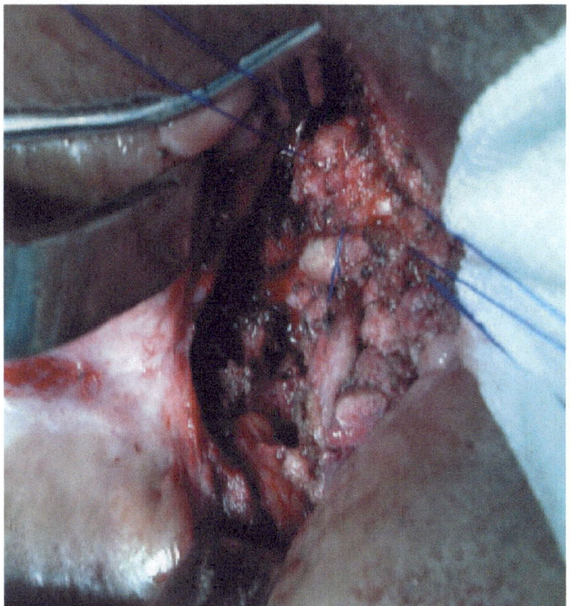

Fig. 3.10 d A gauze was positioned in the rectum. In the central part of the cavity, the right end of the external sphincter is seen to be whiter than the contralateral one. The front side shows the internal sphincter plasty, performed with prolene stitches

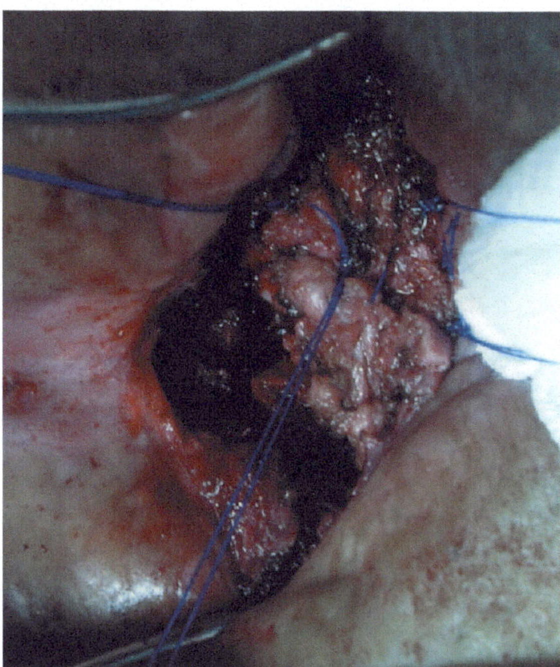

Fig. 3.10 e The plasty was finished with the overlapping technique reconstructing the external sphincter

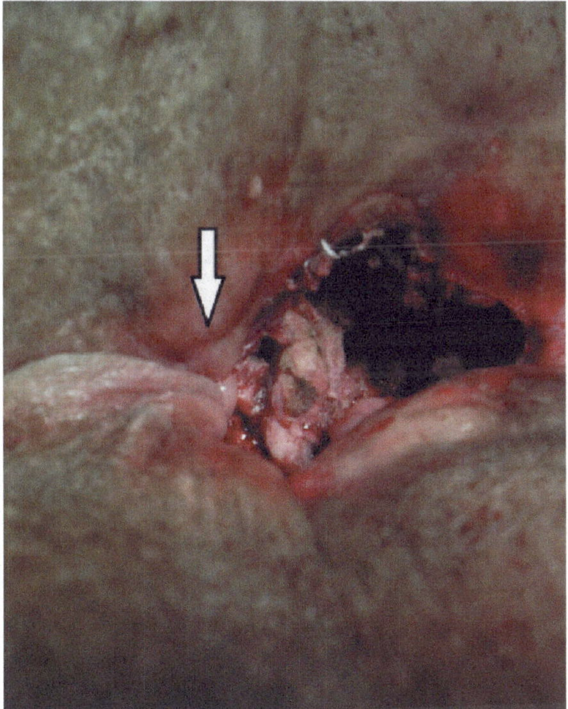

Fig. 3.10 f Reconstruction of the internal and external sphincter has been completed. The anal canal, an important continence factor, was lengthened. *Arrow* indicates the closed anus, showing that the preoperative gaping has been repaired

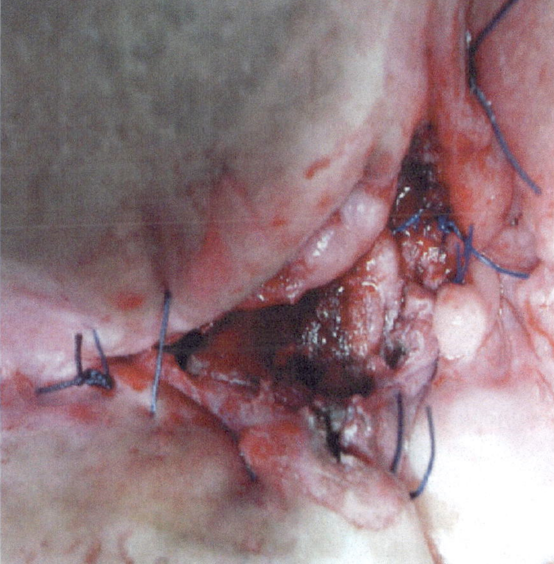

Fig. 3.10 g The surgical wound was partially closed by cross stitches

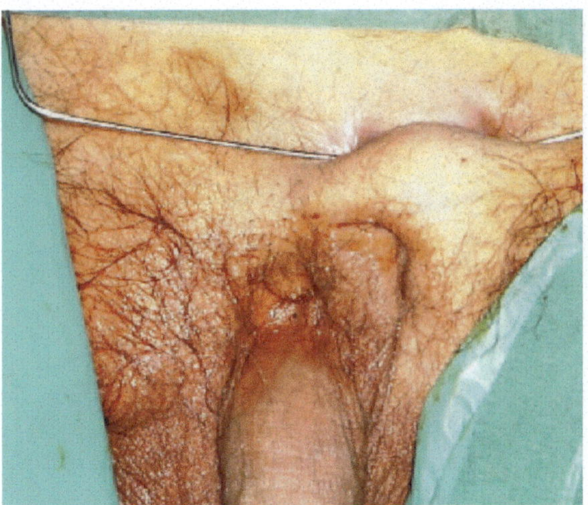

Fig. 3.11 A patient with hidradenitis suppurativa. A suprapubic superficial fistula is present

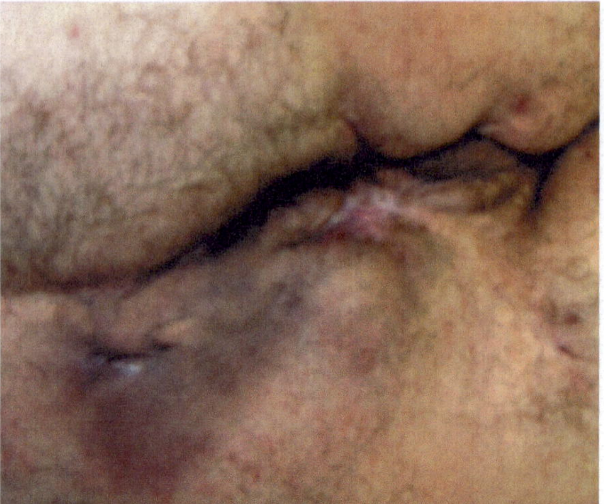

Fig. 3.12 Recurrence fistula in a smoker patient with hidradenitis suppurativa who already underwent perineoplasty

Table 3.6 Complications in hidradenitis suppurativa or acne inversa

Dermal retraction after wound healing
Systemic or local sepsis
Erysipelas (rare in the anogenital area)
Rectal or urethral fistulae (often iatrogenic)
Osteomyelitis, nephrotic syndrome, lymphedema
Symmetrical polyarteritis, systemic amyloidosis
Bacterial meningitis, bronchitis, pneumonia
Anemia due to chronic infection
Squamous cell carcinoma (Marjolin ulcer)

the rectum and recording the volumes that elicit first sensation, urge to pass stool, and maximal urgency.

If the anal sphincters are markedly injured or atrophic, an encirclement procedure using either the bulbocavernosus or the gracilis muscle may be indicated. Alternatives are the artificial bowel sphincter (ABS), which as reported in Chap. 9 (Anal Incontinence) has numerous drawbacks, and the novel Dacron ring (Devesa et al., 2011). Overlapping sphincter reconstruction is performed at our unit in these cases (Bondurri et al., 2011).

More information may be found in the ASCRS guidelines for anal incontinence (Tjandra et al., 2007).

3.8 Complications After Surgery for Hidradenitis Suppurativa

In these patients, sepsis is limited to the apocrine glands and is unlikely to deepen below the skin. As the anal sphincters are rarely involved, the risk of postoperative anal incontinence is low. In purulent lesions, the best treatment is lay-open of the fistula tract (Fig. 3.11). A potential complication is delayed wound healing, due to either new-onset infection or the persistence of causative factors, i.e., smoking, obesity, and diabetes (Fig. 3.12). If wide skin areas are to be excised, with the aim of radically curing the disease, it may be necessary to construct skin fascia or/and muscle advancement flaps. According to Rubin and Chinn (1994) and Buimer et al. (2009), hematomas, seromas, suture dehiscences, and consequent anal strictures may occur postoperatively, as reported after surgery of pilonidal sinus (see Chap. 5).

Other complications, either related to surgery or, more often, to the underlying disease, were reported by Hartschuh (2008) and are detailed in Table 3.6.

3.9 Tricks of the Trade

1. You've just carried out a fistulectomy for a high trans-sphincteric tract and are considering whether to perform a rectal mucosal advancement flap or position a seton. Although aware of the pros and cons of the two procedures, you are not sure which is the better choice in this case. But, there is a third option: both! Pass the seton through the internal orifice and the excised fistula tract, then divide the epithelium of the anal canal and the perianal skin between the internal

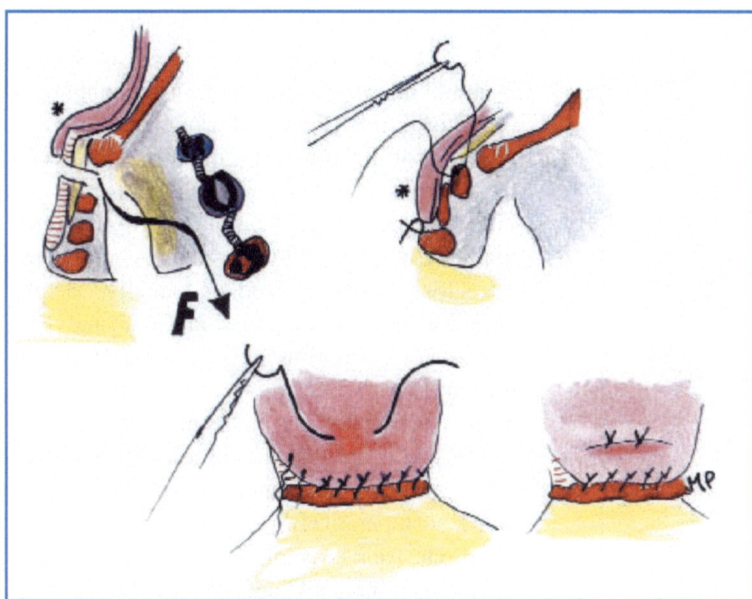

Fig. 3.13 Surgical procedure to reduce the risk of dehiscence of the rectal advancement flap (*) after fistulectomy (F). *Top left*: the removed tissue consists of the high trans-sphincteric fistula and three chronic abscess layers, perianal-*red*, ischiorectal-*purple*, intersphinteric-*blue*. After suturing of the rectal flap as usual, to the subcutaneous portion of the external sphincter (*top right*), two extra stitches are positioned at the flap center. Anchored to the underlying muscles, the two stitches are likely to prevent detachment of the flap in case of dehiscence of the suture, as shown in the *bottom* drawings

and external openings and tighten the seton around the underlying muscle, using a bit less tension than you normally apply for a cutting seton. The knot will be positioned a few millimeters below the tissue, so the seton is a bit loose. Then perform the flap as you usually do, ignoring the presence of the seton below it. Leave a small space between two of the flap sutures to the subcutaneous part of the external sphincter, thus making room for the distal end of the seton, i.e., the knot, to protrude outside the anus. In case of flap suture dehiscence, after a few days the flap procedure can be easily converted into a seton procedure, by tightening the seton over the muscle, as is normally done when using the cutting seton. I used this trick in two patients. In the first, the flap did not cause any problem and I cut the seton after a week. The small perianal wound healed in due time. The second patient had a flap dehiscence. After the seton was tightened as suggested above, there were no further complications. The procedure has been illustrated in *The Last Image Section, Techniques in Coloproctology* (Pescatori et al., 2002).

2. In a patient with a high trans-sphincteric fistula, treated with a rectal mucosal advancement flap following fistulectomy, there may be concern about the risk of flap breakdown, perhaps because the rectal mucosa is a bit inflamed and/or the patient is a heavy smoker. One solution (I have used it twice, successfully) is to stitch the central part of the flap to the underlying internal sphincter with one or two 2/0 vicryl sutures, at the level of the internal orifice of the excised fistula. In case of a breakdown, this suture is likely to hold the flap in its position (Fig. 3.13).
3. After draining a supralevator abscess, you prefer not to perform vigorous curettage, in order to avoid a lesion of the rectum, or you are concerned about the risk of bleeding from the levator muscles. While you don't want to divide much of the levator ani, you are concerned about possibly entrapping residual sepsis above it. In this case, the tip of a Foley catheter can be positioned in the supralevator space, followed by inflation of the balloon, which is left in place for a couple of days, maybe irrigating with disinfectant. This will help to achieve better drainage and will indicate whether there is bleeding (Fig. 3.14).
4. This is a simple maneuver used after the excision of a large chronic ischiorectal abscess. Perhaps you have intensively used diathermy (or scissors excision) to remove the upper part of the mass from the inferior aspect of the levator plane and are thus concerned about bleeding at the time of the first dressing. Or maybe the patient is hypersensitive, tense, and unlikely to tolerate a potentially painful dressing.

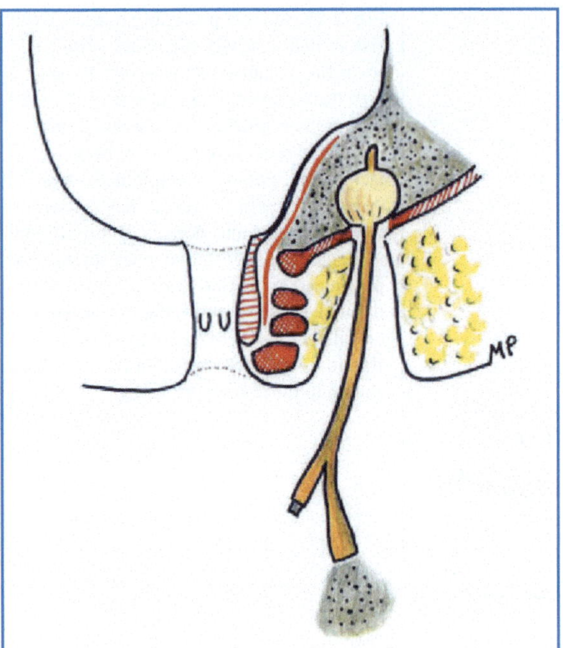

Fig. 3.14 After surgical drainage of an abscess above the levators muscles, a Foley catheter may be placed in the pelvic rectal space for postoperative irrigations in case of residual sepsis

One approach to minimize problems is to wrap the gauze with a Tabbotamp and insert it into the patient's ischiorectal cavity. This will prevent early postoperative bleeding and pain, as the Tabbotamp becomes a semi-fluid substance that will prevent adhesions between the gauze and the ischiorectal cavity, thus making the first dressing almost bloodless and painless.

5. You are going to start a fistulectomy. The tract should be cannulated by means of a probe. This common maneuver avoids the creation of false tracts and keeps the probe inside the fistula. Once the probe has been gently pushed until the proximal end of the tract, firmly secure a Kocher forceps around the base of the probe, at the level of the external orifice, grabbing the divided skin together with the fistula and the probe. This will prevent the probe from becoming dislocated, allowing the fistulectomy to proceed more rapidly and securely. During fistula excision, the risk of incidentally pulling the probe out of the tract, thereby losing the correct direction of dissection, will be minimized.
6. This is another trick aimed at not leaving secondary tracts behind when examining the ischiorectal space. Inserting an Eisenhammer retractor in this space will provide better visualization of the structures, i.e., the ischiorectal fat, outer surface of the external sphincter, and inferior aspect of the levator ani, all structures that may be crossed by a secondary tract. This retractor, usually placed endoanally, clearly demonstrates the ischiorectal fossa and permits the cannulation of secondary tracts, if present (Fig. 3.15).
7. Your patient has an intersphincteric fistula, which you have treated with a lay-open procedure, and internal hemorrhoids, which might bleed postoperatively (I recently had a similar case). The trick is as follows: when marsupializing the fistulotomy wound, wider portions of tissue at the edges of the wound in the anal canal should be used during suturing of the submucosal hemorrhoidal plexus. This simple maneuver will prevent bleeding and cure the hemorrhoids, similar to a Farag procedure (see Chap. 2).
8. Again, your patient has an anal fistula, primary and secondary intersphincteric tracts, and internal and external hemorrhoids. The treatment of both diseases must be delayed, as the piles are symptomatic and have not responded to conservative measures. Then, after fistulotomy and hemorrhoidectomy, it becomes clear that the anal canal is almost completely denuded of its epithelium, such that you are concerned about the occurrence of a postoperative stricture. A good option in this case is to harvest a cutaneous flap and advance it towards the anal canal to partly fill the defect (Fig. 3.16). The criteria for preparing and advancing the flap are described in Chap. 7 (Anorectal Strictures). We published this procedure in 1996.
9. The following maneuver is aimed at stopping intraoperative and preventing postoperative bleeding when the wound is left unsutured in either the anal canal or the lower rectum. It also may be useful after adenoma and hemorrhoid excision, as already illustrated in Chap. 2 (Fig. 2.24). After removal of a fistula tract containing a chronic abscess, oozing is sometimes observed in the anal canal at the site of the surgical wound. This is likely to happen in patients who

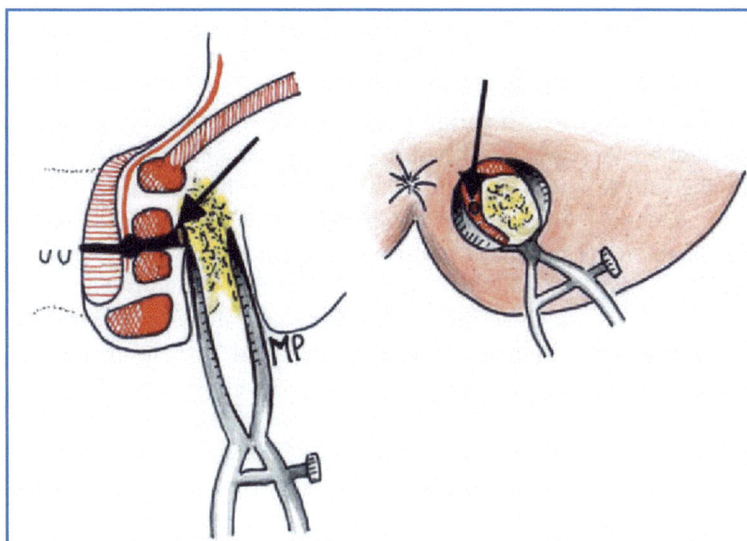

Fig. 3.15 An Eisenhammer's bivalve retractor allows better exploration of the ischiorectal space. *Left*: sagittal view; *right*: frontal view. The patient has been placed in the lithotomy position. The fat of the ischiorectal space and a fistula crossing the external sphincter are seen (*arrow*)

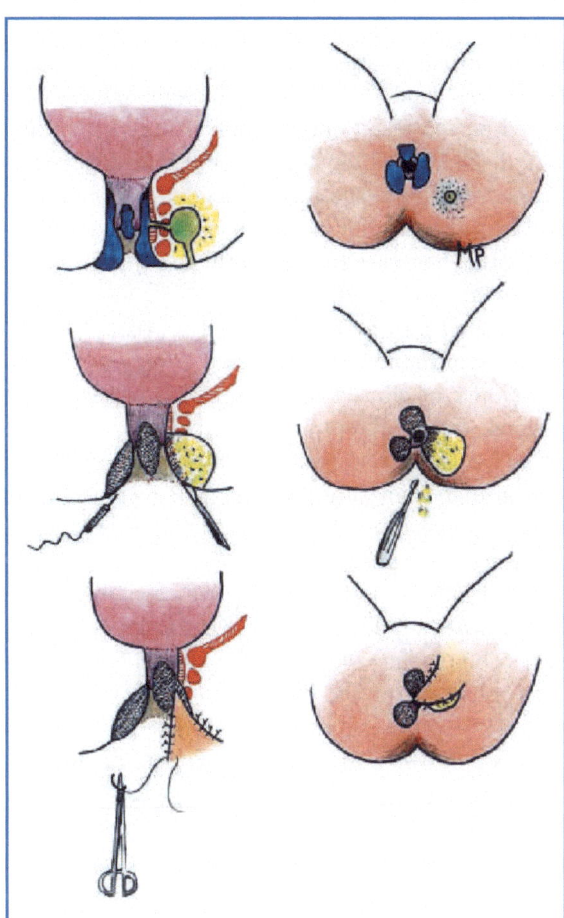

Fig. 3.16 Skin flap advanced into the anal canal to prevent stenosis after extensive de-epithelialization following simultaneous hemorrhoidectomy and fistulotomy. Hemorrhoids are shown in *blue*, surgical wounds in *gray* and *yellow*

have already had anal surgery. It becomes clear that compression with gauze that is left "in situ" is not an effective means to stop the bleeding whereas diathermy is ruled out to avoid excessive tissue necrosis, which might cause postoperative pain and sepsis. In such cases, the answer lies in the use of a Tabbotamp, suturing it onto the bleeding area with two-three stitches of Vicryl Rapid suture. Most of the time, this will result in effective control of the bleeding.

10. Finally, both pain and bleeding at the time of the first dressing can be prevented with a trick that we usually carry out in the ward on postoperative day two. Prior to removal of the gauze from the surgical cavity, which might be endo- or perianal or both, 10–20 ml of saline, or just water, is injected into the gauze using a needle and syringe. The gauze will become wet and swollen and can then easily be pulled and detached from the wound with minimal discomfort and almost no bleeding.

3.10 An Unforgettable Complication

In 2001, S., a sweet, thin, 23-year-old girl, came to our unit after two operations for anal fistula, the first performed by a vascular surgeon, the second by a colorectal surgeon. However, the fistula wound was still unhealed, with some degree of local sepsis and discharge, such that she complained of severe anal pain. According to her history, after the first operation, i.e., drainage of a perianal abscess, the persistent sepsis resulted in the need for nearly 20 consecutive dressings, performed by the vascular surgeon under sacral anesthesia, but they were of no benefit. She then started complaining of severe anal pain. Six months later, the colorectal surgeon carried out a fistulotomy, but healing of the wound was not achieved and pus discharge was noted.

When I saw the patient, she was continent at flatus and stool, and her main complaint was proctalgia, a severe continuous dull pain that was slightly diminished in the prone position and exacerbated by defecations. A discharging perianal wound was noted; at digital exploration, the pain increased upon digital pressure. At anal manometry, resting tone was reduced and the rectal sensitivity threshold was increased, with the patient reporting pain at small-volume inflation of the rectal balloon. Her bowel habit was normal and she did not complain of abdominal pain. However, to exclude Crohn's disease, we performed a colonoscopy. Both the large bowel and the terminal ileum had a normal appearance and the biopsies were negative. At anal ultrasound, carried out with a rotating probe (she had never undergone this examination before), a distal defect of the internal sphincter was seen, together with a low intersphincteric abscess. A psychological consultation was carried out based on the known relationship between stress, immunodeficiency, and anal sepsis, indicating the need for a holistic approach in these cases. However, the patient exhibited only low degrees of anxiety and there had been no stressful event prior to disease onset. The only slightly questionable finding was the strong attachment of the mother, who was constantly present and seemed to be much more anxious than her daughter.

In 2002, S. was operated on under general anesthesia (Fig. 3.17). The intersphincteric abscess seen at anal US was identified and the intersphincteric plane was curetted, apparently removing the abscess. To achieve better drainage, I decided to perform a distal internal sphincterotomy (Park's procedure), despite concern about potential anal continence in a young nulliparous patient. Unfortunately, one month later, S. still had a discharging, unhealed perianal wound and her severe pain was unchanged. However, she was fully continent.

Therefore, I discussed the matter with her mother (I had never seen her father in ten years) and explained that, to eradicate the sepsis, it was necessary to completely divide the internal sphincter and a portion of the external sphincter, which was likely to cause incontinence, and to carry out a covering sigmoidostomy, aimed at achieving complete wound healing and preventing painful defecations. "Once the wound is healed," I said, "before or after the stoma closure, she could try pelvic floor exercises. Alternatively, a sphincter reconstruction might be carried out at the time of stoma closure or prior to it, aimed at preventing fecal incontinence." Both the mother and S. agreed with the surgical plan.

Thus, in 2003, S. underwent a second operation, consisting of a laying-open of the intersphincteric and low trans-sphincteric tracts, followed by the fashioning of a diverting stoma. She was discharged after an uneventful postoperative course. At home, she began successful stoma irrigations, the wound healed completely, and the proctalgia decreased. One month later, when I saw her in my office, the perineum was healed, the anus gaped on traction and, not surprisingly, voluntary contraction was reduced. I suggested that the stoma be closed and a sphincteroplasty performed, but she replied: "Doctor, I'm not concerned with the fistula and incontinence, my problem is that I am sure the pain will increase with normal defecations. I prefer to remain like this."

In 2004, the girl's mother called me on the phone: "Doctor, unfortunately, my daughter's pain increased. I bought her a little dog to make her happier, but she keeps complaining of severe pain all day. She cannot even go out for a walk. Please help us."

What would you do to help this patient? In summary: A 26 year-old female, four operations for anal fistula. Diverting stoma. Fistula healed. Severe proctalgia. No sign of Crohn's disease. No significant mental distress.

Our neurologist performed an EMG study, measuring pudendal motor latency, which was found to be prolonged. This was foreseeable, considering that

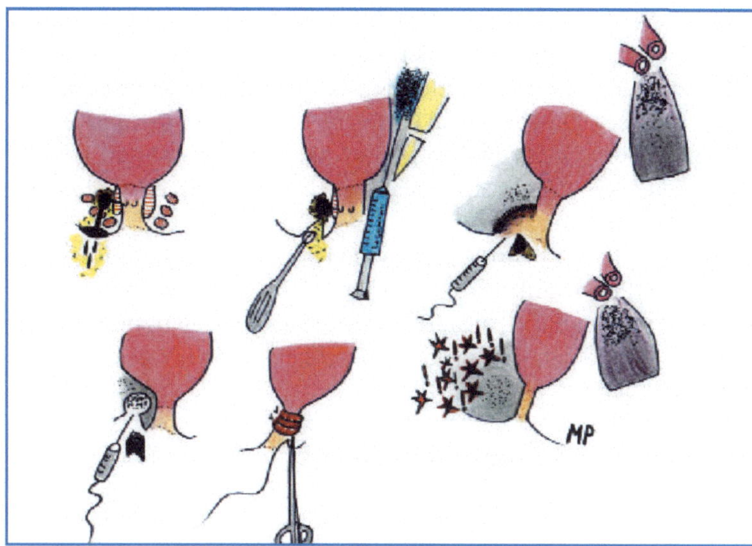

Fig. 3.17 Severe chronic proctalgia after drainage of a perianal abscess, repeated sacral anesthesia and fistulectomy with diverting sigmoidostomy (*top*). The patient also underwent excision of a perirectal granuloma and sphincteroplasty, but without positive outcome (*bottom*)

she had had nearly 20 sacral punctures at the time of the first unhealed fistula wound, following the operation performed by the vascular surgeon. We tried a course of transanal electrostimulation, which is helpful in nearly half of such cases, but she had no improvement. Anal US showed marked fibrosis at the site of anal pain. "Should we remove this fibrosis, do you think that she will be cured?" her mother asked. "It is unlikely," I said, "I would not be in favor of doing that." "Could you advise us where to go? We want to try." At this point, I suggested the name of a very skilled UK surgeon who, after a month, excised the fibrotic tissue close to the anal canal and, as the sphincters were injured after the four fistula surgeries, carried out a sphincter reconstruction.

In 2005, I saw the patient after a few postoperative months. She still had severe anal pain, with no improvement at all.

In 2006, another surgical attempt was made, also abroad. A colorectal surgeon tried to relieve the pudendal neuropathy by carrying out transperineal neurolysis. Again, there was no improvement.

In 2007, I received a telephone call from my patient's mother, with bad news: S. was in Rome, at the Policlinico Gemelli Hospital (where I had worked for several years), where she had just undergone an operation to remove an ovarian carcinoma. When I saw her, she smiled and told me that the operation went well, but she still had anal pain.

The latest news, received in 2010, was that S., now over thirty, is alive, still plays with her dog, and goes out from time to time. Her colostomy continues to function. She still complains of proctalgia.

My thoughts after such a sad case. A vascular surgeon should not operate on an anal fistula. If the anal wound does not heal after fistula surgery, better to perform one, two, or three re-operations than repeated dressings under sacral anesthesia, as they may damage the pudendal nerves and cause chronic proctalgia, which may affect the quality of life for decades.

Summary

The most frequent and feared complication following fistula surgery is anal incontinence, which may be temporary and minor or, more rarely, gross and permanent. Rectal hyposensation may be a negative predictor of postoperative anal incontinence, which is more likely to occur following an extended fistulotomy for a high tract, although this operation is associated with better healing and a lower recurrence rate. If performed using radiofrequency, extended fistulotomy results in less postoperative bleeding and pain. According to surgeons at St. Marks' Hospital, a lay-open is a good option in the management of high fistulae, as it rarely causes permanent and major incontinence.

According to a recent systematic review, distal division of the internal sphincter, popularized by Parks and aimed at better draining of the intersphincteric plane, is of limited value as far as the recurrence rate. However, it is still used at our unit, as continence disorders occur in less than 5% of patients if those with weak sphincters are excluded from the procedure.

Low posterior fistulae may be laid-open without affecting anal continence, whereas care should be taken in the management of high anterior fistulae in women, who are likely to have deficient sphincters, especially if multiparous. Patients with neuropathic sphincters, previous anal surgery, advanced age, Crohn's disease, or diabetes are at greater risk of postoperative incontinence.

Many sphincter-saving procedures have been proposed, especially for trans-sphincteric and high trans-sphincteric fistulae. The seton may cause soiling but not gross incontinence; in rectal mucosal or cutaneous flap advancement, there is a 30% rate of suture dehiscence. Direct suture of the internal orifice following fistulectomy has been proposed as an effective method. Re-routing of the fistula tract is an alternative to reduce the risk of incontinence. The LIFT procedure, first described by Phillips, has been advocated by Rojanasakul and is gaining popularity due to its good results. Among the novel procedures stem cells or platelet-enriched plasma injection, fistula tract destruction using a laser probe, and VAAFT are gaining increasing interest. Plug and fibrin-glue injections have been carried out in several cases, with almost no risk of incontinence; but these approaches are costly and are followed by non healing wounds in one-third of the patients.

When dealing with an acute abscess, the best policy is to insert a loose seton into the fistula tract, if the internal orifice is found, and delay the operation for fistula, which should be carried out by a specialist.

When dealing with iatrogenic incontinence, pelvic floor rehabilitation may be of some help. In rare cases, sacral neuromodulation is indicated. Minor localized defects of the internal sphincter may be successfully treated with bulking agent injection, whereas sphincter reconstruction or, rarely, transposed muscle encirclement may be performed in case of wider injuries to the striated sphincters. Irritable bowel and rectal hyposensation may affect the outcome of sphincter repair.

Rectal bleeding is only occasionally seen following fistula surgery and may be minimized by marsupialization of the wound, which is also aimed at decreasing the healing time by reducing its size.

Hidradenitis suppurativa or acne inversa is unlikely to be followed by fecal incontinence as the sepsis rarely extends to the deep tissues and the anal sphincters are unlikely to be involved.

Suggested Readings

Abarca F, Brand M, Saclarides T (2010) Cutting seton: outcomes, safety, and efficacy for the treatment of anorectal fistulas. Dis Colon Rectum 53:574

Abulian A, Kaji A, Kumar R, CA Torrance (2010) Early results of ligation of intersphincteric fistula tract for fistula-in-ano. Dis Colon Rectum 53:552-553

Adams J, Whitlow C, Beck D et al (2010) Does catheter drainage time affect outcome of perianal abscesses? Dis Colon Rectum 53:570

Adams T, Yang J, Kondylis LA et al (2008) Long-term outlook after successful fibrin glue ablation of cryptoglandular transsphincteric fistula-in-ano. Dis Colon Rectum 51:1488-1490

Alexander SM, Mitalas LE, Gosselink MP et al (2008) Obliteration of the fistulous tract with BioGlue adversely affects the outcome of transanal advancement flap repair. Tech Coloproctol 12:225-228

Altomare DF, Greco VJ, Tricomi N et al (2011) Seton or glue for trans-sphincteric anal fistulae: a prospective randomized crossover clinical trial. Colorectal Dis 13:82-86

Altomare DF, La Torre F, Rinaldi M et al (2008) Carbon-coated microbeads anal injection in outpatient treatment of minor fecal incontinence. Dis Colon Rectum 51:432-435

Amin SN, Tierney GM, Lund JN et al (2003) V-Y advancement flap for treatment of fistula-in-ano. Dis Colon Rectum 46:540-543

Athanasiadis S, Helmes C, Yazigi R et al (2004) The direct closure of the internal fistula opening without advancement flap for transsphincteric fistulas-in-ano. Dis Colon Rectum 47:1174-1180

Atkin GK, Martins J, Tozer P et al (2011) For many high anal fistulas, lay open is still a good option. Tech Coloproctol 15:143-150

Bassi R, Rademacher J, Savoia A (2006) Rectovaginal fistula after STARR procedure complicated by haematoma of the posterior vaginal wall: report of a case. Tech Coloproctol 10:361-363

Bemelman WA (2009) Vacuum assisted closure in coloproctology. Tech Coloproctol 13:261-263

Bernardi C, Pescatori M (1998) Perineal lipofilling: a new surgical treatment for fecal incontinence. Tech Coloproctol 2:46-51

Bernardi C, Pescatori M (2001) Reconstructive perineoplasty in the management of non-healing wounds after anorectal surgery. Tech Coloproctol 5:27-32

Binda GA, Trizi F (2007) Treatment of unhealed wound after anal fistulotomy with full-thickness skin graft. Tech Coloproctol 11:294

Bleier JI, Moloo H, Goldberg SM (2010) Ligation of the intersphincteric fistula tract: an effective new technique for complex fistulas. Dis Colon Rectum 53:43-46

Blumetti J, Quinteros F, Abcarian A et al (2010) The evolution of treatment of fistula-in-ano. Dis Colon Rectum 53:570

Browder LK, Sweet S, Kaiser AM (2009) Modified Hanley procedure for management of complex horseshoe fistulae. Tech Coloproctol 13:301-306

Buchanan GN, Bartram CI, Phillips RK et al (2003) Efficacy of fibrin sealant in the management of complex anal fistula: a prospective trial. Dis Colon Rectum 46:1167-1174

Buchanan GN, Owen HA, Torkington J et al (2004) Long-term outcome following loose-seton technique for external sphincter preservation in complex anal fistula. Br J Surg 91:476-480

Cavanaugh M, Hyman N, Osler T (2002) Fecal incontinence severity index after fistulotomy: a predictor of quality of life. Dis Colon Rectum 45:349-353

Champagne BJ, O'Connor LM, Ferguson M et al (2006) Efficacy of anal fistula plug in closure of cryptoglandular fistulas: long-term follow-up. Dis Colon Rectum 49:1817-1821

Chaudhary BN, Chadwick M, Roe AM (2010) Selecting patients with fecal incontinence for anal sphincter surgery: the influence of irritable bowel syndrome. Colorect Dis 12-750-753

Choi D, Sung KH, Seo HI et al (2010) Patient-performed seton irrigation for the treatment of deep fistulas. Dis Colon Rectum 53:812-816

Christoforidis D, Etzioni DA, Goldberg SM et al (2008) Treatment of complex anal fistulas with the collagen fistula plug. Dis Colon Rectum 51:1482-1487

Christoforidis D, Pieh MC, Madoff RD et al (2009) Treatment of transsphincteric anal fistulas by endorectal advancement flap or collagen fistula plug: a comparative study. Dis Colon Rectum 52:18-22

Chung W, Kazemi P, Ko D et al (2009) Anal fistula plug and fibrin glue versus conventional treatment in repair of complex anal fistulas. Am J Surg 197:604-608

Cintron JR, Park JJ, Orsay CP et al (2000) Repair of fistulas-in-ano using fibrin adhesive: long-term follow-up. Dis Colon Rectum 43:944-999

Cox SW, Senagore AJ, Luchtefeld MA et al (1997) Outcome after incision and drainage with fistulotomy for ischiorectal abscess. Am Surg 63:686-689

Devesa JM, Hervás PL, Vicente R et al (2011) Anal encirclement with a simple prosthetic sling for faecal incontinence. Tech Coloproctol 15:17-22

Eitan A, Koliada M, Bickel A (2009) The use of the loose seton technique as a definitive treatment for recurrent and persistent high trans-sphincteric anal fistulas: a long-term outcome. J Gastrointest Surg 13:1116-1119

Eléouet M, Spiroudhis L, Guillou N et al (2010) Chronic posterior tibial nerve transcutaneous electrical nerve stimulation (TENS) to treat fecal incontinence. Int J Colorectal Dis 25:1127-1132

Ellis CN (2007) Bioprosthetic plugs for complex anal fistulas: an early experience. J Surg Educ 64:36-40

Ellis CN (2010) Management of anal fistulas: what patients want. Dis Colon Rectum 53:571

Ellis CN (2010) Outcomes with the use of bioprosthetics grafts to reinforce the ligation of the intersphincteric fistula tract (BioLIFT procedure) for the management of complex anal fistulas. Dis Colon Rectum 53:1361-1364

Ellis CN (2010) Sphincter-preserving fistula management: what patients want. Dis Colon Rectum 53:1652-1655

Ellis CN, Clark S (2006) Fibrin glue as an adjunct to flap repair of anal fistulas: a randomized, controlled study. Dis Colon Rectum 49:1736-1740

Eykyn SJ, Grace RH (1986) The relevance of microbiology in the management of anorectal sepsis. Ann R Coll Surg Engl 68:237-239

Faucheron JL, Voirin D, Badic B (2010) Sacral nerve stimulation for fecal incontinence: causes of surgical revision from a series of 87 consecutive patients operated on in a single institution. Dis Colon Rectum 53:1501-1507

Filingeri V, Gravante G, Baldessari E et al (2004) Radiofrequency fistulectomy vs. diathermic fistulotomy for submucosal fistulas: a randomized trial. Eur Rev Med Pharmacol Sci 8:111-116

Gaertner W, Finne C, Mellgren A et al (2010) Perianal hidradenitis suppurativa and Crohn's desease: is nonoperative treatment associated with better outcomes? Dis Colon Rectum 53:601

Ganio E, Marino F, Giani I et al (2008) Injectable synthetic calcium hydroxylapatite ceramic microspheres (Coaptite) for passive fecal incontinence. Tech Coloproctol 12:99-102

Garcia-Aguilar J, Belmonte C, Wong WD et al (1996) Anal fistula surgery. Factors associated with recurrence and incontinence. Dis Colon Rectum 39:723-729

Garcia-Olmo D, Herreros D, Pascual I et al (2009) Expanded adipose-derived stem cells for the treatment of complex perianal fistula: a phase II clinical trial. Dis Colon Rectum 52:79-86

Garg P, Song J, Bhatia A et al (2010) The efficacy of anal fistula plug in fistula-in-ano: a systematic review. Colorect Dis 12:965-970

Grace RH, Harper IA, Thompson RG (1982) Anorectal sepsis: microbiology in relation to fistula-in-ano. Br J Surg 69:401-403

Gupta PJ (2003) Radiosurgical fistulotomy; an alternative to conventional procedure in fistula in ano. Curr Surg 60:524-528

Gustafsson UM, Graf W (2002) Excision of anal fistula with closure of the internal opening: functional and manometric results. Dis Colon Rectum 45:1672-1678

Hammond TM, Porrett TR, Scott SM et al (2011) Management of idiopathic anal fistula using cross-linked collagen: a prospective phase 1 study. Colorectal Dis 13:94-104

Hartschuh W (2008) Hidradenitis suppurativa. In: Herold A, Lehur PA et al (eds) Coloproctology. Springer, Berlin Heidelberg New York

Hasegawa H, Radley S, Keighley MR (2000) Long-term results of cutting seton fistulotomy. Acta Chir Iugosl 47:19-21

Hebjørn M, Olsen O, Haakansson T et al (1987) A randomized trial of fistulotomy in perianal abscess. Scand J Gastroenterol 22:174-176

Heidenreich A, Collarini HA, Paladino AM et al (1966) Cancer

in anal fistulas: report of two cases. Dis Colon Rectum 9:371-376
Ho KS, Ho YH (2005) Controlled, randomized trial of island flap anoplasty for treatment of trans-sphincteric fistula-in-ano: early results. Tech Coloproctol 9:166-168
Ho KS, Tsang C, Seow-Choen F et al (2001) Prospective randomized trial comparing ayurvedic cutting seton and fistulotomy for low fistula-in-ano. Tech Coloproctol 5:137–141
Ho YH, Tan M, Chui CH et al (1997) Randomized controlled trial of primary fistulotomy with drainage alone for perianal abscesses. Dis Colon Rectum 40:1435-1438
Ho YH, Tan M, Leong AF et al (1998) Marsupialization of fistulotomy wounds improves healing: a randomized controlled trial. Br J Surg 85:105-107
Holzheimer RG, Siebeck M (2006) Treatment procedures for anal fistulous cryptoglandular abscess-how to get the best results. Eur J Med Res 11:501-515
Hossack T, Solomon MJ, Young JM (2005) Ano-cutaneous flap repair for complex and recurrent supra-sphincteric anal fistula. Colorectal Dis 7:187-192
Johnson EK, Gaw JU, Armstrong DN (2006) Efficacy of anal fistula plug vs. fibrin glue in closure of anorectal fistulas. Dis Colon Rectum 49:371-376
Jongen J, Koepcke A, Peleikis H et al (2010) Results of rectal advancement flap for high anal fistula. Dis Colon Rectum 53:574
Jordán J, Roig JV, García-Armengol J et al (2010) Risk factors for recurrence and incontinence after anal fistula surgery. Colorectal Dis 12:254-260
Kleinübing H Jr, Jannini JF, Campos AC et al (2007) The role of transperineal ultrasonography in the assessment of the internal opening of cryptogenic anal fistula. Tech Coloproctol 11:327-331
Koehler A, Risse-Schaaf A, Athanasiadis S (2004) Treatment for horseshoe fistulas-in-ano with primary closure of the internal fistula opening: a clinical and manometric study. Dis Colon Rectum 47:1874-1882
Lacima G, Pera M, Amador A et al (2010) Long-term results of biofeedback treatment for fecal incontinence: a comparative study with untreated controls. Colorectal Dis 12:742-749
Lenisa L, Espìn-Basany E, Rusconi A et al (2010) Anal fistula plug is a valid alternative option for the treatment of complex anal fistula in the long term. Int J Colorectal Dis 25:1487-1493
Loungnarath R, Dietz DW, Mutch MG et al (2004) Fibrin glue treatment of complex anal fistulas has low success rate. Dis Colon Rectum 47:432-436
Malik AI, Nelson RL (2008) Surgical management of anal fistulae: a systematic review. Colorectal Dis 10:420-430
Mann CV, Clifton MA (1985) Re-routing of the track for the treatment of high anal and anorectal fistulae. Br J Surg 72:134-137
Mitalas LE, van Onkelen RS, Gosselink MP et al (2010) The anal fistula plug as an adjunct to transanal advancement flap repair. Dis Colon Rectum 53:1713
Mizrahi N, Wexner SD, Zmora O et al (2002) Endorectal advancement flap: are there predictors of failure? Dis Colon Rectum 45:1616-1621
Mylonakis E, Katsios C, Godevenos D et al (2001) Quality of life of patients after surgical treatment of anal fistula; the role of anal manometry. Colorectal Dis 3:417-421
Nadal SR, Manzione CR, Horta SH et al (2010) Anal fistulas are associated with condyloma in HIV-infected patients. Int J Colorectal Dis 25:663-664
Nelson RL, Cintron J, Abcarian H (2000) Dermal island-flap anoplasty for transsphincteric fistula-in-ano: assessment of treatment failures. Dis Colon Rectum 43:681-684
Nordenstam JF, Altman DH, Mellgren AF et al (2010) Impaired rectal sensation at anal manometry is associated with anal incontinence one year after primary sphincter repair in primiparous women. Dis Colon Rectum 53:1409-1414
Oberwalder M, Dinnewitzer A, Baig MK et al (2006) Do internal anal sphincter defects decrease the success rate of anal sphincter repair? Tech Coloproctol 10:94-97
Ohana G, Salem L, Arich A et al (2004) Development of epidural abscess following surgical drainage of perianal abscess: report of a case. Dis Colon Rectum 47:392-394
Oliver I, Lacueva FJ, Pérez Vicente F et al (2003) Randomized clinical trial comparing simple drainage of anorectal abscess with and without fistula track treatment. Int J Colorectal Dis 18:107-110
Ortiz H, Marzo J, Ciga MA et al (2009) Randomized clinical trial of anal fistula plug versus endorectal advancement flap for the treatment of high cryptoglandular fistula in ano. Br J Surg 96:608-612
Ozuner G, Hull TL, Cartmill J et al (1996) Long-term analysis of the use of transanal rectal advancement flaps for complicated anorectal/vaginal fistulas. Dis Colon Rectum 39:10-14
Patrlj L, Kocman B, Martinac M et al (2000) Fibrin glue-antibiotic mixture in the treatment of anal fistulae: experience with 69 cases. Dig Surg 17:77-80
Perez F, Arroyo A, Serrano P et al (2005) Fistulotomy with primary sphincter reconstruction in the management of complex fistula-in-ano: prospective study of clinical and manometric results. J Am Coll Surg 200:897-903
Perez F, Arroyo A, Serrano P et al (2006) Randomized clinical and manometric study of advancement flap versus fistulotomy with sphincter reconstruction in the management of complex fistula-in-ano. Am J Surg 192:34-40
Pescatori M (1997) Use of a rubber tube to protect endoanal sutures. Tech Coloproctol 1:32-35
Pescatori M (2011) Ascessi, fistole anali e retto-vaginali. Springer, Milano
Pescatori M, Ayabaca S, Caputo D (2004) Can anal manometry predict anal incontinence after fistulectomy in males. Colorect Dis 6: 97-102
Pescatori M, Ayabaca SM, Cafaro D et al (2006) Marsupialization of fistulotomy and fistulectomy wounds improves healing and decreases bleeding: a randomized controlled trial. Colorectal Dis 8:11-14
Pescatori M, Interisano A, Basso L et al (1995) Management of perianal Crohn's disease. Results of a multicenter study in Italy. Dis Colon Rectum 38:121-124
Pescatori M, Maria G, Anastasio G et al (1989) Anal manometry improves the outcome of surgery for fistula-in-ano. Dis Colon Rectum 32:588-592
Pescatori M, Mungo M, Guarino E (2002) Combined seton-double flap procedure for complex high anal fistula. Tech Coloproctol 6:71
Phillips RKS, Lunniss PJ (1996) Anal fistula: surgical evaluation and management. Chapman & Hall, London
Quah HM, Tang CL, Eu KW et al (2006) Meta-analysis of randomized clinical trials comparing drainage alone vs primary

sphincter-cutting procedures for anorectal abscess-fistula. Int J Colorectal Dis 21:602-609

Queralto M, Portier G, Bonnaud G et al (2010) Efficacy of synthetic glue treatment of high crypoglandular fistula-in-ano. Gastroenterol Clin Biol 34:477-482

Ritchie RD, Sackier JM, Hodde JP (2009) Incontinence rates after cutting seton treatment for anal fistula. Colorectal Dis 11:564-571

Roig JV, García-Armengol J, Jordán JC et al (2010) Fistulectomy and sphincteric reconstruction for complex cryptoglandular fistulas. Colorectal Dis 12:145-152

Roig JV, Jordán J, García-Armengol J et al (2009) Changes in anorectal morphologic and functional parameters after fistula-in-ano surgery. Dis Colon Rectum 52:1462-1469

Rojanasakul A, Pattanaarun J, Sahakitrungruang C, Tantiphlachiva K (2007) Total anal sphincter saving technique for fistula-in-ano; the ligation of intersphincteric fistula tract. J Med Assoc Thai 90:581-586

Rojanasakul A (2009) LIFT procedure: a simplified technique for fistula-in-ano. Tech Coloproctol 13:237-240

Rubin RJ, Chinn BT (1994) Perianal hidradenitis suppurativa. Surg Clin North Am 74:1317-1325

Safar B, Jobanputra S, Sands D et al (2009) Anal fistula plug: initial experience and outcomes. Dis Colon Rectum 52:248-252

Sainio P (1985) A manometric study of anorectal function after surgery for anal fistula, with special reference to incontinence. Acta Chir Scand 151:695-700

Schouten WR, van Vroonhoven TJ (1991) Treatment of anorectal abscess with or without primary fistulectomy. Results of a prospective randomized trial. Dis Colon Rectum 34:60-63

Schouten WR, Zimmerman DD, Briel JW (1999) Transanal advancement flap repair of transsphincteric fistulas. Dis Colon Rectum 42:1419-1422

Schwandner O (2010) Surgery: Are bioprosthetic plugs for complex anal fistulas effective? Nat Rev Gastroenterol Hepatol 7:419-420

Schwartz DA, Wiersema MJ, Dudiak KM et al (2001) A comparison of endoscopic ultrasound, magnetic resonance imaging, and exam under anesthesia for evaluation of Crohn's perianal fistulas. Gastroenterology 121:1064-1072

Sentovich SM (2003) Fibrin glue for anal fistulas: long-term results. Dis Colon Rectum 46:498-502

Shanwani A, Nor AM, Amri N (2010) Ligation of the intersphincteric fistula tract (LIFT): a sphincter-saving technique for fistula-in-ano. Dis Colon Rectum 53:39-42

Shukla NK, Narang R, Nair NGK et al (1991) Multicentric randomized controlled clinical trial of Kshaarasootra (Ayurvedic medicated thread) in the management of fistula-in-ano. Indian J Med Res 94:177–185

Sonoda T, Hull T, Piedmonte MR et al (2002) Outcomes of primary repair of anorectal and rectovaginal fistulas using the endorectal advancement flap. Dis Colon Rectum 45:1622-1628

Stremitzer S, Strobl S, Kure V et al (2011) Treatment of perianal sepsis and long-term outcome of recurrence and continence. Colorect Dis 13:703-707

Subhas G, Gupta A, Balaraman S et al (2011) Non-cutting setons for progressive migration of complex fistula tracts: a new spin on an old technique. Int J Colorectal Dis 26:793:798

Sungurtekin U, Sungurtekin H, Kabay B et al (2004) Anocutaneous V-Y advancement flap for the treatment of complex perianal fistula. Dis Colon Rectum 47:2178-2183

Swinscoe MT, Ventakasubramaniam AK, Jayne DG (2005) Fibrin glue for fistula-in-ano: the evidence reviewed. Tech Coloproctol 9:89-94

Takesue Y, Ohge H, Yokoyama T et al (2002) Long-term results of seton drainage on complex anal fistulae in patients with Crohn's disease. J Gastroenterol 37:912-915

Tan JJ, Chan M, Tjandra JJ (2007) Evolving therapy for fecal incontinence. Dis Colon Rectum 50:1950-1967

Tan K, Tan I, Ko D,Tsang C (2010) Long term results of ligation of intersphincteric fistula tract (LIFT) technique in the management of anal fistula. Dis Colon Rectum 53:576-577

Tang CL, Chew SP, Seow-Choen F (1996) Prospective randomized trial of drainage alone vs. drainage and fistulotomy for acute perianal abscesses with proven internal opening. Dis Colon Rectum 39:1415-1417

Terra MP, Deutekom M, Beets-Tan RG et al (2006) Relationship between external anal sphincter atrophy at endoanal magnetic resonance imaging and clinical, functional, and anatomic characteristics in patients with fecal incontinence. Dis Colon Rectum 49:668-678

Thekkinkattil DK, Botterill I, Ambrose NS et al (2009) Efficacy of the anal fistula plug in complex anorectal fistulae. Colorectal Dis 11:584-587

Thornton M, Solomon MJ (2005) Long-term indwelling seton for complex anal fistulas in Crohn's disease. Dis Colon Rectum 48:459-463

Tjandra JJ, Dykes SL, Aumar RR et al (2007) Practice parameters for the treatment of fecal incontinence. Dis Colon Rectum 50:1497-1507

Tjandra JJ, Lim JF, Hiscock R et al (2004) Injectable silicone biomaterial for fecal incontinence caused by internal anal sphincter dysfunction is effective. Dis Colon Rectum 47:2138-2146

Toyonaga T, Matsushima M, Kiriu T et al (2007) Factors affecting continence after fistulotomy for intersphincteric fistula-in-ano. Int J Colorectal Dis 22:1071-1075

Toyonaga T, Matsushima M, Tanaka Y et al (2007) Non-sphincter splitting fistulectomy vs conventional fistulotomy for high trans-sphincteric fistula-in-ano: a prospective functional and manometric study. Int J Colorectal Dis 22:1097-1102

Tyler KM, Aarons CB, Sentovich SM (2007) Successful sphincter-sparing surgery for all anal fistulas. Dis Colon Rectum 50:1535-1539

van der Hagen SJ, Baeten CG, Soeters PB et al (2011) Autologous platelet-derived growth factors (platelet-rich plasma) as an adjunct to mucosal advancement flap in high cryptoglandular perianal fistulae: a pilot study. Colorectal Dis 13:215-218

van Koperen PJ, Safiruddin F, Bemelman WA et al (2009) Outcome of surgical treatment for fistula in ano in Crohn's disease. Br J Surg 96:675-679

van Koperen PJ, ten Kate FJ, Bemelman WA et al (2009) Histological identification of epithelium in perianal fistulae: a prospective study. Colorectal Dis 12:891-895

van Koperen PJ, Wind J, Bemelman WA et al (2008) Fibrin glue and transanal rectal advancement flap for high transsphincteric perianal fistulas; is there any advantage? Int J Colorectal Dis 23:697-701

van Tets WF, Kuijpers HC (1994) Continence disorders after anal fistulotomy. Dis Colon Rectum 37:1194-1197

Vial M, Parés D, Pera M et al (2010) Faecal incontinence after seton treatment for anal fistulae with and without surgical division of internal anal sphincter: a systematic review. Colorectal Dis 12:172-178

Wang JY, Garcia-Aguilar J, Sternberg JA et al (2009) Treatment of transsphincteric anal fistulas: are fistula plugs an acceptable alternative? Dis Colon Rectum 52:692-697

Westerterp M, Volkers NA, Poolman RW et al (2003) Anal fistulotomy between Skylla and Charybdis. Colorectal Dis 5:549-551

Whiteford MH, Kilkenny J 3rd, Hyman N et al (2005) Practice parameters for the treatment of perianal abscess and fistula-in-ano (revised). Dis Colon Rectum 48:1337-1342

Wilhelm A (2011) New technique for sphincter-preserving anal fistula repair using a novel radial emitting laser probe (FilacTM). Tech Coloproctol (Epub ahead of print)

Zbar AP, Pescatori M (2005) Internal anal sphincter preservation with seton rerouting in high transsphincteric anal fistula. Dis Colon Rectum 48:1666-1667

Zbar AP, Ramesh J, Beer-Gabel M et al (2003) Conventional cutting vs. internal anal sphincter-preserving seton for high trans-sphincteric fistula: a prospective randomized manometric and clinical trial. Tech Coloproctol 7:89-94

Zimmermann DDE, Delemarre JB, Gosselink MP et al (2003) Smoking affects the outcome of transanal mucosal advancement flap repair of trans-sphinteric fistulas. Br J Surg 90:351-354

Zmora O, Neufeld D, Ziv Y et al (2005) Prospective, multicenter evaluation of highly concentrated fibrin glue in the treatment of complex cryptogenic perianal fistulas. Dis Colon Rectum 48:2167-2172

Rectovaginal Fistulae

4

4.1 Introduction

Rectovaginal fistulae (RVF) may be considered as "border-line" disease, in that they may be managed by the gynecologist, colorectal surgeon, or, more rarely, by the general surgeon. RVF may be iatrogenic, as they may occur following surgical procedures, such as anterior resection of the rectum, Delorme mucosectomy, stapled transanal rectal resection (STARR), Altemeier perineal proctosigmoidectomy, Transanal Endoscopic Microsurgery (TEM), or rectocele repair. Rex and Khubchandani (1992), in a survey carried out among members of the American Society of Colon and Rectal Surgeons, found that 3.5% of anterior resections (7% when including female patients) were followed by RVF.

However, most RVF, those with the best prognosis after surgical repair, are post-obstetric (Fig. 4.1). According to Rothenberger (1993), RVF may be classified into two categories: 1) simple RVF, which are low, small, and involve a healthy rectum, and 2) complex RVF, which are high, larger than 2.5 cm, and involve a diseased rectum (usually in patients with Crohn's disease or who have received radiotherapy) and/or are recurrent after failed surgical repair. Complex RVF, which may require an abdominal procedure that includes rectal resection and coloanal anastomosis, are more likely to be followed by postoperative complications and recurrences. By contrast, simple RVF are usually managed by a transanal, transvaginal, or perineal route.

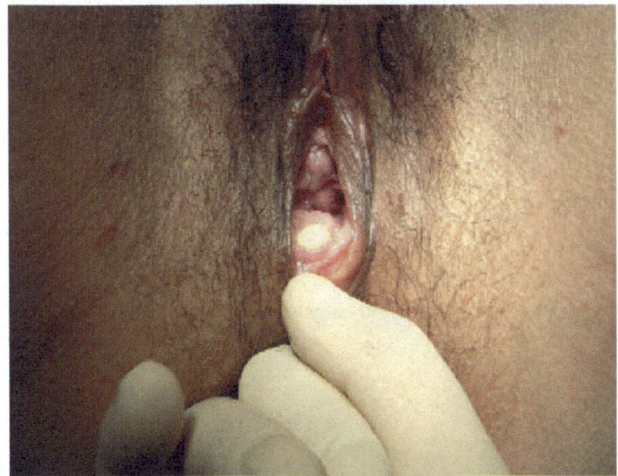

Fig. 4.1 a The patient came to our observation with a diverting colostomy. She is in the lithotomy position. A low rectovaginal fistula is observed

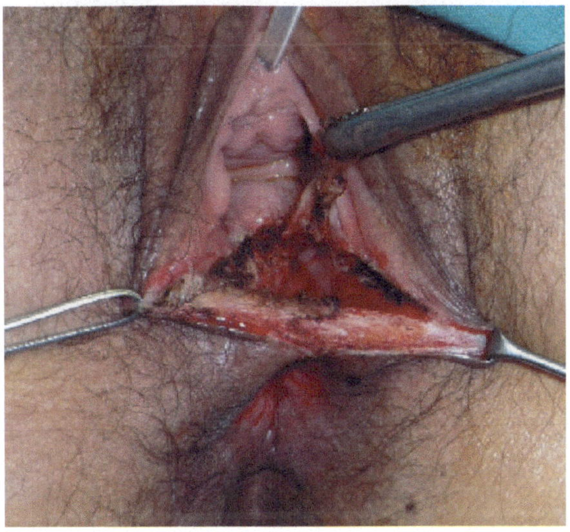

Fig. 4.1 b Low transvaginal incision and removal of the vaginal tract of the fistula

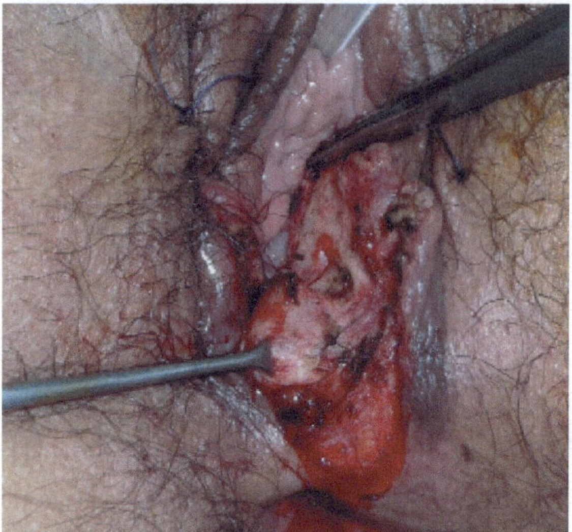

Fig. 4.1 c Removal of the rectal tract of the fistula

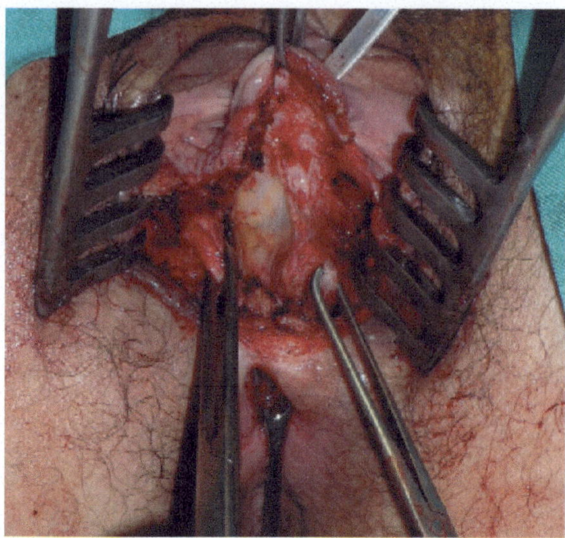

Fig. 4.1 d Lateral branches of the puborectalis muscle are seen

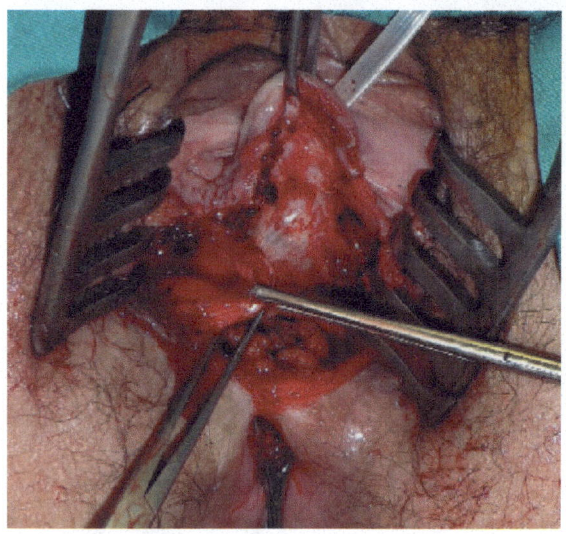

Fig. 4.1 e The right lateral branch of the muscle is clearly visible

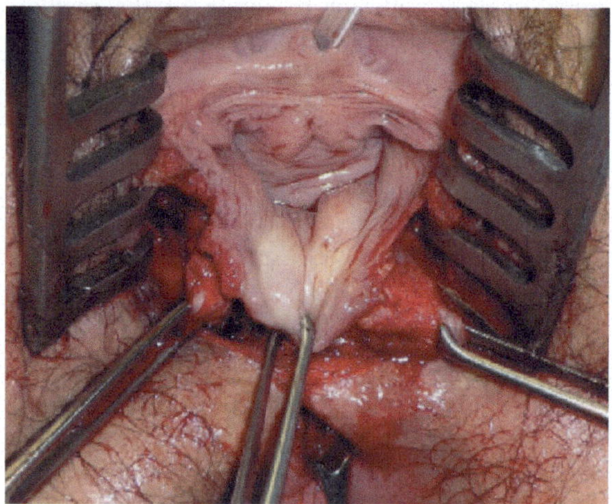

Fig. 4.1 f The posterior wall of the vagina and, at the sides, the puborectalis muscle, which will be used for the plasty

4.2 Types of Operations and Postoperative Complications

The types of surgical procedures and the most frequent postoperative complications are listed in Table 4.1.

I have personal experience with nine of these procedures. I used graciloplasty just once, in a patient with an ileal pouch-vaginal fistula after restorative proctocolectomy. I have never performed Schouten's trans-sacral operation but I did carry out a lay-open procedure in a patient with Crohn's disease, who fortunately remained continent. I have also never performed gluteoplasty, bulbo-cavernosus muscle interposition, or plug procedures. Most of my patients (Gagliardi and Pescatori, 2007) have been treated with an episiotomy with layered closure, puborectalis muscle interposition, fistulectomy with rectal advanced flap through the anus, and an inversion and layered closure through the vagina. I was taught these four types of surgery by

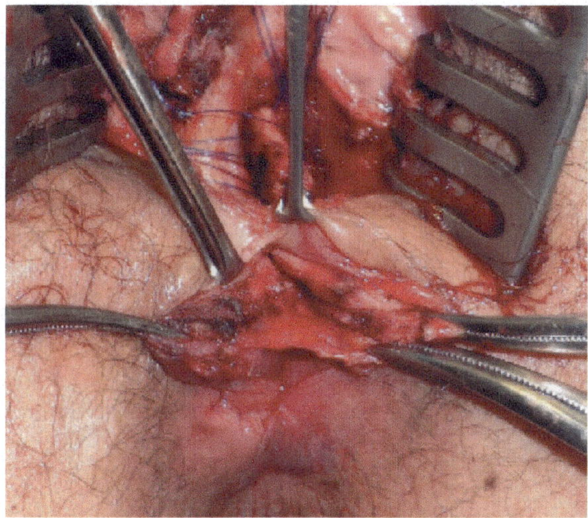

Fig. 4.1 g An advancement rectal flap is constructed "to cover" the fistula rectal orifice

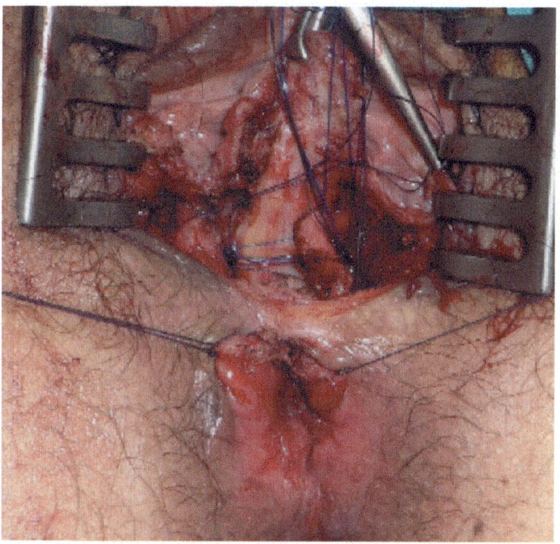

Fig. 4.1 h Prolene U-shaped sutures of the levatorplasty are passed through the puborectalis muscle

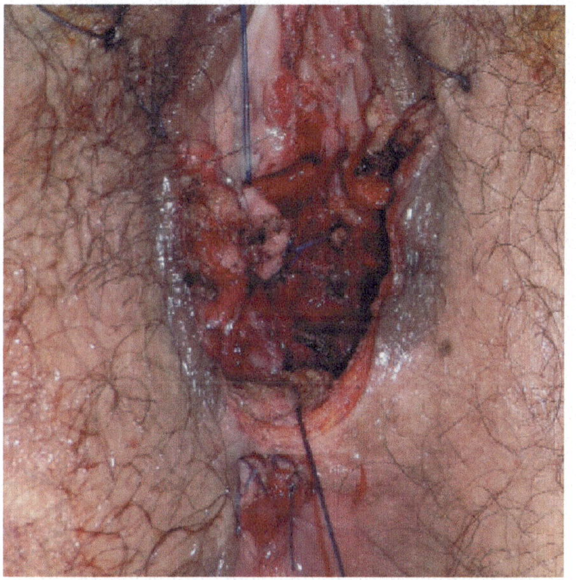

Fig. 4.1 i After the rectal flap is sutured to the subcutaneous part of the external sphincter, the stitches of the levatorplasty are woven

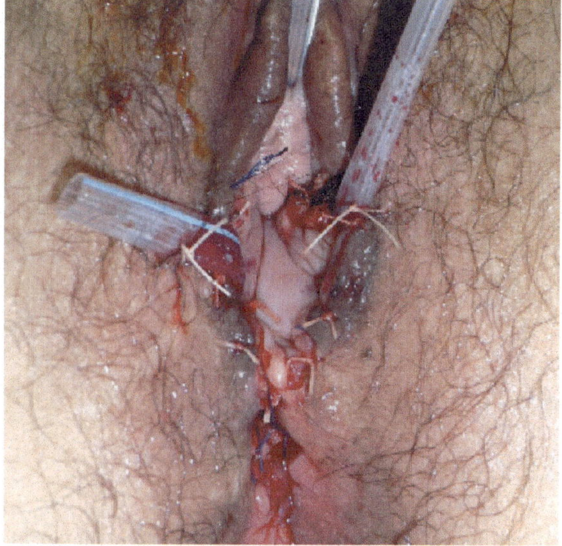

Fig. 4.1 k Two laminar drainages are placed and a cutaneous anovulvar plasty is performed

Sir Alan Parks, in the early 1980s. Previously, I covered complex RVFs with more than one flap. In repairs carried out in patients with a diseased rectum, I performed a diverting sigmoidostomy. In my opinion, the colorectal surgeon must have all these procedures in his or her surgical armamentarium for the following reasons: 1) RVF surgery must be tailored to the patient's anatomy and symptoms, e.g., a transanal approach, requiring a sphincter stretch, should be avoided in a multiparous female with a weak pelvic floor; 2) one should be prepared to carry out more than one operation in the same patient, as in one third of the cases cure is achieved only after multiple procedures; 3) alternative, more sophisticated surgical options should be available for recurrent-complex RVF.

Table 4.1 Surgical procedures for RVF and the most frequent postoperative complications, as reported in the literature (abdominal procedures are excluded)

Operation	Author and year	Reported complication
Transanal route		
Rectal advancement flap	Goldberg, 1990	Suture dehiscence
	Hoexter, 1990	Sepsis and dehiscence
	Lowry, 1992	Suture dehiscence
	Marchesa, 1998	Sepsis and dehiscence
TEM plasty	Darwood, 2008[a]	
Surgisis plug	Gonsalves, 2009	Plug detachment
Perineal route		
Lay-open	Belt 1969,	Anal incontinence
	Francois, 1990	Anal incontinence
Fistulotomy and layered suture	Hudson, 1977	Rectal bleeding
Puborectalis muscle interposition	Oom, 2006	Local sepsis
Excision, suture, and sphincteroplasty	Gagliardi, 2007	Suture dehiscence
	Pinto, 2010	Dehiscence, bleeding
Bulbocavernosus muscle interposition	Cui, 2009	Dyspareunia
Graciloplasty	Lefèvre, 2009	Loss of libido
Gluteoplasty	Lefèvre, 2009	Dyspareunia
Transvaginal route		
Inversion and layered closure	Given, 1970	Suture dehiscence
Episiotomy and layered closure	Tancer, 1990	Bleeding, cellulitis
Vaginal advancement flap	Ruffolo, 2009	Suture dehiscence
Transcoccygeal route		
Rectal advancement flap	Schouten, 2009[b]	Suture dehiscence

[a]Only one case.
[b]All complex RVF recurring after previous repair.

4.3 Bleeding and Dyspareunia

4.3.1 Bleeding

Bleeding rarely occurs after RVF repair (Tancer et al., 1990) but when it does it may be dramatic and require emergency re-intervention, as discussed at the end of the chapter. It is likely to be successfully managed by suturing the bleeding area, but may also require a diverting stoma. In a series of 184 patients treated at the Cleveland Clinic in Florida, Pinto et al. (2010) reported three cases of severe bleeding in which re-operation was required.

4.3.2 Dyspareunia

Dyspareunia may follow anterior levatorplasty or, more often, puborectalis muscle interposition. It is due to the fact that the bulk of the muscle tissue sutured at the level of the rectovaginal septum can hinder sexual intercourse. Dyspareunia has been also reported in association with either a loss or a reduction of libido following graciloplasty for recurrent RVF (Lefèvre, 2009). This complication is prevented by a rectal flap advancement performed via the transcoccygeal route, as reported by Schouten and Oom (2009). Only one of the nine patients operated upon by Cui (2009) using bulbocavernosus muscle interposition complained of dyspareunia after surgery.

4.4 Local Sepsis and Suture Dehiscence

This complication has occurred in 10% of our patients after RVF repair (Gagliardi and Pescatori, 2007). Similar findings were reported by Pinto et

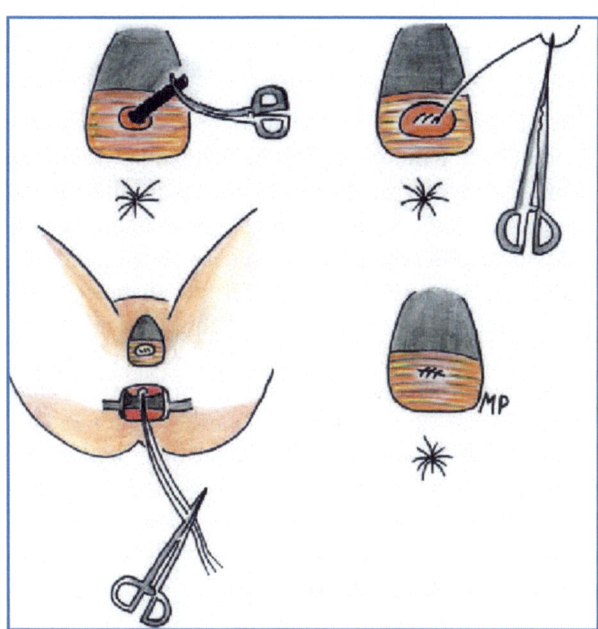

Fig. 4.2 Surgical procedure of reverse suturing after excision of a transvaginal high rectovaginal fistula (*black*). The reversed stitches, translocated to the rectal side, prevent problems with the sutures and facilitate an effective plasty

al. (2010) in patients treated at the Cleveland Clinic in Florida, with sepsis and suture breakdown occurring in 13 out of 125 patients. When confined to the bowel, the dehiscence may either heal spontaneously following the application of local healing ointments/gels or in response to systemic antibiotics. Alternatively, treatment may require a diverting sigmoidostomy, with or without re-suture of the dehiscent wound, depending on its dimension and provided that the local infection has subsided.

A method to prevent (or minimize the risk of) anastomotic breakdown when performing complex procedures, e.g., a Martius flap or layered closure with sphincter reconstruction, is to prolong the administration of antibiotics beyond the typical antibiotic prophylaxis and to give the patient a course of intravenous feeding with enough calories to favor tissue healing. Alternatively, it may be preferable to perform a temporary diverting stoma, usually a sigmoidostomy, which does not increase the risk of RVF recurrence. The latter may be carried out to prevent fecal contamination in more complex repairs, such as the inverted layered closure with a rectal advancement flap (Fig. 4.2).

According to Wexner (in Pinto et al., 2010), heavy smokers, as previously reported by the Schouten group for anal fistula surgery (see Chap. 3), are at risk for anastomotic dehiscence, as smoke stimulates the production of catecholamines and thus causes vasoconstriction, with the decreased blood supply in turn affecting the healing properties of the tissues. Crohn's disease is another condition that increases the risk of suture breakdown after RVF repair, with a dehiscence rate of 60% reported in these patients by Lowry and Goldberg in 1992. Fry and Kodner (1989) reported a much lower dehiscence rate of 20% in their Crohn's patients. Interestingly, Garcia Olmo et al. (2003) suggested the therapeutic use of stem cells in patients with RVF and Crohn's diseases.

The construction of a flap offers several advantages for patients with anal continence, which is more often seen in patients with Crohn's disease. These patients may have a less compliant, inflamed rectum and a reduced stool consistency due to diarrheal episodes. By carrying out a flap, one may avoid the formation of a perineal wound, possibly affecting the sensory component of anal continence, and an anal deformity, which is likely to favor postoperative soiling. The question then becomes whether the surgical strategy should include a vaginal or a rectal flap. After reviewing the literature, Ruffolo et al. (2010) recommended the vaginal flap, the main reason being that the construction of a rectal flap requires a transanal procedure with stretching of the sphincter. Regarding the need for a stoma, Marchesa et al. (1998) preferred the use of a diverting colostomy when dealing with Crohn's RVF in patients treated at the Cleveland Clinic in Ohio.

Darwood and Borley (2008) successfully treated a patient with a rectovaginal fistula following an anterior resection of the rectum using TEM. As the latter technique is minimally invasive, it is less likely than conventional procedures to cause postoperative complications. However, this remains to be confirmed in larger series.

4.5 Re-interventions

A surgeon dealing with RVF patients should be prepared to re-operate, mostly due to dehiscences or recurrences. About one-third of RVF patients need more than one operation to be cured, underlining the importance of alternative procedures, as noted above.

The crucial point is that a patient who needs a re-intervention is at greater risk of complications and failures, namely, local sepsis, suture dehiscences, bleeding, and incontinence. In fact, the patient's tissues are less vascularized, the anal sphincters are weaker, etc., due to the previous operation. This is true also for other proctological diseases, such as hemorrhoids (see Chap. 2). It is known that re-interventions for either complicated or recurrent hemorrhoids, namely, after procedures for prolapsing hemorrhoids, are more likely to cause postoperative bleeding (Brusciano et al., 2004). Based on these considerations, surgically treated tissues are less vascularized and surgically treated sphincters are weaker and more prone to causing anal incontinence. Schouten and Oom (2009) recommended the avoidance of a perineal/transanal/transvaginal route in these cases, instead re-operating by another approach, through tissues with a good vascular supply and leaving intact the anal sphincters. They operated on a number of patients with recurrent RVF via a trans-sacral approach, with successful outcome. There was only one local infection in eight cases managed with a mucosal advancement flap. It should be noted, however, that most of the RVF in this Dutch series were post-obstetric, i.e., the patients with the best prognosis. The local sepsis rate was as high as 42% after another type of RVF repair, interposition of the puborectalis muscle, carried out by the same authors (Oom et al., 2006).

4.6 Drains

Beck and Wexner (1992) recommend the use of a drain in repairs of high RVF with long tracts, in order to decrease the risk of sepsis and dehiscences. The Surgisis plug (Biodesign, Cook Medical, Bloomington, USA) has been used for the management of RVF, but it was displaced due to suture dehiscence in 42% of the patients in one series, with the fistula tract open within 4 weeks and requiring the implantation of another plug (Gonsalves et al., 2009). However, infection did not occur in any of the patients operated on by these surgeons.

4.7 Fecal Incontinence

Postoperative fecal incontinence was a complaint in 15% of the patients I operated upon for RVF (Gagliardi and Pescatori, 2007). When graded according to our validated system (Pescatori et al., 1992), incontinence was due to liquid stool in all cases, occurring at least once a week (B2, score 4) in two-thirds and occasionally (B1, score 3) in one-third of the cases. However, some of these patients already suffered from incontinence prior to surgery, due to either diarhea or, more rarely, an inflamed rectal reservoir (in cases of Crohn's disease) or an obstetric injury to the anal sphincters.

In an earlier report Belt (1969) found that fecal incontinence always occurred after laying open RVF. Francois et al. (1990) reported fecal incontinence in three out of nine surgically treated patients. I carried out a fistulotomy in a 35-year-old patient with Crohn's disease. While she remained continent, the tract was very low, anovulvar rather than rectovaginal. The risk of postoperative incontinence may be minimized by using a tailored approach, i.e., avoiding transanal repair, which is likely to stretch the anal sphincters, in patients with weak pelvic floor. The use of a Martius flap, transposing the bulbocavernosus muscle, might be a good option in these patients (Cui, 2009). Alternatively, as suggested by Lowry in Beck and Wexner's book (1993), anterior sphincter reconstruction may be required in case of injured anal sphincters. Annaway and Hull (2008) reported good results using this procedure, and a

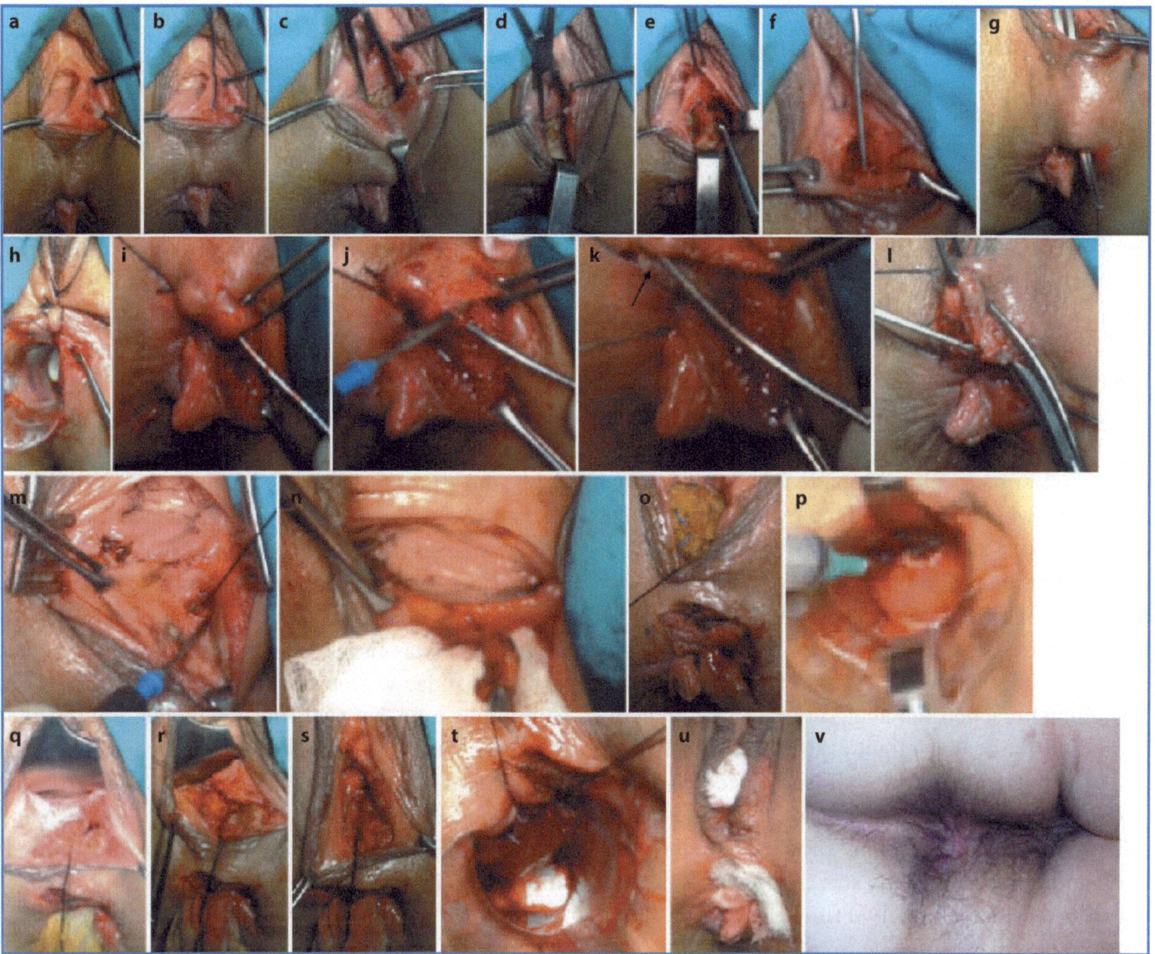

Fig. 4.3 Sphincter-sparing procedure, aimed at preventing potoperative incontinence, in a patient with recurrent anal and rectovaginal fistula **a** Patient in the lithotomy position. *On the left*: external opening of a vulvar fistula (images by N. Clemente); **b** probing of the fistulous track; **c** lay-open of a chronic abscess at the site of a Bartolini's gland; **d** the cavity is completely laid-open after the partial division of both the bulbo-cavernosus and the superficial transverse muscle of the perineum; **e** the cavity is curetted with a Volkman spoon; **f** the underlying recto-vaginal fistula is probed; **g** a seton is inserted in the fistula; **h** the external orifice of a concomitant anal fistula is found and the small perianal abscess is curetted; **i** the horse-shoe anterior perianal fistula is probed; **j** the fistula is laid-open, dividing just a few fibers of the subcutaneous part of the external sphincter, anteriorly; **k** the fistulotomy has been carried out (*arrow*); **l** anal trimming; **m** the recto-vaginal fistula is excised; **n** it will be sent for histological examination; **o** a gauze soaked with Betadine is inserted in the vagina; **p** endoanal view: a Beak Sapimed anoscope has been inserted and a rectal mucosal advancement flap is prepared, injecting adrenaline and saline 1:200,000 under the submucosal layer; **q** vaginal aspect: the post-fistulectomy cavity is shown; **r** suture of the vaginal wall: 1) reconstruction of the bulbo-cavernosus muscle using 2/0 vicryl; **s** 2) the superficial layer of the vaginal wall has been sutured; **t** endoanal view: the rectal flap is sutured without tension to the subcutaneous part of the external sphincter, to cover the surgical defect in the lower rectum; **u** end of the surgical procedure; **v** two months later, the wounds are healed and the patient, in the Sims position, is fully continent

similar positive experience was obtained in our series, as noted above.

Anal and vaginal ultrasound (US) may be helpful to detect anterior occult lesions of the external sphincter in patients who do not present with clinically evident anal incontinence. When anal US and manometry are not available, a careful anamnesis and physical examination will allow surgeons to easily identify patients at risk for postoperative incontinence, i.e., those who are multiparous, have a perineal descent and a short anal canal, suffer from irritable bowel syndrome, and have already undergone proctological surgery. However, an operation aimed at preserving anal sphincters may be carried out even when a fistula-in-ano is associated to RVF, as illustrated in Fig. 4.3.

4.8 An Unforgettable Complication

The patient is a friendly, smiling, but rather nervous 42-year-old woman who came to my office accompanied by her husband and daughter. One year before, in 2001, she had undergone a STARR procedure, performed for obstructed defecation, but she was still constipated, with the constant need to strain, unable to empty her bowel, and spending hours at the toilet, self-digitating. During digital exploration, when I asked her to strain, I clearly felt a paradoxical contraction of the puborectalis muscle. Pushing my finger towards the vagina, I also felt a modest rectocele. The patient had two vaginal deliveries, which had caused the rectocele. She then had undergone a stapled rectotomy, aimed at its correction, but, due to the repeated excessive straining against a contracted puborectalis, it had, not surprisingly, recurred. At proctoscopy, a prevalently anterior rectal internal mucosal prolapse was detectable that almost reached the anal verge on straining. At this point, the reader might ask how all this relates to RVF, but the answer will soon become clear. "Your main problem is the non-relaxing muscle," I said to the anxious woman, showing her the contracted puborectalis on the screen of the US device. "You need a course of pelvic floor exercises." A few months later, after seeing a physiotherapist, she returned for a follow-up exam, still constipated despite several sessions of biofeedback training. The muscle tended to relax but the rectocele and the prolapse of course persisted. The woman was even more distraught and agitated. She pleaded for a repair operation, to which I did not agree. But when I saw her again, 2 months later, she was still very upset and said that her obstructed defecation had worsened. I agreed that surgery was necessary and scheduled her for a Sarles mucosectomy to repair both the rectocele and the prolapse. Three weeks later, I performed the operation, which was technically demanding due to the fibrosis of the lower rectum caused by the previous operation. On postoperative day two, the patient had her first, albeit painful, bowel movement, with some pus discharge. Her temperature rose to 39°C and she was very uncomfortable. Two days later, at digital exploration, I felt a small gap in the rectoanal suture; moreover, the patients told me that she felt air coming out through the vagina. "The same feeling I had sometimes after the STARR operation" she added. "But you never reported this symptom to me before!" I said. "Well, doctor, you never asked me if I felt a loss of air through the vagina!" she replied. I discussed with her the need for re-intervention, explaining that in case of suture breakdown and RVF, a diverting stoma should have been carried out, but she strongly refused a possible stoma formation.

What did I find? What did I do in the operating theatre? Please provide your own hypotheses.

The patient was returned to the operating theatre, with the findings shown in Fig. 4.4. A Foley catheter was positioned in the bladder and the anal canal was gently stretched with a dilator. The rectoanal anastomosis of the Sarles (a type of anterior Delorme) appeared to be almost completely dehiscent. There was tissue ischemia, pus discharge, and a high fistula was clearly detectable, with a wide communication between the lower rectum and the vagina. After a complex perineal, transanal, and transvaginal repair, as a stoma could not be fashioned due to the patient's refusal, a course of parenteral nutrition was started and the bowel confined to prevent fecal contamination of the sutures. One week later, the patient was doing well, with the wounds sutures apparently healed, but as she was not allowed to eat and had to stay in bed, she became increasingly agitated, until one afternoon she violently pulled out the Foley catheter, with the balloon inflated, causing bleeding from the perineum. Despite perineal compression with gauze, the hemorrhage did not stop. It was late in the evening, the patient was pale and tachycardic, and it was not possible to admit her to the operating room to administer anesthesia and suture the bleeding site; therefore, I had her transferred to a better-equipped, larger hospital, where an urgent reoperation was carried out, with suturing of the bleeding area, i.e., part of the surgical wound at the vaginal side. In addition, a diverting colostomy was performed. The patient was discharged one week later. The stoma was closed after a few months. After 8 years, she still suffers from obstructed defecation. In conclusion: postoperative bleeding is rare but may be dramatic after RVF repair. And never operate on a very anxious patient with anismus and obstructed defecation.

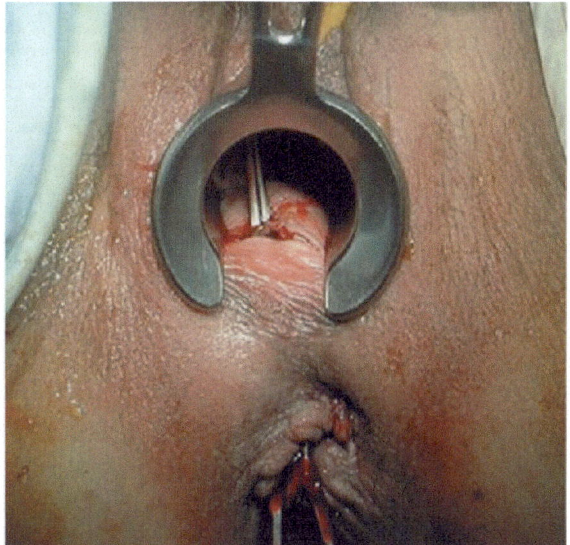

Fig. 4.4 a "Unforgettable complication:" a mildly symptomatic rectovaginal fistula, after STARR, that usually becomes clinically evident as a result of anastomotic dehiscence for local sepsis after Delorme prolapsectomy. At re-operation, a fistula excision with levatorplasty was performed. The patient refused a covering stoma and instead underwent peripheral total parenteral nutrition. A second operation became necessary because of an acute hemorrhage from the surgical wound, as a result of local trauma, i.e., forced removal of the Foley catheter by the patient, who suffered from high levels of anxiety

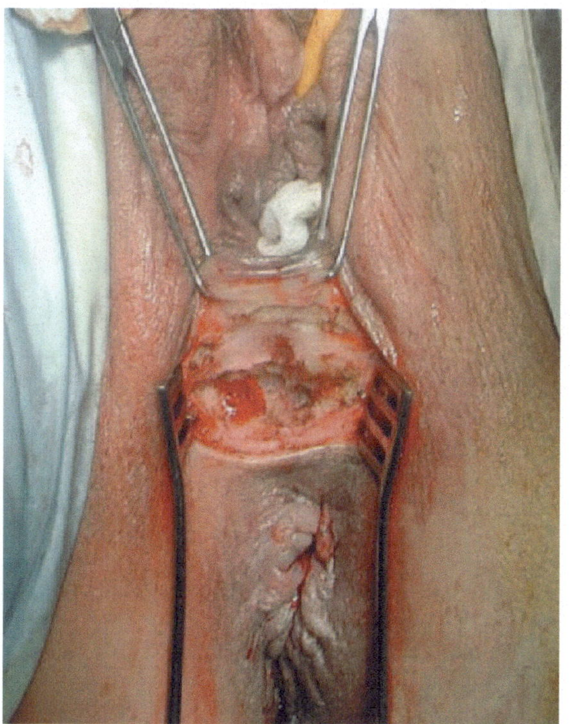

Fig. 4.4 b Transverse incision between the rectum and vagina. The subcutaneous portion of the external sphincter is seen below and the superficial transverse perineal muscles (*pink*) above. The patient is in the lithotomy position

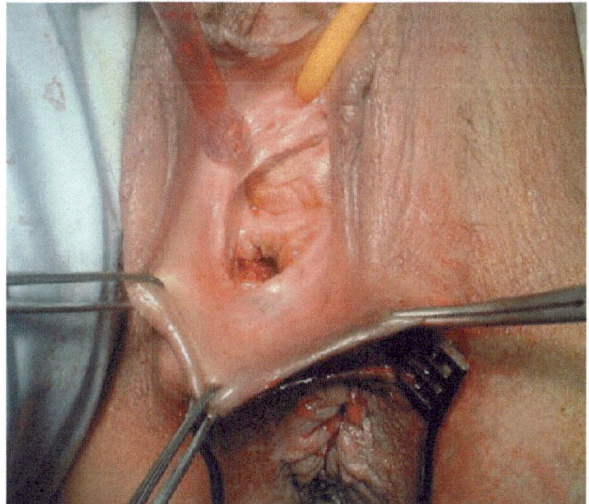

Fig. 4.4 c The posterior distal portion of the vagina is intact, with the vaginal orifice of the fistula situated above

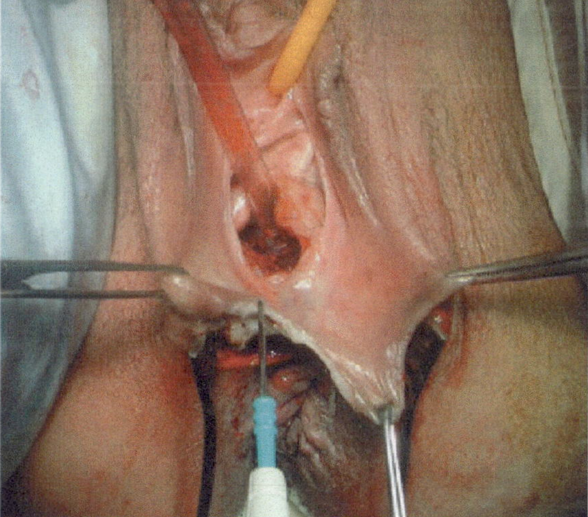

Fig. 4.4 d Vertical incision on the vaginal side

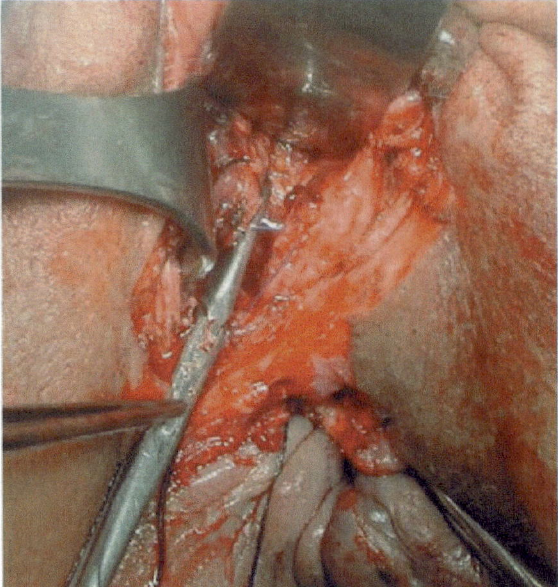

Fig. 4.4 e Traction stitches are placed to better view the operative field, which, from anus to vagina, includes the subcutaneous portion of the external sphincter, the transverse superficial and deep perineal muscles, and the bulbocavernosus muscle

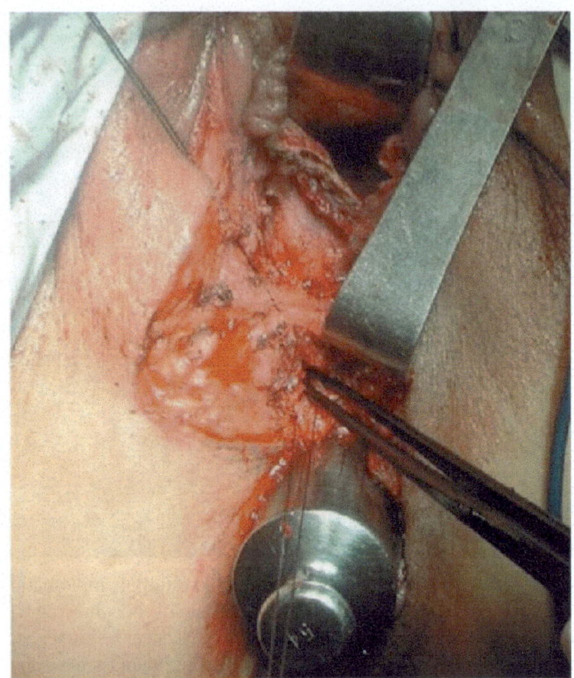

Fig. 4.4 f Clamp tips are inserted in the fistula orifice

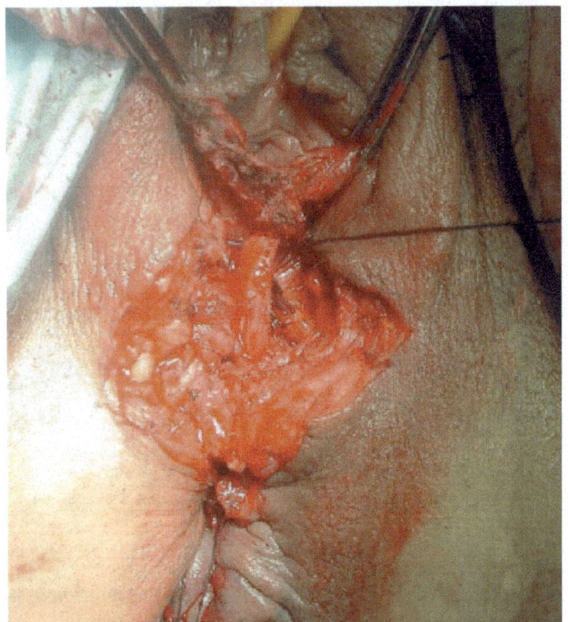

Fig. 4.4 g Both lateral branches of the puborectal muscle are placed on the medial side and sutured, performing an anterior levatorplasty, to interpose vital and well vascularized tissue between the rectum and vagina

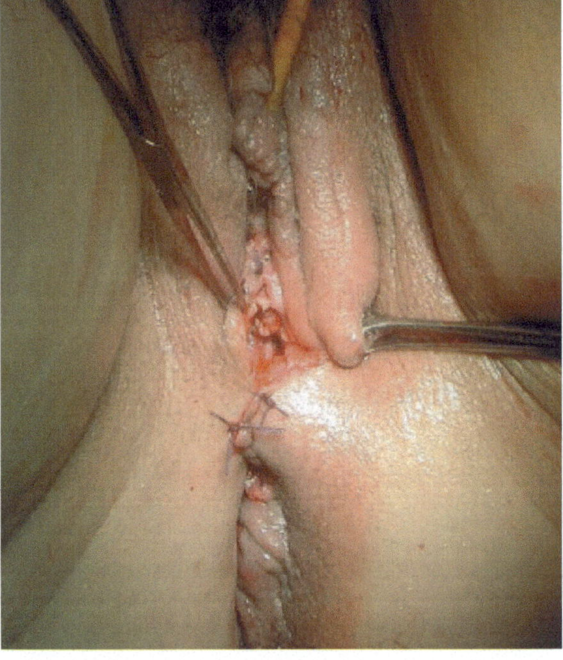

Fig. 4.4 h Cutaneous plasty was performed to create more space between the anus and the vulva

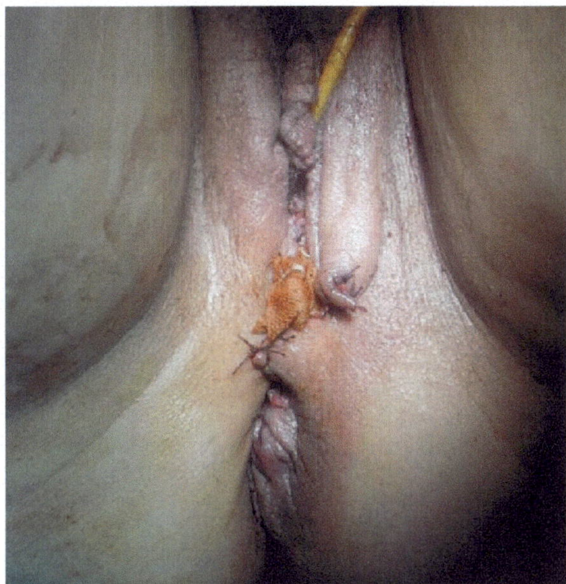

Fig. 4.4 i The surgical wound is incompletely sutured, to prevent sepsis. The patient refused a covering stoma. Seven days later, bleeding from the depth of the surgical wound occurred, requiring an urgent hemostatic suture, followed by a diverting colostomy that was closed after a few months (from Pescatori, 2011)

Summary

The most feared complication after RVF repair is local sepsis, with suture dehiscence, which may occur in around 10% of patients. It may be prevented, or its consequences minimized, by performing a diverting stoma at the end of the fistula repair. Dehiscences are more prone to occur (up to 40%) in patients with Crohn's disease or in those with recurrent RVF, who are operated on with a rectal advancement flap. Postoperative bleeding is rare, but may require re-intervention. Dyspareunia may follow levatorplasty and graciloplasty.

Fecal incontinence is more likely in patients operated upon via a transanal route, due to excessive stretching of the sphincters, but may be prevented by means of sphincter reconstruction following fistulectomy in patients with weak pelvic floor muscles. Alternatively, a transvaginal or a trans-sacral approach may be used.

The best clinical and functional results are achieved in low post-obstetric RVF, as the rectum is healthy and the patient is young. Patients with Crohn's or post-radiation RVF have the worst prognosis.

The surgeon who deals with RVF should be a specialist able to perform more than one procedure, as approximately one-third of the patients require repeated interventions to achieve cure.

Suggested Readings

Athanasiadis S, Yazigi R, Köhler A et al (2007) Recovery rates and functional results after repair for rectovaginal fistula in Crohn's disease: a comparison of different techniques. Int J Colorectal Dis 22:1051-1060

Bassi R, Rademacher J, Savoia A (2006) Rectovaginal fistula after STARR procedure complicated by haematoma of the posterior vaginal wall: report of a case. Tech Coloproctol 10:361-363

Belt RL Jr (1969) Repair of anorectal vaginal fistula utilizing segmental advancement of the internal sphincter muscle. Dis Colon Rectum 12:99-104

Chu M, Crist H, Zaino RJ (2010) Adenocarcinoma arising in a rectovaginal fistula in Crohn's disease. Int J Gynecol Pathol 29:497-500

Cui L, Chen D, Chen W et al (2009) Interposition of vital bulbocavernosus graft in the treatment of both simple and recurrent rectovaginal fistulas. Int J Colorectal Dis 24:1255-1259

Darwood RJ, Borley NR (2008) TEM: an alternative method for the repair of benign recto-vaginal fistulae. Colorectal Dis 10:619-620

de Parades V, Dahmani Z, Blanchard P et al (2010) Endorectal advancement flap with muscular plication: a modified technique for rectovaginal fistula repair. Colorectal Dis 13:921-925

Devesa JM, Devesa M, Velasco GR et al (2007) Benign rectovaginal fistulas: management and results of a personal series. Tech Coloproctol 11:128-134

El-Gazzaz G, Hull TL, Mignanelli E et al (2010) Obstetric and cryptoglandular rectovaginal fistulas: long-term surgical outcome; quality of life; and sexual function. J Gastrointest Surg 14:1758-1763

Ellis CN (2008) Outcomes after repair of rectovaginal fistulas using bioprosthetics. Dis Colon Rectum 51:1084-1088

Francois Y, Descos L, Vignal J (1990) Conservative treatment of low rectovaginal fistula in Crohn's disease. Int J Colorectal Dis 5:12-14

Fry RD, Shomesh EI, Kodner IS, Timmcke A (1989) Techniques and results in the management of anal and perianal Crohn's disease. Surg Gynaecol Obstet 168:42-48

Gagliardi G, Pescatori M (2007) Clinical and functional results after tailored surgery for rectovaginal fistula. Perineology 26:78-81

Gagliardi G, Pescatori M, Altomare DF et al (2008) Results, outcome predictors, and complications after stapled transanal rectal resection for obstructed defecation. Dis Colon Rectum 51:186-195

García-Olmo D, García-Arranz M, García LG et al (2003) Autologous stem cell transplantation for treatment of rectovaginal fistula in perianal Crohn's disease: a new cell-based therapy. Int J Colorectal Dis 18:451-454

Giordano A, della Corte M (2008) Non-operative management of a rectovaginal fistula complicating stapled haemorrhoidectomy. Int J Colorectal Dis 23:727-728

Given FT Jr (1970) Rectovaginal fistula. A review of 20 years' experience in a community hospital. Am J Obstet Gynecol 108:41-46

Gonsalves S, Sagar P, Lengyel J et al (2009) Assessment of the efficacy of the rectovaginal button fistula plug for the treatment of ileal pouch-vaginal and rectovaginal fistulas. Dis Colon Rectum 52:1877-1881

Hannaway CD, Hull TL (2008) Current considerations in the management of rectovaginal fistula from Crohn's disease. Colorectal Dis 10:747-755

Hull TL, El-Gazzaz G, Gurland B et al (2011) Surgeons should not hesitate to perform episioproctotomy for rectovaginal fistula secondary to cryptoglandular or obstetrical origin. Dis Colon Rectum 54:54-59

Ijaiya MA, Mai AM, Aboyeji AP et al (2009) Rectovaginal fistula following sexual intercourse: a case report. Ann Afr Med 8:59-60

Jalim SL, McKinnon AO (2010) Surgical correction of rectovaginal fistula in mares and subsequent fertility. Aust Vet J 88:211-214

Kaymakcioglu N, Yagci G, Can MF et al (2006) An unusual complication of the use of stapler after Hartmann's procedure. West Afr J Med 25:289-291

Lee RC, Rotmensch J (2004) Rectovaginal radiation fistula repair using an obturator fasciocutaneous thigh flap. Gynecol Oncol 94:277-282

Lefèvre JH, Bretagnol F, Maggiori L et al (2009) Operative results and quality of life after gracilis muscle transposition for recurrent rectovaginal fistula. Dis Colon Rectum 52:1290-1295

Lowry AC, Thorson AG, Rothenberger DA, Goldberg SM (1988) Repair of simple rectovaginal fistulas. Influence of previous repairs. Dis Colon Rectum 31:676-678

Marchesa P, Hull TL, Fazio VW (1998) Advancement sleeve flaps for treatment of severe perianal Crohn's disease. Br J Surg 85:1695-1698

McDonald PJ, Bona R, Cohen CR (2004) Rectovaginal fistula after stapled haemorrhoidopexy. Colorectal Dis 6:64-65; Comment on: Colorectal Dis. 2003; 5:304-310

McNevin MS, Lee PY, Bax TW (2007) Martius flap: an adjunct for repair of complex, low rectovaginal fistula. Am J Surg 193:597-599

Mirnezami AH, Gonsalves S, Gatt M et al (2009) Ileal pouch-vaginal fistula: treatment with the new Surgisis Biodesign fistula plug. Tech Coloproctol 13:259-260

Mitalas LE, Gosselink MP, Oom DM et al (2009) Required length of follow-up after transanal advancement flap repair of high transsphincteric fistulas. Colorectal Dis 11:726-728

Neely DT, Minford EJ (2011) Nicorandil-induced rectovaginal fistula. Am J Obstet Gynecol epub ahead of print

Onodera H, Nagayama S, Kohmoto I et al (2003) Novel surgical repair with bilateral gluteus muscle patching for intractable rectovaginal fistula. Tech Coloproctol 7:198-202

Oom DM, Gosselink MP, Van Dijl VR et al (2006) Puborectal sling interposition for the treatment of rectovaginal fistulas. Tech Coloproctol 10:125-130

Penninckx F, Moneghini D, D'Hoore A et al (2001) Success and failure after repair of rectovaginal fistula in Crohn's disease: analysis of prognostic factors. Colorectal Dis 3:406-411

Pescatori M (2011) Ascessi, fistole anali e retto-vaginali. Springer, Milan

Pescatori M, Dodi G, Salafia C et al (2005) Rectovaginal fistula after double-stapled transanal rectotomy (STARR) for obstructed defaecation. Int J Colorectal Dis 20:83-85

Pescatori M, Anastasio G, Bottini C et al (1992) New grading and scoring for anal incontinence. Evaluation of 335 patients. Dis Colon Rectum 35:482-487

Pinto RA, Peterson TV, Shawki S et al (2010) Are there predictors of outcome following rectovaginal fistula repair? Dis Colon Rectum 53:1240-1247

Rabau M, Zmora O, Tulchinsky H et al (2006) Recto-vaginal/urethral fistula: repair with gracilis muscle transposition. Acta Chir Iugosl 53:81-84

Rex JC Jr, Khubchandani IT (1992) Rectovaginal fistula: complication of low anterior resection. Dis Colon Rectum 35: 354-356

Ruffolo C, Scarpa M, Bassi N et al (2010) A systematic review on advancement flaps for rectovaginal fistula in Crohn's disease: transrectal vs transvaginal approach. Colorectal Dis 12:1183-1191

Ruffolo C, Penninckx F, Van Assche G et al (2009) Outcome of surgery for rectovaginal fistula due to Crohn's disease. Br J Surg 96:1190-1195

Ruiz D, Bashankaev B, Speranza J et al (2008) Graciloplasty for rectourethral, rectovaginal and rectovesical fistulas: technique overview, pitfalls and complications. Tech Coloproctol 12:277-281

Sathappan S, Rica MA (2006) Pudendal thigh flap for repair of rectovaginal fistula. Med J Malaysia 61:355-357

Shelton AA, Welton ML (2006) Transperineal repair of persistent rectovaginal fistulas using an acellular cadaveric dermal graft (AlloDerm). Dis Colon Rectum 49:1454-1457

Stone JM, Goldberg SM (1990)The endorectal advancement flap procedure. Int J Colorectal Dis 5:232-235

Schouten WR, Oom DM (2009) Rectal sleeve advancement for the treatment of persistent rectovaginal fistulas. Tech Coloproctol 13:289-294

Schwandner O, Fuerst A (2009) Preliminary results on efficacy in closure of trans-sphincteric and rectovaginal fistulas associated with Crohn's disease using new biomaterials. Surg Innov 16:162-168

Singhal SR, Nanda S, Singhal SK (2007) Sexual intercourse: an unusual cause of rectovaginal fistula. Eur J Obstet Gynecol Reprod Biol 131:243-244

Tañag MA, Kubo T, Yano K et al (2004) Simple repair of complex rectovaginal fistulas. Scand J Plast Reconstr Surg Hand Surg 38:121-124

Tancer ML, Lasser D, Rosenblum N (1990) Rectovaginal fistula or perineal and anal sphincter disruption, or both, after vaginal delivery. Surg Gynecol Obstet 171:43-46

Tsang CB, Madoff RD, Wong WD et al (1998) Anal sphincter integrity and function influences outcome in rectovaginal fistula repair. Dis Colon Rectum 41:1141-1146

Ulrich D, Roos J, Jakse G et al (2009) Gracilis muscle interposition for the treatment of recto-urethral and rectovaginal fistulas: a retrospective analysis of 35 cases. J Plast Reconstr Aesthet Surg 62:352-356

Vavra P, Dostalik J, Vavrova M et al (2009) Transanal endoscopic microsurgery: a novel technique for the repair of benign rectovaginal fistula. Surgeon. 7:126-127

Yodonawa S, Ogawa I, Yoshida S et al (2010) Rectovaginal fistula after low anterior resection for rectal cancer using a double stapling technique. Case Rep Gastroenterol 4:224-228

Zimmerman DD, Briel JW, Gosselink MP et al (2001) Anocutaneous advancement flap repair of transsphincteric fistulas. Dis Colon Rectum 44:1474-1480

Zimmermann MS, Hoffmann M, Hildebrand P et al (2011) Surgical repair of rectovaginal fistulas—a challenge. Int J Colorectal Dis 26:817:819

Zmora O, Tulchinsky H, Gur E et al (2006) Gracilis muscle transposition for fistulas between the rectum and urethra or vagina. Dis Colon Rectum 49:1316-1321

5 Sacrococcygeal Pilonidal Sinus

5.1 Introduction

I was a 25-year-old trainee at the Department of Surgery of the Catholic University in Rome when I operated on my first patient with sacrococcygeal pilonidal sinus. The only such procedure I had seen until then had been carried out at our institution, i.e., excision of the infected sinus, leaving the wound open after suturing of the gluteal to the presacral fascia. This is the procedure I performed, packing the wound with a wad of gauze anchored with several plasters to the iliac crest. The patient was then returned to his room, where he remained, immobile in bed in a prone position with a heavy bag of sand compressing the surgical wound.

Two hours later, as I walked along the corridor of the ward, I saw the nurses nervously running in and out of my patient's room. He was pale and sweaty, turned on his flank, with the gauzes wet and red and a drip of plasma-expander in his arm. He was bleeding and tachycardic, nearly in shock. Following prolonged manual compression at the bleeding site, he promptly recovered but the young Pescatori's reputation was compromised for months. I thought I had performed an adequate hemostasis at the end of the operation, but the oozing had started as the patient's blood pressure had risen while he gradually recovered from general anesthesia. Consequently, a severe hemorrhage had occurred at the wound site despite the compressive dressing.

On that occasion, decades ago, I learned that even a minor surgical procedure may be followed by a life-threatening complication and that management of a sacrococcygeal pilonidal sinus, the "Cinderella of surgery," could be very risky.

Many years later, in 2006, I was comforted by reading a paper in which Kement et al. reported the same complication after the same operation. Their patient was returned to the operating room and the authors performed a diathermy to stop the bleeding.

5.2 Types of Operations

Prior to discussing the postoperative complications, I will list the operations that may be carried out when dealing with a patient suffering from a pilonidal sinus. At the end of the chapter, it will become clear that Table 5.1 is mainly of historical value, as the number of procedures that can actually be used and are thus worth knowing is much lower. Nevertheless, the one I perform more often is the first in the list, i.e. the oldest, just to remind us that not always innovations replace the classic procedures.

5.3 Postoperative Bleeding

Kement et al. (2006), in the procedure already cited, had one case of severe hemorrhage out of 62 patients managed with the open technique. This patient required a surgical hemostasis 18 h postoperatively. Petersen et al. (2007) operated on 91 patients using a similar procedure and reported only a single case of significant bleeding. Hematoma occurred in four out of nearly 100 patients managed by the same authors using the Karydakis operation, possibly due to the more extended dissection needed to harvest the flaps. Buckzaki et al. (2009) had only two hematomas in 100 patients who underwent the Bascom procedure. Senapati et al. (2011) excised the natal cleft and performed an asymmetric suture; they reported 10 hematomas in 150 patients. By contrast, no

Table 5.1 Type of operation for the management of sacroccygeal pilonidal sinus, listed in chronological order with the names of the authors who first reported them in the literature and the year in which the report was published

Operation	Author	Year
Excision and marsupialization	McFee	1942
Excision and rhomboid flap	Limberg	1946
Excision and lay-open	Palombo[a]	1951
Excision and skin graft	Boger	1951
Excision and suture	Goodall	1961
Excision and flap without a sharp angle	Defurmentel	1962
Excision and "Z" plasty	Monro	1965
Lay-open	Notaras[b]	1970
Excision and myocutaneous flap	Minami	1977
Lateral incision and follicle removal	Bascom	1983
Excision and gluteal fascia flap	Karydakis	1992
Excision and V-Y fasciocutaneous flap	Khatri	1994
Excision and cleft closure with asymmetric flap	Bascom	2002
Excision, lateral flap, and fibrin glue	Greenberg	2004
Excision and double rhomboid flap	El-Tawil	2008
Excision and alternate sutures	Muzi	2008
Excision and V-Y fascio-adipose cutaneous flap	Ekci & Gokce	2009

[a]With an elastomer foam.
[b]First randomized trial between closed and open technique.

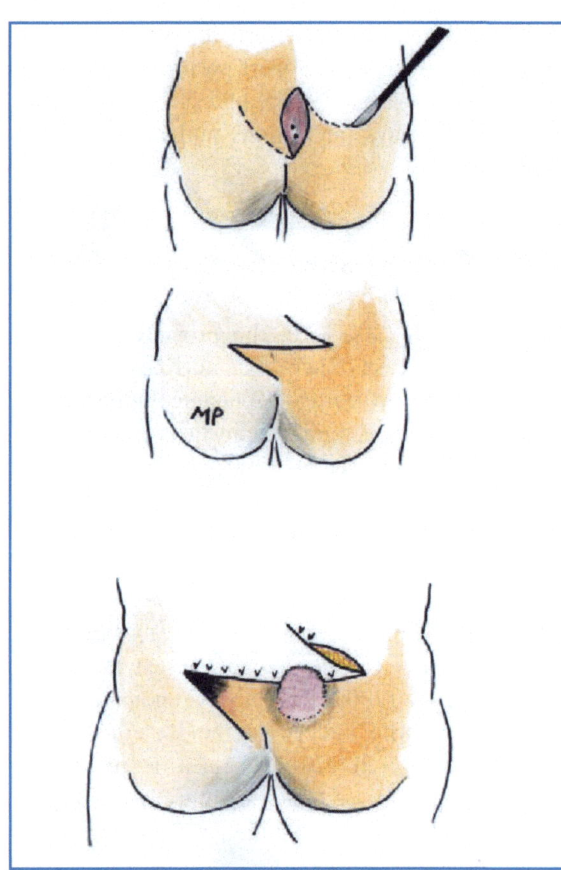

Fig. 5.1 Possible complication of "Z" plasty (*below*). Apex skin ischemia, seroma, and suture dehiscence

Table 5.2 Complications after the open procedure and "Z" plasty

Postoperative complication	Open technique	"Z" plasty	*P*
Bleeding	2.8%	0	< 0.05
Hematoma	5.6%	5.6%	n.s.
Local sepsis	13.9%	9.7%	< 0.05

bleeding occurred at all in 278 patients operated on by Krand et al. (2009), who used a closed procedure, i.e., suture of the gluteal to the presacral fascia bilaterally, followed by complete suturing of the skin.

The postoperative complication rate reported by Fazeli et al. (2006) in a study comparing two techniques, the open procedure and the "Z" plasty, is shown in Table 5.2. There were 72 patients in each group. The closed operation is depicted in Fig. 5.1.

Bleeding, albeit a rare event, is possible when an open technique is performed. Although hematoma is likely to occur in patients undergoing the closed procedure using flaps, sepsis is more frequent following the open technique.

5.4 Local Sepsis and Suture Dehiscence

As shown in Fig. 5.2, infiltration with local anesthetic may favor infection. Kement et al. (2006), using the open technique, did not report any case of local sepsis. However, superficial infection occurred in 3.2% of the patients operated upon by Krand (2009) using the closed procedure. Another 3.2% had a seroma, which was drained using a sterile needle and a syringe. Infection and seroma were the cons of a technique whose pro was the absence of bleeding. Akin et al. (2008) reported infections in 3.6% and seromas in 2.9% of 411 patients operated on using a rhomboid incision and a Limberg flap. The same authors reported a 4.1% rate of permanent cutaneous hypoesthesia, a complication that may follow the construction of large flaps.

Faux et al. (2005) reported a minor dehiscence of the wound suture in six out of 120 patients operated upon with the Limberg procedure.

A simpler flap operation, the "cleft lift," avoids wide and unaesthetic flaps and has a very low recurrence rate. The procedure was performed by Tezel et al. (2009), who reported postoperative complications of local sepsis (13.2%), partial dehiscence (14.5%), and total wound suture breakdown (5.3%).

Ekci and Gokce (2009) had no complications at all in 17 patients operated upon with an original technique consisting of excision and a V-Y fascio-adipose cutaneous flap. The procedure was performed with patients placed under general anesthesia.

5.5 The Prevention of Local Sepsis

Regardless of the use of antibiotic prophylaxis, a closed procedure should be performed with caution in patients with an infected sinus. Doll et al. (2008) sutured the skin wound in 11% of the patients with an acute abscess and in about 50% of those with a chronic abscess. Tension on the suture should be avoided to minimize the risk of dehiscence. A recent Cochrane meta-analysis by Al-Khamis et al. (2010) showed that a wound positioned along the midline is more likely to be followed by suture dehiscence than an off-midline suture in which either a rhomboid flap or a Z-plasty is used. For this reason, Petersen et al. (2007) favor the Karydakis flap and are convinced that the use of the procedure can be extended to selected patients with an infected sinus, based on the results of an evaluation of the bacterial overgrowth at the lesion site. According to these authors, the Karydakis procedure is less costly, because it is associated with reductions in both the complication rate and hospital stay. Lynch et al. (2004) successfully used the VAC suction system following a flap proce-

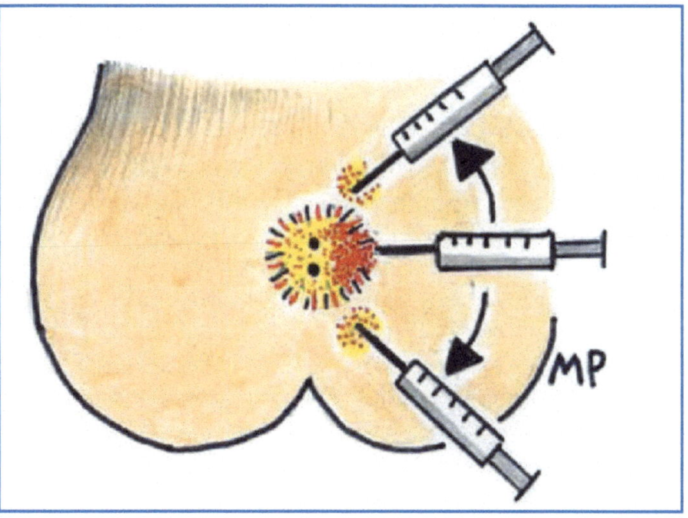

Fig. 5.2 During surgery, moving the needle containing local anesthesia can transfer sepsis to the adjacent tissues

dure. Greenberg et al. (2004) and Lund (2005) used fibrin glue to minimize the risk of dehiscence after flap construction, without significant postoperative complications. The use of a Jackson-Pratt drain did not reduce the occurrence of local sepsis in patients undergoing closed procedures, according to Milone et al. (2011).

The wound gauzes have to be changed on a regular basis, with adequate disinfection and periodic curettage of second-intention healing wounds performed using a Volkmann spoon. The suture stitches have to stay in place for at least 10 days if flaps have been constructed, and even longer if the primary suture was made along the midline with some degree of tension. Lorant et al. (2011), who did not use flap reconstruction, removed the mass sutures encompassing the subcutis fascia and skin after 5–7 days; the skin sutures were removed after 2 weeks. The patients were allowed to shower, with an endosponge inserted in the cavity of the wound, as long as there was no primary suture.

5.6 The Treatment of Local Sepsis and Suture Dehiscence

Antibiotic therapy should be administered after the infectious agent has been identified and drug allergy excluded. Simple drainage of the seroma, which is a pre-septic condition, using a sterile needle and a syringe, prevents infection in two-thirds of patients. Partial opening of the wound by removal of a few stitches may be necessary; patients with deep or extended sepsis possible typically require a more aggressive type of drainage.

Dehiscence of the sutured Karydakis flap occurred in 12% of the patients, as reported by Petersen et al. (2007), with a few flaps requiring reopening of the wound with a toilette of the infected cavity, performed with the patient under anesthesia. The positioning of a Penrose drain was required in one patient. The same authors reported only one case of cellulitis and no sepsis at all in a group of patients operated upon using the open technique.

Therefore, each of the two options has its pros and cons. The flap procedure avoids painful dressing of the wound and ensures a faster recovery, but carries a higher risk of sepsis and hematoma formation. However, the aforementioned Cochrane meta-analysis (Al-Khamis et al. 2010) of 2530 patients did not report any significant differences between the open and closed methods in terms of postoperative complications. Indeed, the time-consuming flap construction might not reduce the complication rate! Moreover, according to the same authors, a wound sutured along the midline is at greater risk of complications. Similar conclusions were reported after another review of 1573 cases, published in the Journal of the American College of Surgeons in 2010: the wound healed more rapidly if a midline approach was not used. Finally, you can find some interesting data in Table 5.3. According to a randomized prospective trial carried out by Lorant et al. (2011), sinus excision followed by primary closure results in faster healing than is achieved with a lay-open technique, but there is no difference in healing rate after one year. The postoperative bleeding rate was similar: 7/39 cases after excision vs. 6/41 cases after the lay-open technique. Pain was reported by approxi-

Table 5.3 Suture dehiscence rate after a closed procedure for pilonidal sinus

Author	Year	Cases (N)	Technique hospitalization (days)	Dehiscence (%)	Median (range)
Kapan	2002	85	Limberg flap	5.3 (3-12)	1.2
Anmugam	2003	53	Rhomboid flap	4 (3-10)	13
Daphan	2004	147	Limberg flap	5.9[a] (1-10)	4.1
Akca	2005	100	Excision and suture	5 (4-6)	5
Mentes	2006	493	Excision and suture	5.5 (2-17)	1
Muzi	2009	152	Excision and suture	8 (7-10)	5.3
Lorant	2011	39	Excision and suture	1[b]	11

[a]Mean.
[b]All patients were discharged the same day of surgery.

mately one-third of the patients in each group. Three patients had sepsis after excision and one after the lay-open procedure, but the difference was not statistically significant. Re-interventions were rare: one in each group. The lay-open and curettage procedure is minimally invasive, with a small risk of complications, and might therefore be considered as the treatment of choice.

5.7 Sinus Pilonidalis Associated with Anal Fistula or Abscess

The first time I operated upon a patient with a combination of the two conditions was 20 years ago. The case consisted of a recurrence of sacrococcygeal sepsis, as I had failed to diagnose anal sepsis, which occurred due to an intersphincteric and a retroanal abscess (Fig. 5.3). Based on that experience, in a patient presenting with anal fistula, I carefully examine the sacroccygeal region. Needless to say, when a patient comes to my office with a pilonidal sinus, I examine the perineum and, after performing a digital rectal exploration and a proctoscopy, carry out an anal ultrasound examination using a 7-mHz rotating probe, which provides a good view up to a few centimeters behind the anal canal.

Therefore, when operating on a patient with a pilonidal sinus who is placed in either a prone or jack-knife position, it is advisable to have a large operative field, extended well below the coccyx, with the buttocks pulled apart by plasters, as this allows accurate anorectal exploration if necessary. Four of my patients required re-operation, because the anal sepsis had been either undiagnosed or not adequately managed. One of these patients was a 23-year-old man from the south of Italy, who was a bit rebellious and had not followed the postoperative advice, i.e., to keep the sacral region shaved and to stop smoking. It was necessary to re-open the previously sutured sacrococcygeal wound, which had become infected, and to lay-open a concomitant, low posterior intersphincteric abscess, in a procedure performed using local anesthesia. Heavy smoking by patients with anal fistula managed with a rectal advancement flap might have contributed to the partial dehiscence of the sacral wound, but the main cause of wound infection was probably persistent anal sepsis. As for sacral depilation, according to Petersen et al. (2009), using a razor may be insufficient and laser depilation may be more effective to prevent infection recurrences.

In conclusion, Hartschuh, who wrote the chapter on pilonidal sinus in the Springer-Verlag book *Coloproctology*, sponsored by the ESCP (2008), stated that flap procedures for pilonidal sinus carry a high complication rate and are not cosmetic; therefore, they should be considered as overtreatment. Indeed, based on the series published by Tawil and Carapeti (2009), who reported several suture dehiscences, and the figures presented in their paper, showing wide non-aesthetic wounds after double rhomboid flap operations, we might agree with Hartschuh. Williams and Keighley, in their well-known book published by Saunders in 1993, also stated that "major reconstructive surgery" should be avoided when dealing with pilonidal sinus.

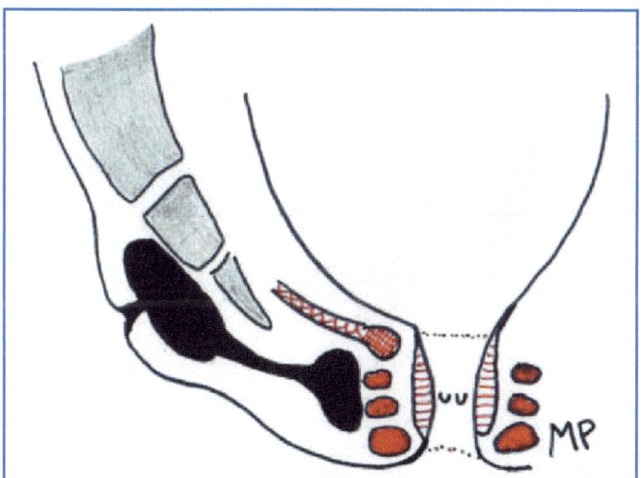

Fig. 5.3 Combination of cyst and sacrococcygeal fistula with retroanal abscess

5.8 An Unforgettable Complication

Recently, I saw a 26-year-old man in my office. His mother had given me a thick folder containing his clinical records, which revealed that he had been operated on for pilonidal sinus 5 years earlier by a general surgeon. Six months later, he had a recurrence and went to another surgeon, the head of a Department of Thoracic Surgery, who excised the infected sinus with laser. After a few months, the patient still had a sacrococcygeal abscess, in addition to complaining of rectal bleeding and tenesmus. A rigid sigmoidoscopy revealed a polypoid lesion in the posterior aspect of the lower rectum. The biopsies showed granulomatous tissue. The same surgeon performed a re-intervention, using a combined trans-sacral and trans-anal route. At the end of the operation, the surgeon told the patient's mother that he was rather skeptical about the outcome and that the son might need a colostomy in the near future, due to persisting disease. As the woman looked very concerned, he encouraged her to trust him, saying that, being a surgeon accustomed to operating on the lungs, he was used to dealing with difficult cases and severe disease.

What do you think I found when I examined the patient? In summary: recurrent pilonidal disease, sacrococcygeal sepsis, rectal bleeding, tenesmus, and rectal granulomata

The findings are illustrated in Figs. 5.4 and 5.5. A wound, 8 x 6-cm-wide and characterized by granulation tissue, was detectable in the sacrococcygeal region. The distal end of the wound seemed to have an external orifice, which could be probed for about 5 cm. Proctoscopy showed a posterior internal orifice, just above the anorectal ring, which I probed for 1-2 cm. Leaving the proctoscope inserted, I injected Betadine through the external orifice. The solution passed into the lumen through the internal orifice. At anal ultrasound using the 7-mHz rotating probe and following the injection of peroxide water through the sacrococcygeal external orifice, I saw a contrasted tract at the level of the superficial retrorectal space, close to a small hyperechogenic spot, 1 cm in diameter, similar to a chronic abscess. Using the 10-mHz probe, I detected a small interruption of the smooth muscle of the rectum, just above the puborectalis muscle and the upper edge of the internal sphincter. This gap was likely to be the internal orifice of the sacral-rectal fistula. The tract appeared to be extrasphincteric, above the anococcygeal raphe, and was clearly related to the multiple surgeries previously carried out for the management of the pilonidal sinus. These operations had been performed using a laser and were followed by rectal bleeding and tenesmus.

How would you treat this patient?

Well, of course, the patient was concerned about the need for a stoma, which I felt might be avoided. I planned an operation which I have not performed yet, as the case is very recent, i.e., excision of the fistula via a combined posterior, trans-anal (and possibly perineal) approach, followed by a rectal mucosal advancement flap and a 2-week course of parenteral nutrition with constipating agents and nil per os. This strategy is aimed at preventing fecal contamination and minimizing the risk of suture dehiscence.

However, let me finish by saying that a thoracic surgeon should not operate on patients with complex perineal diseases (I would not operate on a patient with a lung abscess) and that sometimes the use of laser in proctology may act as a "looking-glass."

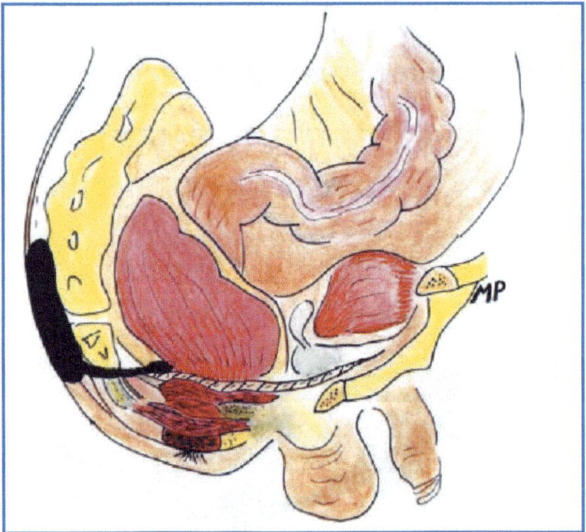

Fig. 5.4 a Sacrorectal fistula (*black*) after repeated laser surgery for a cyst, sacrococcygeal fistula, and subsequent granulomatous rectal polyp. Five years of complications and recurrences

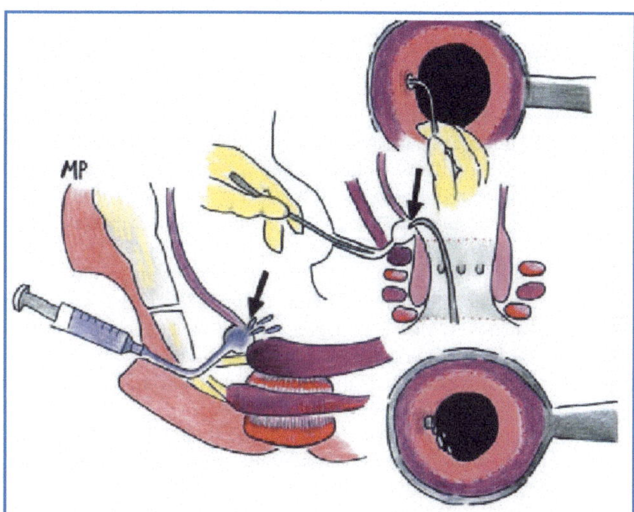

Fig. 5.4 b Postoperative sacrorectal fistula with a low, small perirectal abscess. *Arrows* indicate the internal opening of the fistula, located just above the puborectalis muscle. *Top* A probe is inserted in the tract of the sacrococcygeal wound through the proctoscope. *Below* Injected dye shows the communication with the rectum

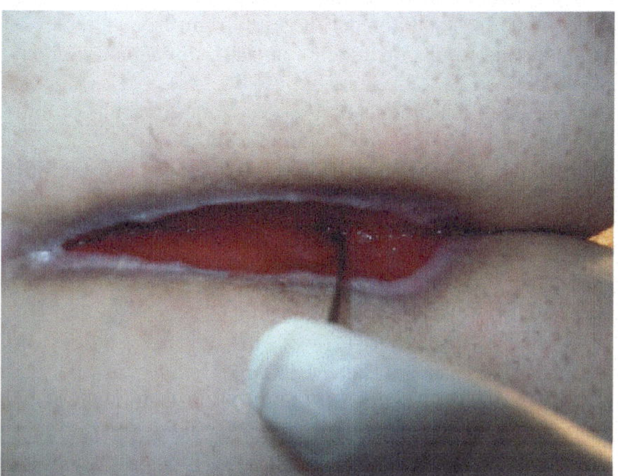

Fig. 5.5 a A probe is inserted in the fistula tract of the sacrococcygeal wound

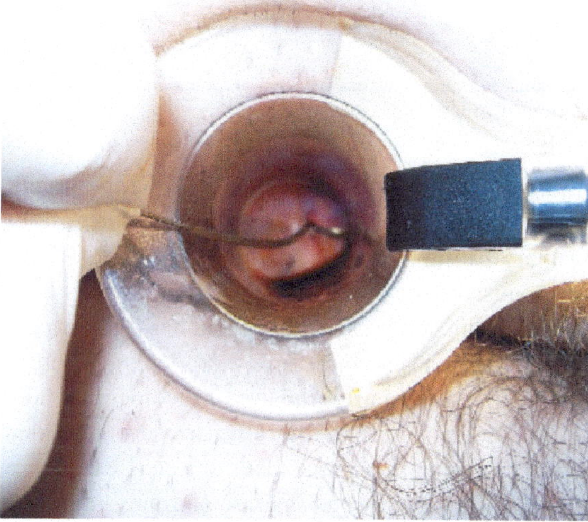

Fig. 5.5 b A probe is inserted in the fistula's internal opening

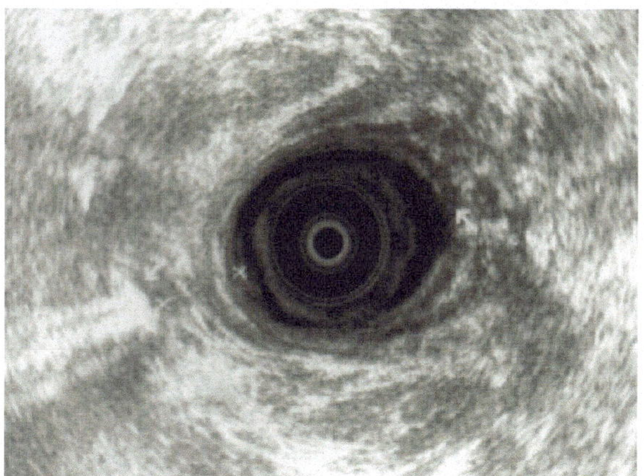

Fig. 5.5 c Transanal ultrasonography with rotating probe. The patient is in the Sims position. Posterior sacrorectal fistula is shown by the injection of hydrogen peroxide through the sacrococcygeal orifice

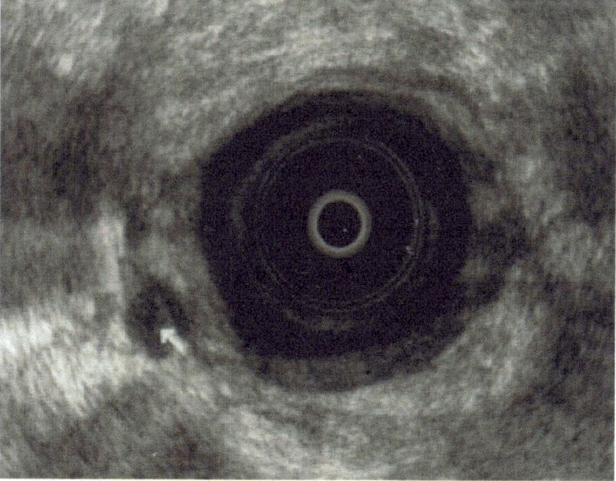

Fig. 5.5 d Above and behind the puborectalis muscle, a hypoechogeneic roundish area (*arrow*) is attributable to an abscess in the superficial retrorectal space

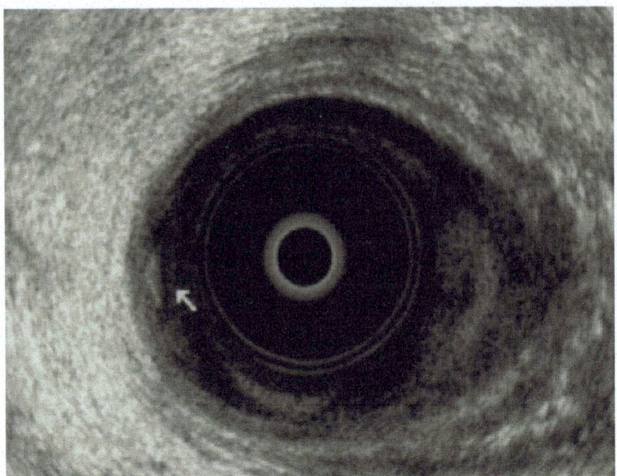

Fig. 5.5 e Below, at the puborectalis muscle, the *arrow* indicates a small spot that partially interrupts the internal sphincter and is related to the fistula's internal orifice

Summary

The most frequent complication following surgery for pilonidal sinus is local sepsis, which, in case of primary closure, with or without the use of flaps, may cause suture dehiscence. Infection is less likely to occur if the surgical wound is left open. Hematoma and seroma are more frequent after wound suture than after the use of the open method. A seroma may be successfully drained, provided that the procedure is carried out in a sterile environment. Severe hemorrhage is rare and may require a re-intervention, which in most cases consists of a simple diathermy of the bleeding area performed under local anesthetic.

Two recent meta-analyses did not show any significant difference between the open and the closed methods in term of postoperative complications. By contrast, an off-midline incision is less likely than a midline incision to be followed by dehiscence. Patients with acute pilonidal abscess do better if operated on by means of the open procedure.

One must be careful when dealing with the association of pilonidal sinus and anal sepsis, which, if misdiagnosed, is likely to cause a recurrence of the sacrococcygeal disease. A wide operative field should be used in these cases to allow adequate exploration of both the sacral and the perineal region.

Suggested Readings

Akin M, Gokbayir H, Kilic K et al (2008) Rhomboid excision and Limberg flap for managing pilonidal sinus: long-term results in 411 patients. Colorectal Dis 10:945-948

Al-Homoud SJ, Habib ZS, Abdul Jabbar AS, Isbister WH (2001) Management of sacrococcygeal pilonidal disease. Saudi Med J 22:762–764

Al-Jaberi TM (2001) Excision and simple primary closure of chronic pilonidal sinus. Eur J Surg 167:133-135

Al-Khamis A, McCallum I, King PM, Bruce J (2010) Healing by primary versus secondary intention after surgical treatment for pilonidal sinus. Cochrane Database Syst Rev 20:CD006213

Al-Khayat H, Al-Khayat H, Sadeq A et al (2007) Risk factors for wound complication in pilonidal sinus procedures. J Am Coll Surg 205:439-444

Armstrong JH, Barcia PJ (1994) Pilonidal sinus disease. The conservative approach. Arch Surg 129:914-917

Bascom JU (1980) Pilonidal disease: origin from follicles of hairs and results of follicle removal as treatment. Surgery 87:567–572

Bascom JU (1983) Pilonidal disease: long-term results of follicle removal. Dis Colon Rectum 26:800-807

Bascom JU (2008) Surgical treatment of pilonidal disease. BMJ 336:842–843

Bascom JU, Bascom T (2002) Failed pilonidal surgery: new paradigm and new operation leading to cures. Arch Surg 137:1146-1150

Bascom JU (1996) Procedures for Pilonidal Sinus. In: Pitt HA, Carter DC, Russell RCG (eds) Atlas of general surgery, 3rd edn. Chapman and Hall, Melbourne

Bessa SS (2007) Results of the lateral advancing flap operation (modified Karydakis procedure) for the management of pilonidal sinus disease. Dis Colon Rectum 50:1935-1940

Bissett IP, Isbister WH (1987) The management of patients with pilonidal disease-a comparative study. Aust N Z J Surg 57:939–942

Borges VF, Keating JT, Nasser IA, Cooley TP, Greenberg HL, Dezube BJ (2001) Clinicopathologic characterization of squamous-cell carcinoma arising from pilonidal disease in association with condylomata acuminatum in HIV-infected patients: report of two cases. Dis Colon Rectum 44:1873-1877

Brasel KJ, Gottesman L, Vasilevsky CA; Members of the Evidence-Based Reviews in Surgery Group (2010) Meta-analysis comparing healing by primary closure and open healing after surgery for pilonidal sinus. J Am Coll Surg 211:431-434

Brook I, Anderson KD, Controni G, Rodriguez WJ (1980) Aerobic and anaerobic bacteriology of pilonidal cyst abscess in children. Am J Dis Child 134:679–680

Can MF, Sevinc MM, Hancerliogullari O et al (2010) Multicenter prospective randomized trial comparing modified Limberg flap transposition and Karydakis flap reconstruction in patients with sacrococcygeal pilonidal disease. Am J Surg 200:318-327

Can MF, Sevinc MM, Yilmaz M (2009) Comparison of Karydakis flap reconstruction versus primary midline closure in sacrococcygeal pilonidal disease: results of 200 military service members. Surg Today 39:580-586

Cavanagh CR, Schnug GE, Girvin GW, McGonigle DJ (1970) Definitive marsupialization of the acute pilonidal abscess. Am Surg 36:650–651

Cihan A, Mentes BB, Tatlicioglu E, Ozmen S, Leventoglu S, Ucan BH (2004) Modified Limberg flap reconstruction compares favourably with primary repair for pilonidal sinus surgery. ANZ J Surg 74:238-242

Collazo E, Luna M (1994) Obeid's technique for treatment of pilonidal sinus. Dis Colon Rectum 37:731-732

Courtney SP, Merlin MJ (1986) The use of fusidic acid gel in pilonidal abscess treatment: cure, recurrence and failure rates. Ann R Coll Surg Engl 68:170–171

Darwish AM, Hassanin A (2010) Reconstruction following excision of sacrococcygeal pilonidal sinus with a perforator-based fasciocutaneous Limberg flap. J Plast Reconstr Aesthet Surg 63:1176-1180

Doll D, Friederichs J, Dettmann H, Boulesteix AL, Duesel W, Petersen S (2008) Time and rate of sinus formation in pilonidal sinus disease. Int J Colorectal Dis 23:359-364

Doll D, Krueger CM, Schrank S, Dettmann H, Petersen S, Duesel W (2007) Timeline of recurrence after primary and secondary pilonidal sinus surgery. Dis Colon Rectum 50:1928-1934

Ekçi B, Gökçe O (2009) A new flap technique to treat pilonidal sinus. Tech Coloproctol 13:205-209

El-Tawil S, Carapeti E (2009) Use of a double rhomboid transposition flap in the treatment of extensive complex pilonidal sinus disease. Colorectal Dis 11:313-317

Ersoy E, Devay AO, Aktimur R, Doganay B, Ozdo an M, Gündo du RH (2009) Comparison of the short-term results after Limberg and Karydakis procedures for pilonidal disease: randomized prospective analysis of 100 patients. Colorectal Dis 11:705-710

Faux W, Pillai SC, Gold DM (2005) Limberg flap for pilonidal disease: the "no-protractor" approach, 3 steps to success. Tech Coloproctol 9:153-155

Fazeli MS, Adel MG, Lebaschi AH (2006) Comparison of outcomes in Z-plasty and delayed healing by secondary intention of the wound after excision of the sacral pilonidal sinus: results of a randomized, clinical trial. Dis Colon Rectum 49:1831-1836

Füzün M, Bakir H, Soylu M, Tansu T, Kaymak E, Ha mancio lu O (1994) Which technique for treatment of pilonidal sinus—open or closed? Dis Colon Rectum 37:1148-1150

Gencosmanoglu R, Inceoglu R (2005) Modified lay-open (incision, curettage, partial lateral wall excision and marsupialization) versus total excision with primary closure in the treatment of chronic sacrococcygeal pilonidal sinus: a prospective, randomized clinical trial with a complete two-year follow-up. Int J Colorectal Dis 20:415-422

Gidwani AL, Murugan K, Nasir A, Brown R (2010) Incise and lay open: an effective procedure for coccygeal pilonidal sinus disease. Ir J Med Sci 179:207-210

Goodall P (1961) The aetiology and treatment of pilonidal sinus. A review of 163 patients. Br J Surg 49:212-218

Greenberg R, Kashtan H, Skornik Y, Werbin N (2004) Treatment of pilonidal sinus disease using fibrin glue as a sealant. Tech Coloproctol 8:95-98

Gupta PJ (2003) Radiofrequency incision and lay open technique of pilonidal sinus (clinical practice paper on modified technique). Kobe J Med Sci 49:75-82

Hanley PH (1980) Acute pilonidal abscess. Surg Gynecol Obstet 150:9–11

Hosseini SV, Bananzadeh AM, Rivaz M et al (2006) The comparison between drainage, delayed excision and primary closure with excision and secondary healing in management of pilonidal abscess. Int J Surg 4:228–231

Jensen SL, Harling H (1988) Prognosis after simple incision and drainage for a first-episode acute pilonidal abscess. Br J Surg 75:60–61

Kayaalp C, Aydin C (2009) Review of phenol treatment in sacrococcygeal pilonidal disease. Tech Coloproctol 13:189-193

Keighley MA (2001) Anorectal Disorders. In: Baker RJ, Fischer JE (eds) Mastery of surgery, 4th edn. Lippincott Williams & Kilkins, Sydney

Kement M, Oncel M, Kurt N, Kaptanoglu L (2006) Sinus excision for the treatment of limited chronic pilonidal disease: results after a medium-term follow-up. Dis Colon Rectum 49:1758-1762

Kepenekci I, Demirkan A, Celasin H, Gecim IE (2010) Unroofing and curettage for the treatment of acute and chronic pilonidal disease. World J Surg 34:153-157

Khan MN, Vidya R, Lee RE (2006) The limited role of microbiological culture and sensitivity in the management of superficial soft tissue abscesses. Scientific World Journal 6:1118–1123

Khatri VP, Espinosa MH, Amin AK (1994) Management of recurrent pilonidal sinus by simple V-Y fasciocutaneous flap. Dis Colon Rectum 37:1232-1235

Kitchen P (2010) Pilonidal sinus - management in the primary care setting. Aust Fam Physician 39:372–375

Korownyk C, Allan GM (2007) Evidence-based approach to abscess management. Can Fam Physician 53:1680–1684

Krand O, Yalt T, Berber I et al (2009) Management of pilonidal sinus disease with oblique excision and bilateral gluteus maximus fascia advancing flap: result of 278 patients. Dis Colon Rectum 52:1172-1177

Lee SL, Tejirian T, Abbas MA (2008) Current management of adolescent pilonidal disease. J Pediatr Surg 43:1124-1127

Licheri S, Pisano G, Erdas E, Farci S, Pomata M, Daniele GM (2004) Radical treatment of acute pilonidal abscess by marsupialization. G Chir 25:414–416

Lorant T, Ribbe I, Mahteme H, Gustafsson UM, Graf W (2011) Sinus excision and primary closure versus laying open in pilonidal disease: a prospective randomized trial. Dis Colon Rectum 54:300-305

Lukish JR, Kindelan T, Marmon LM, Pennington M, Norwood C (2009) Laser depilation is a safe and effective therapy for teenagers with pilonidal disease. J Pediatr Surg 44:282-285

Lund JN, Leveson SH (2005) Fibrin glue in the treatment of pilonidal sinus: results of a pilot study. Dis Colon Rectum 48:1094-1096

Lynch JB, Laing AJ, Regan PJ (2004) Vacuum-assisted closure therapy: a new treatment option for recurrent pilonidal sinus disease. Report of three cases. Dis Colon Rectum 47:929-932

Maghsoudi H, Nezami N, Ghamari AA (2011) Ambulatory treatment of chronic pilonidal sinuses with lateral incision and primary suture. Can J Surg 54 epub ahead of print

Mahdy T (2008) Surgical treatment of the pilonidal disease: primary closure or flap reconstruction after excision. Dis Colon Rectum 51:1816-1822

Marrie TJ, Aylward D, Kerr E, Haldane EV (1978) Bacteriology of pilonidal cyst abscesses. J Clin Pathol 31:909
Matter I, Kunin J, Schein M, Eldar S (1995) Total excision versus non-resectional methods in the treatment of acute and chronic pilonidal disease. Br J Surg 82:752–753
McCallum I, King PM, Bruce J (2007) Healing by primary versus secondary intention after surgical treatment for pilonidal sinus s: systematic review and meta-analysis. BMJ 336:868–871
McLaren CA (1984) Partial closure and other techniques in pilonidal surgery: an assessment of 157 cases. Br J Surg 71:561–562
Menteş BB, Leventoğlu S, Cihan A et al (2004) Modified Limberg transposition flap for sacrococcygeal pilonidal sinus. Surg Today 34:419-423
Menteş O, Bagci M, Bilgin T et al (2006) Management of pilonidal sinus disease with oblique excision and primary closure: results of 493 patients. Dis Colon Rectum 49:104-108
Monro RS (1967) A consideration of some factors in the causation of pilonidal sinus and its treatment by Z-plasty. Am J Proctol 18:215-225
Monro Rs, Mcdermott FT (1965) The elimination of causal factors in pilonidal sinus treated by Z-plasty. Br J Surg 52:177-181
Muzi MG, Milito G, Nigro C, Cadeddu F, Farinon AM (2009) A modification of primary closure for the treatment of pilonidal disease in day-care setting. Colorectal Dis 11:84-88
Notaras MJ (1970) A review of three popular methods of treatment of postanal (pilonidal) sinus disease. Br J Surg 57:886-890
Payne CJ, Walker TW, Karcher AM, Kingsmore DB, Byrne DS (2008) Are routine microbiological investigations indicated in the management of non-perianal cutaneous abscesses? Surgeon 6:204–206
Perruchoud C, Vuilleumier H, Givel JC (2002) Pilonidal sinus: how to choose between excision and open granulation versus excision and primary closure? Study of a series of 141 patients operated on from 1991 to 1995. Swiss Surg 8:255-258
Petersen S, Aumann G, Kramer A, Doll D, Sailer M, Hellmich G (2007) Short-term results of Karydakis flap for pilonidal sinus disease. Tech Coloproctol 11:235-240
Petersen S, Wietelmann K, Evers T et al (2009) Long-term effects of postoperative razor epilation in pilonidal sinus disease. Dis Colon Rectum 52:131-134
Pope CE, Hudson HW (1946) Pilonidal sinus; a review of 130 consecutive cases in which patients were treated by closure; a new closed operative method and management. Arch Surg 52:690-700
Rabie ME, Al Refeidi AA, Al Haizaee A, Hilal S, Al Ajmi H, Al Amri AA (2007) Sacrococcygeal pilonidal disease: sinotomy versus excisional surgery, a retrospective study. ANZ J Surg 77:177-180
Rushfeldt C, Bernstein A, Norderval S, Revhaug A (2008) Introducing an asymmetric cleft lift technique as a uniform procedure for pilonidal sinus surgery. Scand J Surg 97:77-81
Sakr M, El-Hammadi H, Moussa M, Arafa S, Rasheed M (2003) The effect of obesity on the results of Karydakis technique for the management of chronic pilonidal sinus. Int J Colorectal Dis 18:36-39
Schoeller T, Wechselberger G, Otto A, Papp C (1997) Definite surgical treatment of complicated recurrent pilonidal disease with a modified fasciocutaneous V-Y advancement flap. Surgery 121:258-263
Seleem MI, Al-Hashemy AM (2005) Management of pilonidal sinus using fibrin glue: a new concept and preliminary experience. Colorectal Dis 7:319-322
Senapati A, Cripps NP, Flashman K, Thompson MR (2011) Cleft closure for the treatment of pilonidal sinus disease. Colorectal Dis 13:333-336
Shpitz B, Kaufman Z, Kantarovsky A, Reina A, Dinbar A (1990) Definitive management of acute pilonidal abscess by loop diathermy excision. Dis Colon Rectum 33:441–442
Søndenaa K, Andersen E, Nesvik I, Søreide JA (1995) Patient characteristics and symptoms in chronic pilonidal sinus disease. Int J Colorectal Dis 10:39–42
Stephens FO, Stephens RB (1995) Pilonidal sinus: management objectives. Aust N Z J Surg 65:558-560
Stewart A, Donoghue J, Mitten-Lewis S (2008) Pilonidal sinus: healing rates, pain and embarrassment levels. J Wound Care 17:468-470
Tezel E (2007) A new classification according to navicular area concept for sacrococcygeal pilonidal disease. Colorectal Dis 9:575–576
Tezel E, Bostanci H, Anadol AZ, Kurukahvecioglu O (2009) Cleft lift procedure for sacrococcygeal pilonidal disease. Dis Colon Rectum 52:135-139
Tinsley P (2002) The management of a pilonidal sinus and its follow-up care. Br J Nurs 11:S31-S36
Tocchi A, Mazzoni G, Bononi M et al (2008) Outcome of chronic pilonidal disease treatment after ambulatory plain midline excision and primary suture. Am J Surg 196:28-33
Topgül K, Ozdemir E, Kiliç K et al (2003) Long-term results of Limberg flap procedure for treatment of pilonidal sinus: a report of 200 cases. Dis Colon Rectum 46:1545-1548
Vahedian J, Nabavizadeh F, Nakhaee N, Vahedian M, Sadegh-pour A (2005) Comparison between drainage and curettage in the treatment of acute pilonidal abscess. Saudi Med J 26:553–555
Webb PM, Wysocki AP (2011) Does pilonidal abscess heal quicker with off-midline incision and drainage? Tech Coloproctol 15 (in press)
Yalcin S, Ergul E (2010) A single-surgeon, single-institute experience of 59 sinotomies for sacrococcygeal pilonidal disease under local anesthesia. Bratisl Lek Listy 111:284-285
Petersen S, Wietelmann K, Evers T et al (2009) Long-term effects of postoperative razor epilation in pilonidal sinus disease. Dis Colon Rectum 52:131-134

6 Tumors of the Rectum and Anus

6.1 Introduction

As this book deals with complications in proctological surgery, this chapter will not cover anterior resection and abdomino-perineal excision of the rectum. Nevertheless, there is much to discuss, since, with the increasing popularity of transanal endoscopic mucosectomy (TEM) and increased knowledge on the oncological indications for local excision (LE) of a rectal tumor, numerous studies have been carried out and many patients undergoing colorectal surgery may now be effectively cured.

For example, there is sound evidence that a Dukes A adenocarcinoma of the rectum or, better, a T1 Sm1 tumor can be adequately treated by means of LE. However, when dealing with T1 Sm3 neoplasms, which invade the deeper third of the submucosal layer, the results achieved by LE are less encouraging, as the recurrence rate is 11.3% and distant metastases will develop in 24% of the patients, with a tumor-free survival rate of 49.8% (Nascimbeni et al., 2004).

The palliation of small tumors with disseminated disease represents another indication for LE, which also may be carried out in fragile elderly patients with a rectal neoplasm but who are not fit for an anterior resection (Nicholls, 2007).

Finally, large sessile adenomas may be also effectively and safely removed by LE.

This chapter discusses the prevention and the treatment of postoperative complications following either transperineal, transanal, trans-sacral, or intersphincteric excision of benign and malignant rectal tumors. These tumors include adenoma, adenocarcinoma, gastrointestinal stromal tumors (GIST), carcinoid, or a granulomatous polyp. The procedures used in the excision of an anal neoplasm and the potential postoperative complications are also described herein. The chapter sections are organized based on the type of surgical procedure rather than on the type of disease.

6.2 TEM or Transanal Endoscopic Mucosectomy

We begin with a question: Does the TEM device, 40 mm in diameter, cause anal incontinence? The answer is: rarely and if so then temporarily. According to Dornebosh et al. (2008), the postoperative quality of life in these patients is normal, as far as anal continence. Tsai et al. (2010) reported only a 4% rate of continence disorders in their patients. Morino's group, as reported in Table 6.1, had just one case of incontinence out of 300 patients. Although the anal manometry pattern may be altered postoperatively, it is unlikely that there will be significant incontinence (De Cataldo et al., 2005).

Table 6.1 Complications occurring following TEM in 300 patients with a lesion (adenomas, early cancer, GIST, leiomyosarcomas, and rectal ulcers) preoperatively diagnosed as located above the peritoneal reflection (from Allaix et al., 2009)

Complication (n)	Treatment (n)
Bleeding (11)	Endoscopic hemostasis (3)
	Rectal tamponade (5)
	Hemotransfusion (3)
Suture dehiscence (5)	Medical treatment (3)
	TEM (1)
	Abdominal surgery (1)
Rectovaginal fistula (4)	Trans-vaginal repair (2)
	Total parenteral nutrition (2)
Perirectal abscess (1)	Antibiotic therapy (1)
Fecal incontinence (1)	Bio-feedback training (1)
Rectovesical fistula (1)	Abdominal surgery (1)

Total complication rate: 7.7%. No patient required a stoma. More than one treatment required for bleeding.

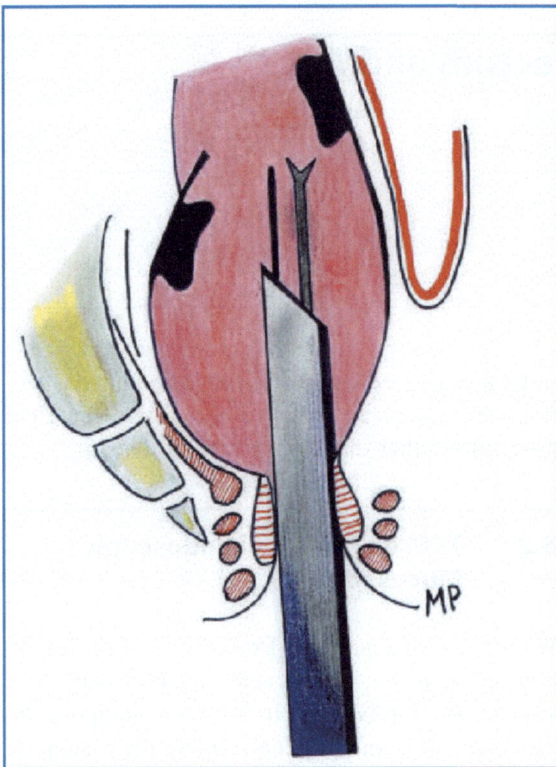

Fig. 6.1 In a lesion of the anterior side of the rectum that must be excised by TEM (*black*), a perforation of the peritoneum may occur because of the anatomic relationships between the rectum and the pouch of Douglas (*red*)

Other complications are more troublesome. Out of 14 cases, Buess, the inventor of the TEM, reported just one bowel perforation, due to a diverticular sigmoid; the patient subsequently underwent a Hartmann procedure (1984). Rectal perforation may be a severe complication if it occurs above the peritoneal reflection, which, in multiparous women with perineal descent, is much less often than expected, especially in case of a previous hysterectomy and a prolapsed pouch of Douglas. Posteriorly, the consequences of a rectal perforation are not significant, as the rectum is below the peritoneal reflection and is adherent to the levator ani muscles (Fig. 6.1). Therefore, especially when the surgeon carries out a full-thickness excision of the tumor, the defect should be sutured along the anterior aspect, whereas posterior defects may be left open. There are skilled surgeons, e.g., Ian Lavery from the Cleveland Clinic, Ohio, who leave the wound open after performing a submucosal excision, in order to avoid the entrapment of exfoliated cancer cells below the suture, at the level of the closed surgical defect.

If there has been an undesired laceration-perforation at the site of tumorectomy, namely, above the peritoneal reflection on the anterior aspect, the defect should be closed immediately. In this case, it is better to keep the patient on intravenous fluids with no enteral feeding for 2-3 days, even if this recommendation appears to be excessive for "fast-track" supporters. Should the surgeon be unaware of an accidental bowel perforation, the patient will complain of abdominal pain and tenderness. If on abdominal plane X-ray a large amount of intraperitoneal air is detected under the diaphragm of a patient whose bowel had been adequately cleaned and who received antibiotic prophylaxis prior to the TEM, i.v. fluids and nil per os will be sufficient. Metronidazole and last-generation cephalosporins should be administered as well. The subsequent approach, whether conservative or (more rarely) surgical, will be determined by the clinical monitoring results, supported by periodic plane X-ray and computed tomography (CT) scan. However, if the bowel was not adequately cleaned such that there is the consistent risk of fecal contamination, a Hartmann procedure might be advisable. In the absence of peritonitis in a patient with a low defect, a transanal suture may be successful.

Lebedyev et al. (2009) had two patients with rectal perforation, one was managed with conservative treatment and the other needed a diverting stoma. The authors also reported fever in four patients and urinary retention in two. Overall, the complication rate was 16%.

A somewhat higher post-TEM complication rate of 21% (59 out of 269 patients), was reported by University of Minnesota surgeons (Tsai et al., 2010): urinary retention 11%, anal incontinence 4%, fever 4%, suture dehiscence 1.5%, and severe bleeding 1.5%.

Dias et al. (2009) reported a conversion rate of 5%. The main reason for changing the approach was the occurrence of technical difficulties.

Scala and Simpson (2010) reported on their experience with giant adenomas (at least 5 cm in diameter) involving three or four rectal quadrants. The complication rate was 21%. One of 149 patients died due to peritonitis following bowel perforation, eight had a pelvic abscess, and two had severe rectal bleeding. Fecal impaction, urinary retention, and rectal stricture were among the minor complications.

Is there any difference, as far as complications, between patients who undergo TEM for cancer and those who have the procedure performed for an adenoma? Not according to Ganai et al. (2006). A few deaths were reported among those patients operated on for cancer, but they were related to the advanced disease and to the fragility of the patient. Most cases involved distant metastases and late postoperative deaths.

Kumar et al. (2010) performed TEM to treat 22 patients with rectal carcinoids. Two had intraoperative arterial bleeding, which was immediately stopped, and one had urinary retention. Three complications is a highly satisfactory experience, as most patients were candidates for anterior resection, with tumors 6-12 cm from the anal verge.

Retroperitoneum, pneumomediastinum, and neck emphysema may also occur after TEM, especially following full-thickness excision The treatment is usually conservative.

Bleeding may occur both intra- and postoperatively, but is rare. In the series of Darwood et al. (2008), comprising patients with large adenomas, there was no occurrence of significant hemorrhage. After the bleeding site has been localized, hemorrhage may be managed either by tightening the vessel with a polypectomy snare, coagulating it with diathermy, infiltrating adrenaline, or positioning a hemostatic clip. In case of massive bleeding and impending hypovolemic shock, it is better to aspirate the blood and resuscitate the patient with intensive fluid therapy, if necessary with blood transfusion, followed by reintubation with the operating scope and then carrying out the above-mentioned operative maneuvers aimed at stopping the hemorrhage.

Rectal stricture is likely to occur after excision of circumferential lesions, as occurred in eight out of the 11 patients treated by Barker and Hill (2011), among a total of 354 patients. Three strictures were due to a recurrence of the tumor, eight to postsurgical fibrosis. All were managed conservatively, using either a Hegar dilator or pneumatic dilation.

Paganini et al. (2009) described the TEM excision of posterior rectal carcinoma, followed by a transanal mesorectal excision, limited to the area below the tumor (Fig. 6.2). A laparoscopic port may be used in association to achieve better control of the surgical field, but bleeding is more likely.

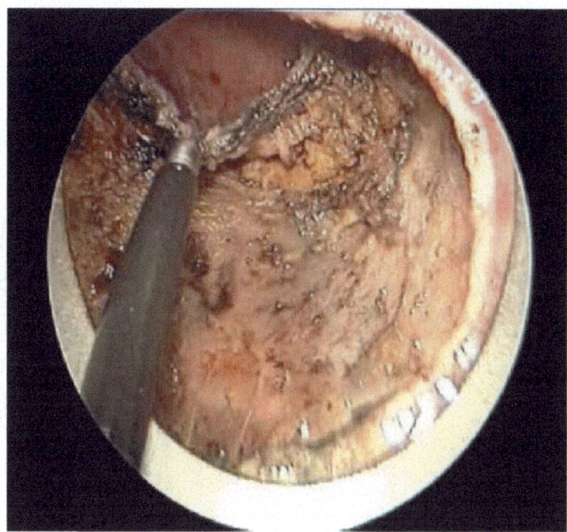

Fig. 6.2 TEM: partial posterior mesorectal excision (from Paganini et al., 2007)

TEM also may be used in the management of retrorectal tumors, as reported by Serra Aracil et al. (2010). As the benignity of the growth may be known only after histological examination of the specimen, the authors recommended refraining from intraoperative biopsies, to avoid the spillage of potentially malignant cells.

According to De Graaf et al. (2003), the postoperative complication rate after TEM is between 4.8 and 9%. The same authors (2011), state that TEM is superior to transanal excision of rectal adenomas, as they had a morbidity of 10% after manual excision and 5.3% after TEM, and recurrence was 28.7% after manual excision and 6.1% after TEM. However, they are much more expert with the latter technique (216 vs 43 cases). The type of complications and the treatment required to manage them, as reported in a recent large Italian series, is discussed in the following sections.

6.3 Transanal Submucosal Excision According to Parks: "Live Surgery"

This is the "classic" operation, which I often use.

The patient, a 70-year-old woman, is ready in the operating theatre, in the lithotomy position, which is fairly advantageous especially when dealing with

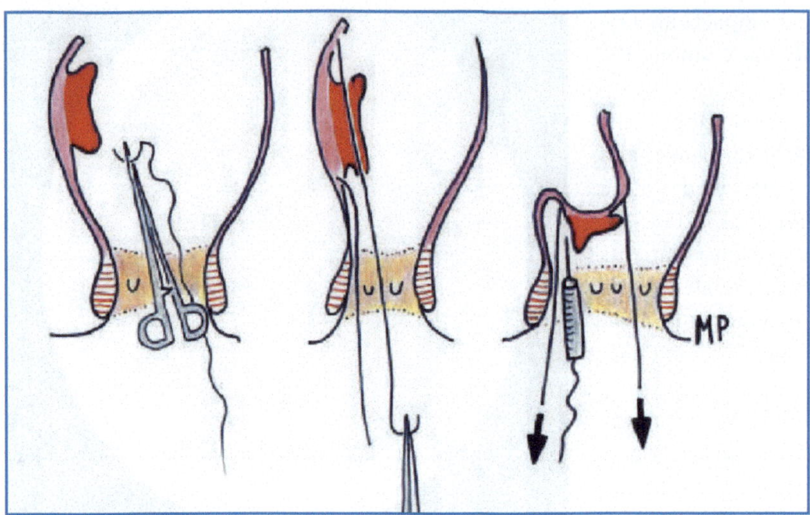

Fig. 6.3 Transanal excision procedure with Francillon's "parachute technique." Traction sutures are placed in the rectal wall around the lesion, which then becomes more accessible to transanal excision

large tumors located in the middle-lower third of the posterior rectum. Alternatively, the jack-knife position may be used; it is more suitable for anterior neoplasms, which are at greater risk of rectovaginal fistula formation. This complication, as reported for PPH and the STARR procedure (Mc Donald et al., Bassi et al.: cited in Chaps. 2 and 8), is not usually due to direct intraoperative injury of the rectovaginal septum but rather to either local ischemia, resulting from stitches or diathermy, or hematoma, followed by a late loss of tissue continuity.

To minimize the risk of postoperative incontinence, it is better to avoid excessive stretching of the sphincter, which is likely to occur using a Park's retractor, as shown by Schouten's group in Rotterdam. Therefore, I instead use a Fansler, an Eisenhammer, or a Sapimed disposable retractor (Alessandria, Italy). The circular anal dilator of the PPH may also be used, provided it is gently inserted, as its diameter is 36 mm, wider than other dilators. The LoneStar retractor has the advantage of offering a good operative view while not stretching the sphincter, but its use should be avoided in rectal carcinoma, as its sharp hooks are likely to cause small lacerations of the anal canal, thus highly increasing the risk of an implant of exfoliated cancer cells.

Melis et al. (2009) reported a 13% incontinence rate following transanal excision.

Returning to the surgical procedure, the anal canal is gently dilated until a good view of the tumor is obtained. Prior to starting the excision, the base of the tumor, below the submucosa, is infiltrated with a 1:200,000 solution of adrenaline in saline. The purpose of this step is twofold: 1) to facilitate the surgical dissection by increasing the space between the mass that has to be removed and the underlying muscular plane, whose integrity has to be preserved (unless a full-thickness excision is planned); 2) to minimize blood loss, thus reducing the risk of hematoma, which might then cause local sepsis and subsequent suture dehiscence. The anesthetist should be informed of the adrenaline infiltration as it may induce vasoconstriction. Although I am not aware of any literature concerning the risks associated with the submucosal injection of adrenaline at such a low concentration, I have seen "liters of juice" infiltrated at St. Mark's Hospital without any adverse events or objections by the attending anesthetist.

If the tumor is located either in the middle or in the upper rectum (in the latter case, transanal manual excision may be contraindicated), i.e., if its lower edge is not easily reachable, I place two stay sutures below the tumor and pull down on them. This will usually cause the mass to be sufficiently displaced downwards. Then, once the dissection has begun, the lower edge of the tumor, if benign, may be grasped with two Babcock forceps and also pulled downwards, thus gaining another 2-3 cm. Alternatively, I perform either the Francillon or the Faivre procedure, using the "parachute" and the "tennis racket" techniques, as illustrated in Figs. 6.3 and 6.4. Again, these procedures move the tumor more distally. Only on one occasion was I unable to change the height of the lesion, which

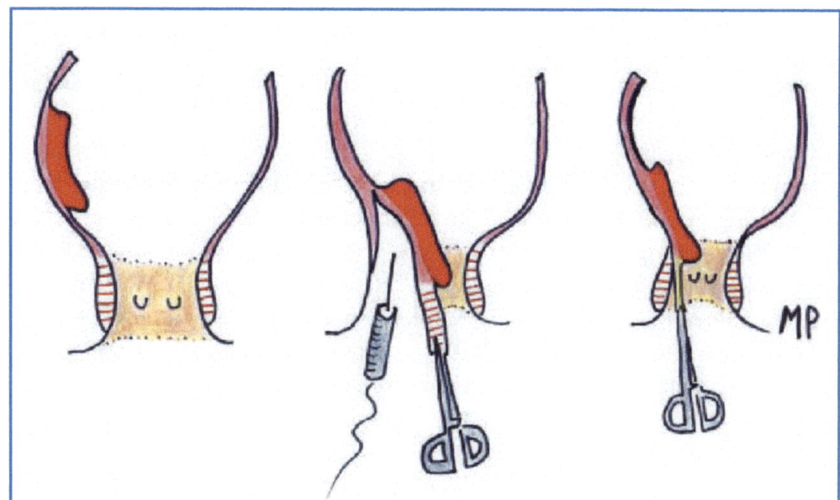

Fig. 6.4 Faivre's "pulling flap" technique. A canal anal "strip" is pulled down to make the lesion accessible to the excision. If flap includes internal sphincter anal incontinence may occur

was not a tumor but a severe post-operative end-to-end anastomosis (EEA) fibrotic stricture, located at the level of the sacral promontory. Having said that, I regret that I never learned to perform a TEM, as it may be superior when dealing with tumors located in the middle rectum. In addition, it is probably the "gold standard" when the mass to be excised is at a relatively high position. In most cases, however, a combination of a favorable anatomy, such as the more lax and intussuscepted rectosigmoid of an elderly male or a multiparous woman with pelvic descensus, and the surgeon's skill and expertise in transanal procedures, makes it possible to reach those tumors that the average surgeon in the average patient would not consider as eligible for manual submucosal excision. After all, it has been known since the late 1980s, when the Int J Colorect Dis published a symposium in which Bartram, Kodner, Kuijpers were included as panelists, that a recto-rectal or even recto-anal invagination is seen in nearly half of the healthy subjects examined by defecography. It is therefore not surprising if a mass located in the lower sigmoid descends into the lower rectal ampulla. Decades ago, I saw Sir Alan Parks perform a full-thickness transanal manual excision to remove a dysplastic large villous adenoma located at the rectosigmoid junction, by entering the peritoneum and then suturing the defect, even though the sigmoid epiploic appendices were sagging downwards, towards the upper edge of the anal retractor and partly obscuring the operative view.

Let's go back to the easy case I have in front of me, i.e., excision of a tumor located in the lower rectum. As the tumor is posterior, the risk of it damaging crucial structures is almost nil. For anterior tumors, attention must be paid not to penetrate too deeply towards the vagina and to avoid rectovaginal fistulae; or, worse, to enter the descended pouch of Douglas and accidentally perforate an enterocele. The generous use of adrenaline-saline solution is mandatory at this level, to better detach the tumor from the underlying tissues and structures. In male patients, care should be taken to avoid lesions to the prostate.

How should we carry out formal dissection of the tumor? Is it better to use scissors or diathermy? Each has its pros and cons. In two cases I found it advantageous to use the harmonic scalpel, but I prefer diathermy to minimize bleeding, using the simple trick described for the Ferguson hemorrhoidectomy in Chap. 2, i.e., sectioning the base of the tumor with forceps touched by the diathermy coagulator, maneuvered by the nurse. Both efficient hemostasis and oncological radicality (in the case of a neoplasm) are critical.

Once the tumor is excised, the decision must be made whether to suture the surgical rectal defect or not. According to Ramirez et al. (2002), it does not make any difference at all. If the wound is small and there is no bleeding, I leave it open, but if it is large or bleeding and I am concerned about the development of a rectal stricture, I prefer to close it, possibly using a transverse suture to minimize the risk of stenosis.

If a full-thickness excision has been performed, excising the muscular layer of the rectum below the tumor, I prefer to suture the wound in two layers, the deep smooth muscle layer and the superficial submucosal and mucosal layer, aimed at decreasing the tension on the latter and minimizing the risk of dehiscence. An endoanal gauze or tampon should not be left behind, as it is likely to cause postoperative pain. If there is a significant risk of postoperative bleeding, I may leave a Foley catheter with the balloon slightly inflated in the lower rectum.

If this operation is carried out in a patient with giant adenoma, especially a tumor that involves more than two-thirds of the rectal circumference, the duration of the procedure will be longer, the sphincter more widely stretched by the anal dilator, and the sutures more broadly extended. Therefore, the risks of anal incontinence, suture breakdown, and rectal stricture will be higher. Orkin et al. (2010) reported a postoperative complication rate of 32% after local excision (either TEM or manual submucosal) in patients with adenomas larger than 5 cm, compared with 8% when the tumor was smaller than 5 cm. These American surgeons operated on 216 patients, of whom 63 had giant adenomas.

Occasionally, like after any other proctological intervention, a Fournier gangrene may occur, especially in patients at higher risk of complications, such as those with diabetes or who are immunocompromised. Following 50 and 52 transanal submucosal excisions, respectively, there were no severe complications in the series of Featherstone et al. (2004), whereas Bergamaschi et al. (1999) had one death and one case of rectal perforation.

6.4 Other Transanal Techniques

6.4.1 Through the Rigid Sigmoidoscope

When located in the proximal rectum or at the level of the rectosigmoid junction, the tumor may be grasped with a biopsy forceps through a rigid sigmoidoscope and then pulled down, even outside the anus, until it can be easily reached by manual excision. The technique was described by Williams and Keighley (1993) and may be suitable in hysterectomized women or in patients with rectoanal intussusceptions. The maneuver avoids both stay sutures and sphincter stretch, as in the Francillon operation, as well as the need for partial internal sphincterectomy, as in the Faivre procedure, thus preventing anal incontinence.

6.4.2 Using an endoGIA or a Urologic Resectoscope

Local excision may also be carried out using an endoGIA stapler or a urologic resectoscope. Maeda et al. (2002) reported only one case of temporary mild incontinence following endoGIA removal of eight small carcinoids, whereas Tsai et al. (2006) operated on 131 patients using a urologic resectoscope and had to re-operate in two cases for pelvic sepsis and in one case for severe bleeding. Another patient needed a transfusion due to hemorrhage and nine had fever, probably related to a small perforation. However, the two patients who underwent a Hartmann procedure for pelvic sepsis were at high risk due to diverticular disease of the sigmoid and previous transanal resections of adenomas.

6.5 Non-transanal Local Excision

6.5.1 The York-Mason Procedure

After a post-anal coccygeal incision, the anal sphincters are divided and the rectum is opened. The operative view of the tumor to be removed is perfect, and no high-risk intraoperative stretching of the sphincter has to be performed. However, after the layered closure of the anal sphincters, a dehiscence may develop, which is likely to affect anal continence. Moreover, as the highly vascularized tissue has to be divided, there is a higher risk of bleeding.

6.5.2 Kraske Operation

The procedure is well-established and well-known. Among the six patients that I operated on using this technique, two had sacral fistulae, the most feared and frequent complication, occurring in 5-70% of the cases (Groebli and Tschanz, 1994). The complication is illustrated in Chap. 5, Fig. 5.3. A two-week course of total parenteral nutrition was needed to manage my patients.

Canessa et al. (2004) described a variation of this technique, using a dorsal approach to preserve both the sacrum and the coccyx, by dividing only the coccygeal muscle, which has no role in maintaining anal continence.

6.5.3 Intersphincteric Resection

According to Pescatori et al. (2005), this approach is indicated in the excision of tumors with an intramural rather than intraluminal localization, such as GISTs. The operation is almost bloodless, since the intersphincteric plane is embryologically avascular. Moreover, there is no sphincter stretch, since the procedure is not endoanal; therefore, postoperative anal incontinence is unlikely to occur.

6.6 Complications Following Surgery for Anal Tumors

Fecal incontinence and anal stricture are the most troublesome complications after surgery for anal neoplasms. Incontinence is likely to develop following local excision of an anal canal tumor, as portions of the internal and external sphincters have to be excised to achieve oncological radicality. This was the case in two of my patients, in whom I performed an associated sphincteroplasty to minimize the risk of postoperative incontinence. If the disepithelialization of the anal circumference is wide, then a stricture is also likely to occur, which may be prevented by carrying out an anoplasty. In the case of a non-healing wound, possibly resulting from suture disruption, that does not respond to either local or systemic cicatrizing drugs, the fibrotic tissue has to be excised and an anoplasty performed, filling the defect with a flap advancement. A cutaneous flap is preferred, either a "house," "diamond," or "torpedo" flap, because a rectal flap is likely to cause soiling and a wet anus due to a mucosal ectropion. The risk of flap dehiscence is high because the anal and perinanal tissues are less elastic and their blood supply is deficient, since in these patients they are often damaged by radiotherapy. Therefore, in these cases it is mandatory to follow the principles of plastic surgery during flap construction: 1) the base of the flap has to be larger than the skin surface, 2) the vascular supply has to be preserved, avoiding diathermy, 3) the flap itself has to be handled with care, without traumatizing it during the surgical maneuvers, and 4) the suture tension should be equally distributed on the layers of the flap, whose base has to be firmly anchored to both the underskin of the anal canal and the residual sphincters by means of introflection stitches. Further technical details are provided in the "Live Surgery" section of the next chapter, which focuses on the complications after surgery for anal strictures. However, better than carrying out excision and suture, Kridel et al. (2011) advocate the use of intra-arterial chemotherapy in the management of post-RT fistulas in patients with squamous carcinoma of the anal canal.

According to O'Connel (Coloproctology, Springer-Verlag, 2008), the local excision of an anal neoplasm should be avoided if it delays radiotherapy.

6.7 Two Unforgettable Complications

6.7.1 Case Number One

Fortunately, this case, which occurred about 10 years ago, ended well. The patient was a woman, about 60-years-old, with no concomitant morbidity. She had a tubulovillous giant sessile adenoma of the posterior aspect of the lower rectum that showed signs of dysplasia, as determined at preoperative biopsy. Therefore, given the size and histology of the tumor, I scheduled a full-thickness excision. During the operation, I considered removing part of the rectal wall, since, based on the mobility of the tumor, its dimensions (5 x 4 cm), smooth surface, absence of ulceration, and soft consistency, as well as the multiple biopsies showing only mild dysplasia and the absence of a familial history of cancer, I was confident that the final histology of the specimen would exclude adenocarcinoma. Dr. Luigi Basso, former member of the Editorial Board of Techniques in Coloproctology, trained in Ireland, and my personal friend, was assisting me in the theatre. As the patient had not undergone a colonoscopy to exclude the presence of further polyps in the rest of the large bowel and wanted to have it performed under anesthesia because she was rather anxious, the endoscopist carried out the exam just prior to surgery, i.e., with the patient in the operating theatre, which was not an unusual policy at our unit. Fortunately, no other polyp was found and I recommended that the endoscopist use suction to remove the air out of the bowel, thus sparing the patient painful abdominal bloating and a "stormy" first defecation.

The operation was a bit difficult, as the upper margin of the tumor was 9 cm from the anal verge; however, the adenoma was fully excised, together with part of the underlying muscular layer and without any additional concern since the growth was located posteriorly, on the levator ani and the presacral plane, well below the peritoneal cavity. The muscle and epithelial defects were sutured at the end of the operation. Nil per os and intravenous fluids during the first 24 hours were prescribed, after which the patient began oral feeding. On postoperative day three, Dr. Basso called me on the phone and told me that the patient looked very anxious and that she was dyspneic, and complained of chest pain. "You should carry out an EKG," I said. One hour later, he called me again: the EKG was normal. "You see, Luigi," I told him, "she was just anxious."

She slept well and I saw her in the morning: no chest pain, normal breathing. Since she had passed a small quantity of soft stool, with no bleeding at all, I was reassured. But early in the afternoon, again, Luigi called me and I heard his concern on the phone. "Listen," he said," the patient still feels chest pain. I've seen her, she is frankly dyspneic, her neck is swollen, and she keeps telling me that she sounds like Donald Duck because of her shrill voice. Something is wrong with her, I'm afraid!" "OK," I answered, "please send her to the radiologist for a chest X-ray." Two hours later, Luigi called me "Come right now Mario, bad news!"

So what did the chest X-ray show? In summary: anxious patient, local excision of a giant rectal adenoma on the posterior wall, bowel function restored after oral feeding, respiratory distress, chest pain, no EKG abnormality.

When I entered the ward, where my colleague was waiting for me, I saw the abdomen, chest, and neck X-rays displayed on the diaphanoscope. The air distribution was clearly abnormal in all the radiograms. "Retro-pneumoperitoneum, pneumomediastinum, and neck emphysema," Luigi said. "What should we do now?" As I had never had this type of complication, I had to think long and hard about it. But suddenly I remembered that, many years before, when I was a university trainee (we were in the pre-CT scan era), I was responsible for injecting air with a syringe just below the coccyx, to fill the retroperitoneum so as to better detect the size and the limits of retroperitoneal masses, namely, kidney tumors, on plane X-ray. None of the patients had died after the puncture! They simply remained in bed for some time after being returned to the ward from the Radiology department. Therefore, I relaxed. We decided to stop oral feeding and re-start i.v. fluids, to put the patient on antibiotics, and confine her to bed rest, with her legs positioned slightly higher than her head in order to prevent the air from traveling upwards. We felt crepitation when palpating her neck, due to the air that had collected below the skin. We asked for the opinion of our thoracic surgeon, who told us that, at the present stage, there was no need to locally insert needles aimed at removing the air. A wait and see approach was recommended. After 24 hours, the patient was feeling much better; she had no temperature and no bowel motion. Two days later, after resuming oral alimentation, she was discharged.

I will never forget her "Donald Duck" voice. The adenoma was indeed benign and the woman was alive and well after two years, with no recurrence of the adenoma in her rectum.

At a Congress held a few months after her discharge, I talked with a colleague who routinely performed TEM; he told me of a similar case. Meanwhile, my friend Luigi had reviewed the literature and found an anecdotal report of (retro)-pneumoperitoneum following colonoscopy. This confirmed that the combination of a trans-rectal incision and a previous colonoscopy, which had left a considerable amount of air in the rectosigmoid despite subsequent suctioning by the endoscopist at the end of the procedure, had caused that unusual postoperative complication.

Various reports on the same complication, which occurred after both PPH and STARR, were published in the literature between 2002 and 2007 by Kanellos, Seow-Choen, Filingeri, and others, in

Dis Colon and Rectum and in Tech Coloproctol. In each case, the complication was due to the infiltration of rectal air through the rectal muscle and then behind, into the retroperitoneal spaces, and upwards into the mediastinum, as occurred after our local excision. In one case, the complication was facilitated by the forced dilation of an anorectal stricture after PPH. Only one patient required a diverting stoma, the others were successfully managed by means of conservative measures. None of them had undergone a colonoscopy prior to the transanal stapling. Our report was published in Surgical Endoscopy (Basso and Pescatori) and the reference is included in the Suggested Reading at the end of this chapter.

When reviewing this chapter, my colleague Dr. Paola De Nardi justly reminded me to mention high-flow oxygen-therapy among the possible treatments of these cases.

My final advice to readers is: (a) never perform a colonoscopy just before local excision of a rectal tumor and (b) be sure to perform further investigations before attributing respiratory distress and chest pain to anxiety, even if the EKG is normal.

6.7.2 Case Number Two

Unfortunately, this case did not have a happy ending like the previous one. However, the patient was at greater risk, because of his advanced age (78 years old), more severe pathology (a rectal cancer), and the presence of concomitant disease (diabetes). He had an ulcerated T2 adenocarcinoma, located in the posterior distal rectum, just above the dentate line. The tumor was 4 x 4 cm in size, as big as half of a tangerine, without distant metastasis. Both resting tone and voluntary contraction were rather weak, due to the patient's advanced age and, to some degree, to the pain caused by the tumor.

We discussed with him and his family the possible therapeutic options. Radiotherapy and intersphincteric anterior resection with colo-anal anastomosis were excluded due to his age and fragility, and to the high risk of incontinence. He refused an abdomino-perineal resection because of the permanent colostomy. Therefore, a palliative local excision was scheduled, to be carried out in a small well-equipped hospital in Tuscany, where I use to operate twice a month. Regarding the choice and potential outcome of the operation, I was encouraged by the already mentioned series of Bergamaschi et al. (1999), in which there was only one death out of 52 patients with rectal cancer, nearly half with the same indication, operated on via a transanal route, and by my previous, more modest but positive experience with that procedure, which I had been carrying out for decades at my unit.

In the operating theatre, I commenced the Parks' operation, a full-thickness excision in this case, removing at least 2 cm around the tumor. Then, as the growth was very low and the residual defect rather wide, extending below the anorectal ring, I thought it wise to harvest a skin flap and partially cover the surgical wound, involving the upper anal canal, to prevent suture tension and dehiscence, with consequent anorectal stricture (Fig. 6.5). The operation was completed after one hour and, as the patient had refused a stoma, and because I was confident that the wound would heal satisfactorily, we started total parenteral nutrition and administered analgesics as well as metronidazole and cephalosporin (Deflamon and Rocephin) to reduce the risk of sepsis.

On postoperative day three, the patient had fever and complained of perineal pain despite the analgesics. I removed the dressing on the wounds and found a swelling of the scrotum and the perineum, with signs of local sepsis. After removal of some of the stitches, an abundant non-purulent secretion leaked out from the underskin. After a few hours the patient had a bowel motion, but only a small quantity of semiformed stools; therefore, we gave him Loperamide to prevent fecal contamination of the wound. The day after, the situation worsened; the patient was confused and tachypneic, his body temperature and his plasma creatinine were elevated, and the flap was necrotic and partly dehiscent. He had Fournier gangrene.

We took him to the operating theatre, where we found that he had severe perineal swelling and necrosis, with complete suture breakdown. Diabetic, almost 80 years old... we were very concerned.

What would have you done at this point?

There were, unfortunately, not many choices. We performed a wide necrosectomy and a sigmoidostomy, after which the patient was stable for 24 hours. I hoped that, as I had read regarding Fournier gangrene, "the improvement is dramatic and unexpected following necrosectomy." Instead, he rapidly worsened and died during the night.

In retrospect, it may have been a mistake to perform a perineal flap, since the patient was diabetic and more prone to local sepsis. Or maybe I should have better protected the sutures with a stoma after the first operation (although he had refused this option). And maybe I should have moved him to the Intensive Care Unit of a large hospital after the re-intervention.

While "one learns from one's mistakes," it was very sad to lose a patient in that manner.

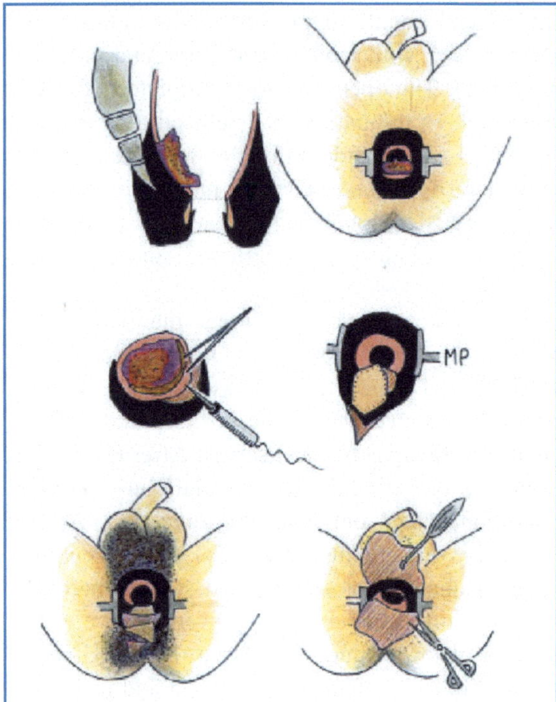

Fig. 6.5 *Top*, distal rectal cancer in an elderly diabetic patient. *Center*, transanal excision of the lesion and anorectoplasty with a cutaneous flap to prevent stenosis. *Below*, Fournier's gangrene and perineal necrosectomy. The patient died

Summary

The local excision of a rectal tumor may be carried out using several procedures. Often, the type of postoperative complication depends on the chosen approach. A troublesome adverse event during TEM is perforation of the bowel, which although rare is more likely to occur when dealing with giant adenomas located anteriorly and above the peritoneal reflection. These can usually be managed with a suture, but in rare cases require a stoma. Rectovaginal fistulae and rectal strictures also have been occasionally reported. The conversion rate with TEM is around 5% and is usually due to technical difficulties.

Retro-pneumoperitoneum, pneumomediastinum, and neck emphysema may occur after TEM as well as after manual transanal excision. These conditions are usually managed conservatively. A sacral fistula may follow the Kraske operation and is likely to heal by placing the patient on total parenteral nutrition. Any type of local excision may be followed by severe rectal bleeding, but this complication seldom occurs. Stretching of the sphincter during manual transanal excision may cause postoperative anal incontinence in up to 13% of patients, but gross incontinence is very rare after TEM (< 0.5%) and may be managed by biofeedback. Instead, this complication is more likely to develop following local excision of anal neoplasms, when preoperative radiotherapy has rendered the sphincters fibrotic.

Suggested Readings

Akin M, Gokbayir H, Kilic K et al (2008) Rhomboid excision and Limberg flap for managing pilonidal sinus: long-term results in 411 patients. Colorectal Dis 10:945-948

Allaix ME, Arezzo A, Caldart M et al (2009) Transanal endoscopic microsurgery for rectal neoplasms: experience of 300 consecutive cases. Dis Colon Rectum 52:1831-1836

Baatrup G, Elbrønd H, Hesselfeldt P et al (2007) Rectal adenocarcinoma and transanal endoscopic microsurgery. Diagnostic challenges, indications and short term results in 142 consecutive patients. Int J Colorectal Dis 22:1347-1352

Bach SP, Hill J, Monson JR et al (2009) A predictive model for local recurrence after transanal endoscopic microsurgery for rectal cancer. Br J Surg 96:280-2

Barker JA, Hill J (2011) Incidence, treatment and outcome of rectal stenosis following transanal endoscopic microsurgery. Tech Coloproctol 15 (in press)

Bergamaschi R, Manunta A, Arnaud JP (1999) Endoscopic trans-anal resection for palliation of acutely obstructed rectal cancer in frail elderly patients. Tech Coloproctol 3:15-17

Betambeau N, Simson JN (2007) Staged anterior resection and TEM to preserve rectal function in synchronous malignant and benign rectal lesions. Colorectal Dis 9:469-471

Bignell MB, Ramwell A, Evans JR et al (2010) Complications of transanal endoscopic microsurgery (TEM): a prospective audit. Colorectal Dis 12:99-103

Bouchoucha M, Devroede G, Arsac M (2004) Anismus: a marker of multi-site functional disorders? Int J Colorectal Dis 19:374-379

Buess G (1998) Complications following transanal endoscopic microsurgery. Surg Technol Int 7:170-173

Buess G, Theiss R, Gunther M et al (1984) Endoscopic operative procedure for the removal of rectal polyps. Coloproctology 6:254-261

Canessa CE, Miegge LM, Bado J (2004) Anatomic study of lateral pelvic lymph nodes: implications in the treatment of rectal cancer. Dis Colon Rectum 47:297-303

Cataldo PA, O'Brien S, Osler T (2005) Transanal endoscopic microsurgery: a prospective evaluation of functional results. Dis Colon Rectum 48:1366-1371

Darwood RJ, Wheeler JM, Borley NR (2008) Transanal endoscopic microsurgery is a safe and reliable technique even for complex rectal lesions. Br J Surg. 95:915-918

de Graaf EJ, Doornebosch PG, Tetteroo GW et al (2009) Transanal endoscopic microsurgery is feasible for adenomas throughout the entire rectum: a prospective study. Dis Colon Rectum 52:1107-1113

de Graaf EJR, Burger JWA, van Ijsseldijk ALA et al (2011) Transanal endoscopic microsurgery is superior to transanal excision of rectal adenomas. Colorect Dis 13:762-767

De Santis G, Gola PS, Lancione L et al (2011) Sigmoid intramural hematoma and hemoperitoneum: an early severe complication after stapled hemorrhoidopexy. Tech Coloproctol in press

Dias AR, Nahas CS, Marques CF et al (2009) Transanal endoscopic microsurgery: indications, results and controversies. Tech Coloproctol 13:105-111

Doornebosch PG, Gosselink MP, Neijenhuis PA et al (2008) Impact of transanal endoscopic microsurgery on functional outcome and quality of life. Int J Colorectal Dis 23:709-713

Duek SD, Issa N, Hershko DD, Krausz MM (2008) Outcome of transanal endoscopic microsurgery and adjuvant radiotherapy in patients with T2 rectal cancer. Dis Colon Rectum 51:379-384

Endreseth BH, Wibe A, Svinsås M et al (2005) Postoperative morbidity and recurrence after local excision of rectal adenomas and rectal cancer by transanal endoscopic microsurgery. Colorectal Dis 7:133-137

Featherstone JM, Grabham JA, Fozard JB (2004) Per-anal excision of large, rectal, villous adenomas. Dis Colon Rectum 47:86-89

Forshaw MJ, Maphosa G, Sankararajah D et al (2006) Endoscopic alternatives in managing anastomotic strictures of the colon and rectum. Tech Coloproctol 10:21-27

Ganai S, Kanumuri P, Rao RS, Alexander AI (2006) Local recurrence after transanal endoscopic microsurgery for rectal polyps and early cancers. Ann Surg Oncol 13:547-556

Gavagan JA, Whiteford MH, Swanstrom LL (2004) Full-thickness intraperitoneal excision by transanal endoscopic microsurgery does not increase short-term complications. Am J Surg 187:630-634

Gervaz P, Huber O, Bucher P et al (2008) Trans-sacral (Kraske) approach for gastrointestinal stromal tumour of the lower rectum: old procedure for a new disease. Colorectal Dis 10:951-952

Groebli Y, Tschantz P (1994) Should the posterior approach to the rectum be forgotten?. Helv Chir Acta 60:599-604

Guerrieri M, Baldarelli M, de Sanctis A et al (2010) Treatment of rectal adenomas by transanal endoscopic microsurgery: 15 years' experience. Surg Endosc 24:445-449

Heintz A, Mörschel M, Junginger T (1998) Comparison of results after transanal endoscopic microsurgery and radical resection for T1 carcinoma of the rectum. Surg Endosc 12:1145-1148

Jeong WK, Park JW, Choi HS et al (2009) Transanal endoscopic microsurgery for rectal tumors: experience at Korea's National Cancer Center. Surg Endosc 23:2575-2579

Keighley MA (2001) Anorectal Disorders. In: Baker RJ, Fischer JE (eds) Mastery of surgery, 4 edn. Lippincott Williams & Wilkins, Sydney

Kosciñski T, Malinger S, Drews M (2003) Local excision of rectal carcinoma not-exceeding the muscularis layer. Colorectal Dis 5:159-163

Kreissler-Haag D, Schuld J, Lindemann W et al (2008) Complications after transanal endoscopic microsurgical resection correlate with location of rectal neoplasms. Surg Endosc 22:612-616

Kridel R, Cochet S, Roche B et al (2011) Successful closure of anal cancer-related fistulas with upfront intra-arterial chemotherapy: a report of 8 cases. Dis Colon Rectum 54:566-569

Kumar A, Stahl T, Fitzgerald J et al (2010) Rectal carcinoid tumors resected by transanal endoscopic microsurgery (TEM): first reported U.S. series. ASCRS Meeting Abstracts, Dis Colon Rectum 53:639

Langer C, Liersch T, Süss M et al (2003) Surgical cure for early rectal carcinoma and large adenoma: transanal endoscopic microsurgery (using ultrasound or electrosurgery) compared to conventional local and radical resection. Int J Colorectal Dis 18:222-229

Lebedyev A, Tulchinsky H, Rabau M et al (2009) Long-term results of local excision for T1 rectal carcinoma: the experience of two colorectal units. Tech Coloproctol 13:231-236

Lev-Chelouche D, Margel D, Goldman G, Rabau MJ (2000) Transanal endoscopic microsurgery: experience with 75 rectal neoplasms. Dis Colon Rectum 43:662-667

Lezoche G, Baldarelli M, Guerrieri M et al (2008) A prospective randomized study with a 5-year minimum follow-up evaluation of transanal endoscopic microsurgery versus laparoscopic total mesorectal excision after neoadjuvant therapy. Surg Endosc 22:352-358 Epub 2007 Oct 18. Erratum in: Surg Endosc. 2008 Jan 22:278

Lezoche G, Guerrieri M, Baldarelli M et al (2010) Transanal endoscopic microsurgery for 135 patients with small nonadvanced low rectal cancer (iT1-iT2, iN0): short- and long-term results. Surg Endosc 25:1222-1229

Maeda K, Maruta M, Utsumi T et al (2002) Minimally invasive transanal surgery for localized rectal carcinoid tumors. Tech Coloproctol. 6:33-36

Melis M, Gruel R, Darwin P et al (2009) Full thickness transanal re-excision following endoscopic removal of malignant rectal polyps. Int J Colorectal Dis 24:531-536

Meng WC, Lau PY, Yip AW (2004) Treatment of early rectal tumours by transanal endoscopic microsurgery in Hong Kong: prospective study. Hong Kong Med J 10:239-243

Middleton PF, Sutherland LM, Maddern GJ (2005) Transanal endoscopic microsurgery: a systematic review. Dis Colon Rectum 48:270-284

Moore JS, Cataldo PA, Osler T, Hyman NH (2008) Transanal endoscopic microsurgery is more effective than traditional transanal excision for resection of rectal masses. Dis Colon Rectum 51:1026-1030

Moraes Rda S, Malafaia O, Telles JE et al (2008) Transanal en-

doscopic microsurgery in the treatment of rectal tumors: a prospective study in 50 patients. Arq Gastroenterol 45:268-274
Nano M, Ferronato M, Solej M, D'Amico S (2006) T1 adenocarcinoma of the rectum: transanal excision or radical surgery? Tumori 92:469-473
Nascimbeni R, Nivatvongs S, Larson DR, Burgart LJ (2004) Long-term survival after local excision for T1 carcinoma of the rectum. Dis Colon Rectum 47:1773-1779
Nicholls J (2007) Local excision of rectal carcinoma. Colorectal Dis 9:771-772
Orkin BA, Sinykin SB, Lloyd PC (2010) The digital rectal examination scoring system (DRESS). Dis Colon Rectum 53:1656-1660
Paganini AM, Guerrieri M, Rotundo A, Lezoche E (2007) When can local excision be considered adequate for treatment of non advanced low rectal cancer (NALRC)? Tech Coloproctol 11:378
Palma P, Freudenberg S, Samel S, Post S (2004) Transanal endoscopic microsurgery: indications and results after 100 cases. Colorectal Dis 6:350-355
Palma P, Horisberger K, Joos A et al (2009) Local excision of early rectal cancer: is transanal endoscopic microsurgery an alternative to radical surgery? Rev Esp Enferm Dig 101:172-178
Pescatori M, Brusciano L, Binda GA, Serventi A (2005) A novel approach for perirectal tumours: the perianal intersphincteric excision. Int J Colorectal Dis 20:72-75
Ramirez JM, Aguilella V, Arribas D, Martinez M (2002) Transanal full-thickness excision of rectal tumours: should the defect be sutured? a randomized controlled trial. Colorectal Dis 4:51-55
Ramwell A, Evans J, Bignell M et al (2009) The creation of a peritoneal defect in transanal endoscopic microsurgery does not increase complications. Colorectal Dis 11:964-966
Saclarides TJ (2007) TEM/local excision: indications, techniques, outcomes, and the future. J Surg Oncol 96:644-650
Seman M, Bretagnol F, Guedj N et al (2010) Transanal endoscopic microsurgery (TEM) for rectal tumor: the first French single-center experience. Gastroenterol Clin Biol 34:488-493
Serra Aracil X, Gómez Díaz C, Bombardó Junca J et al (2010) Surgical excision of retrorectal tumour using transanal endoscopic microsurgery. Colorectal Dis 12:594-595
Stanley JD, Bell C, Hinkle N et al (2010) The Ferguson Operating Anoscope as a minimally invasive option for the treatment of rectal tumors. Am Surg 76:850-856
Tsai BM, Finne CO, Nordenstam JF et al (2010) Transanal endoscopic microsurgery resection of rectal tumors: outcomes and recommendations. Dis Colon Rectum 53:16-23
Tsai JA, Hedlund M, Sjoqvist U et al (2006) Experience of endoscopic transanal resections with a urologic resectoscope in 131 patients. Dis Colon Rectum 49:228-232
van den Broek FJ, de Graaf EJ, Dijkgraaf MG et al (2009) Transanal endoscopic microsurgery versus endoscopic mucosal resection for large rectal adenomas (TREND-study). BMC Surg 13:4
Zieren J, Paul M, Menenakos C (2007) Transanal endoscopic microsurgery (TEM) vs. radical surgery (RS) in the treatment of rectal cancer: indications, limitations, prospectives. A review. Acta Gastroenterol Belg 70:374-380

Anal Condylomata and Anorectal Stricture

7

7.1 Introduction

Anal condylomata and anal stricture are dealt with in the same chapter because an anal stricture may follow the excision of condylomata, especially if they are giant and/or invade the circumference of the anal canal. The patient with condylomata is often difficult to manage due to concomitant diseases that cause immunodepression and is more prone to complications and recurrences.

As far as rectal stricture, this may be the consequence of a low rectal anastomotic dehiscence and may concern not only specialists, but also general surgeons, e.g., after anterior resection of the rectum. Indeed, anterior resection syndrome, in which there is fecal urgency and anal incontinence, possibly with proctalgia, is seen in up to two thirds of these patients, especially those receiving neoadjuvant radiotherapy prior to surgery, and is usually related to a deficient reservoir, weak sphincters, and post-dehiscence stricture and fibrosis. The following case illustrates the complexity of these patients. A skilled general gastrointestinal surgeon, able to perform both open and laparoscopic procedures, referred a 55-year-old woman to my unit. She had undergone a stapled ultra-low anterior resection of the rectum, performed by a specialist in the USA, after a course of radiochemotherapy. She was rather depressed and complained of anal incontinence and obstructed defecation. Her history revealed a supra-anastomotic diverticulum, the consequence of a suture breakdown, an injured internal sphincter, possibly due to intra-operative stretching, a deficient pelvic floor from two vaginal deliveries, an anorectal stricture, related to the post-dehiscence fibrosis, and a coloanal mucosal intussusception, causing fractioned defecation (Fig. 7.1). The reason for the referral was the need for anal sphincter rehabilitation, and my Italian colleague knew that we had a good physiotherapist at our unit. However, since apart from the sphincter dysfunction, the above-mentioned organic lesions were also present, a surgical re-intervention was indicated, aimed at treating the sphincter disruption, anorectal stricture, supra-anastomotic diverticulum, and internal mucosal prolapse. I told my colleague that the insertion of a probe in the anal canal, to carry out either biofeedback or electrostimulation, would not only have been painful for the patient but was likely to worsen the associated organic lesions. He wisely admitted that, being a general surgeon, he lacked experience to properly deal with such a case, and therefore asked me to carry out the re-operation and manage the rehabilitation. After the injection of bulking agents (Durasphere) to "reinforce" the internal sphincter, I operated on the patient via a transanal route, avoiding excessive sphincter stretch with the anal retractor. The mucosal prolapse was excised, the diverticulum closed by means of a layered suture to obliterate the cavity, and the stricture managed with an anoplasty. After one month, when the surgical wounds had fully healed, the patient underwent a course of pelvic floor rehabilitation. Meanwhile, she had taken advantage of the opportunity to see our psychologist for a couple of months and had markedly improved. This is an example of a multidisciplinary approach to deal with a complex case of anterior resection syndrome.

In addition to following condylomata excision and anterior resection, anorectal stricture may also occur after other surgeries, such as hemorrhoidectomy and prolapsectomy, and may be managed by either abdominal, transanal, or combined procedures. This chapter discusses both the prevention and the treatment of this troublesome complication.

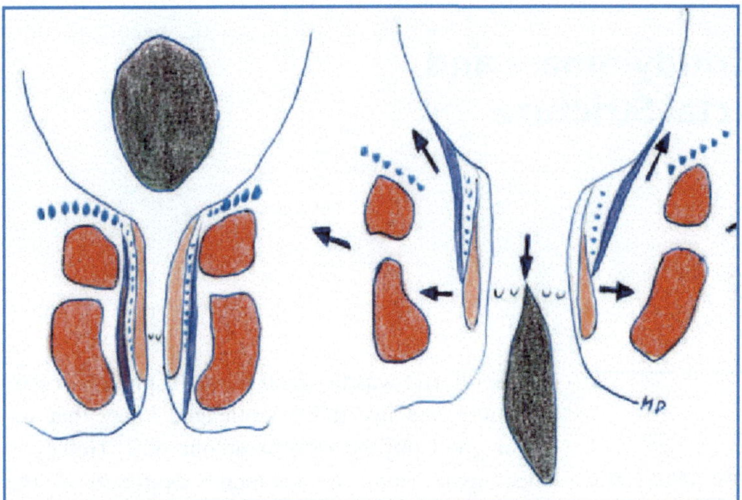

Fig. 7.1 a The dynamic relationships of the normal anatomy of the levators ani, puborectalis muscle, external sphincter, longitudinal muscle of the rectum, and internal sphincter. During defecation, the relationship between these structures changes as shown

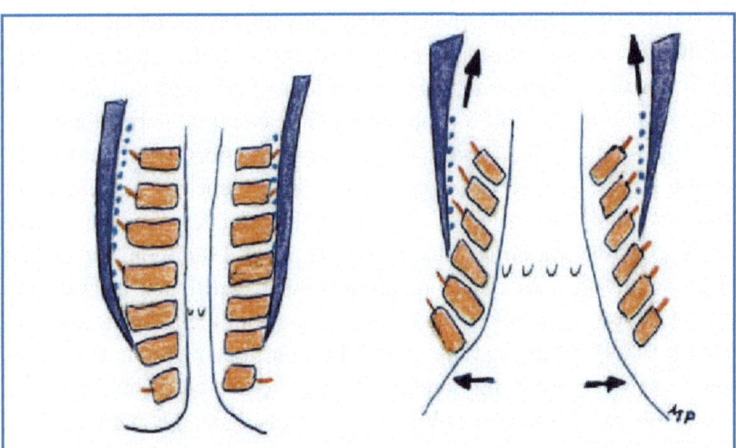

Fig. 7.1 b The lamellar structure of the internal sphincter, with a shift in the orientation of the lamellae from horizontal to oblique during opening of the anal canal. Lateral to the internal sphincter are the neural structures and the longitudinal muscle of the rectum, which pops up

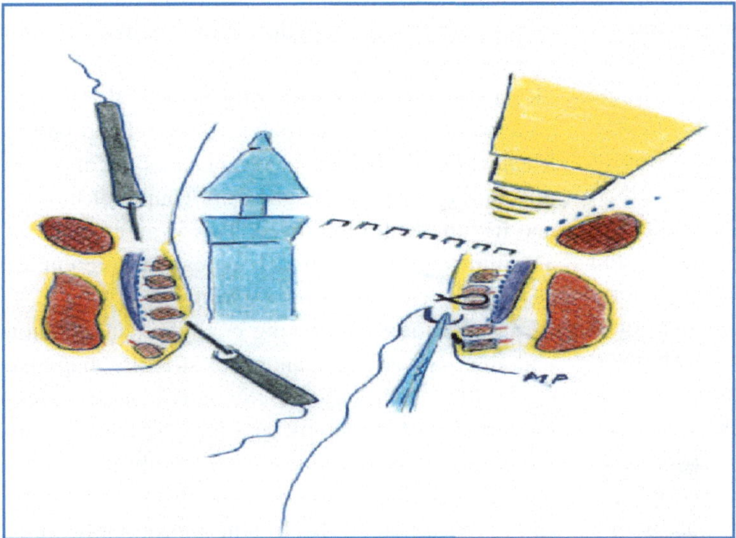

Fig. 7.1 c Anterior resection, in its various phases, in a patient receiving pre-or post-operative radiotherapy, would clearly damage the delicate structures and mechanisms described above. In particular, radiotherapy causes fibrosis; transanal dilatation causes sphincter stretching; colo-anal suturing can result in internal sphincter damage; and dissection between the rectum and elevators muscles, through the abdomen, may damage the sacral nerve endings. These events give rise to anterior resection syndrome, which is characterized by proctalgia, tenesmus, defecatory urgency, and anal incontinence

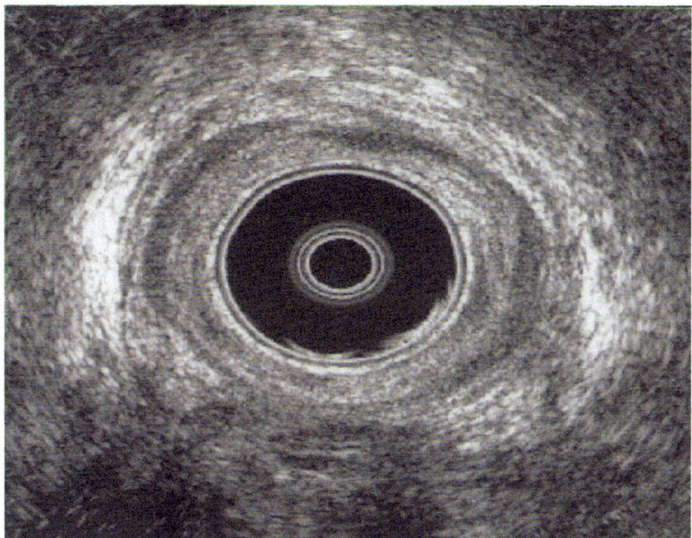

Fig. 7.1 d Transanal ultrasonography with a rotating probe in a patient who underwent ultralow anterior resection for rectal cancer. The patient is in the Sims position. Below, to the left of the patient, thinning is seen until both sphincters are greatly diminished, especially the internal one, as a consequence of the surgical trauma

7.2 Complications After Surgery for Anal Condylomata

Nearly two decades ago, Keighley and Williams, in their already cited text, recommended that laser- and cryotherapy of anal condylomata be abandoned. Nonetheless, I am aware that some dermatologists and some proctologists still use these procedures. Ablative techniques, including cryotherapy and laser treatment, were used by dermatologists for 55 and 40% of the patients compared with, respectively, 7.6 and 14% of patients for colorectal surgeons (Dindo et al., 2011). Therefore, the weak points and the complications of such outmoded procedures deserve review. As is well known (and as clearly illustrated in the "Unforgettable Complication," at the end of this chapter), condylomata may also affect the anal canal and, occasionally, the rectum. Since dermatologists do not perform proctoscopy, after treating the anal lesions, they will leave behind the endoanal-rectal ones, if any, and the patient will not be cured. Moreover, rather than "destroy" the condylomata with cryo- or laser-therapy, it is better to excise them and send them for histological evaluation, as a squamocellular carcinoma may be present. Most condylomata are due to human papilloma virus (HPV) infection. Some species of HPV are oncogenic, and in these cases a persistent infection may result first in dysplasia and then cancer. This is another good reason to examine the removed condylomata. Billingham and Lewis (1982) showed that laser-therapy is more costly and painful than other procedures, and that condylomata particles may be diffused in the air during the procedure, resulting in infection to the respiratory tree of both the physician and the nurses.

However, it should be noted that the technique most commonly used by specialists, and the one that I use, is local excision by scissors after infiltration of the base of the lesion with adrenaline and saline, to facilitate removal and to decrease bleeding. If the number of condylomata is low and they are located perianally, it is very unlikely that excision will be followed by significant complications; but if they are giant or numerous and located also in the anal canal, thus requiring a wide skin removal, an anoplasty may be carried out, aimed at preventing postoperative stricture. Uribe et al. (2004) published a small series of six immunodepressed patients with giant anal condylomata (one case involved a malignancy) who underwent immediate V-Y anoplasty, with no postoperative complications. Those patients were lucky, because Consten et al. (1995) previously reported that immunodepressed patients are more prone to failed healing of the surgical wound. Therefore, the immunological pattern, and especially CD4 lymphocytes, of these patients should be preoperatively evaluated. Nadal et al. (1998) confirmed that the evaluation of CD4 lymphocytes may predict the surgical prognosis. According to Wexner

(*Fundamentals of anorectal surgery*, Beck and Wexner eds., 1992), the procedure of James Thompson, of St. Mark's, i.e., infiltration with adrenaline followed by scissors excision of the condylomata, is the most radical management, as it allows a histological evaluation aimed at excluding cancer. Thompson and Grace (1978) reported the positive outcome of this procedure in 75 patients, with only four cases of bleeding (5%).

Alternatively, diathermy may be carried out, which has the disadvantage that it does not allow histological examination. Furthermore, if performed too deeply, it may cause anal spasm, pain, burning, and bleeding. However, pain may also follow scissors excision, as reported by Khawaja et al. (1989) in 11 out of their 16 patients. A careful hemostasis should be carried out to minimize the risk of intra- and postoperative bleeding, and loss of anoderma should be likewise avoided to prevent anal stricture.

In case severe anal stricture occurs, it may be treated with the operation described in the "Live Surgery" section of this chapter.

7.3 Complications After Surgery for Anal Stricture

The most frequent cause of anal stricture in a proctologist's experience is the Milligan-Morgan hemorrhoidectomy (Fig.7.2). It is well known that stenosis is likely to occur when, upon completion of the procedure, the skin-mucosal bridges are insufficient and disepithelialization of the anal canal is overly extensive. In most cases, anal dilations are sufficient to manage stricture, but if not then an anoplasty may be required. The rectal flap anoplasty, according to Martin, is an easy procedure, albeit infrequently used as it is likely to cause soiling due to mucosal ectropion (Rosen 1988). Instead, flatus and mucus anal incontinence occurred in only five out of 60 patients following cutaneous anoplasty (Farid et al., 2010). Suture dehiscence, due to either sepsis or, more often, to ischemia, was reported by the same authors in 20% of their patients after Y-V and rhomboid anoplasty. Y-V anoplasty may be performed by means of a single flap, as in Farid's series, or using two flaps, which causes less tension on the suture and is the

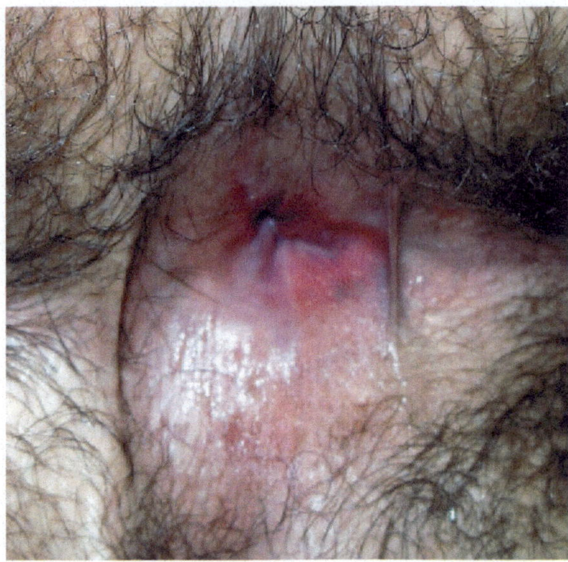

Fig. 7.2 Anal stenosis after hemorrhoidectomy

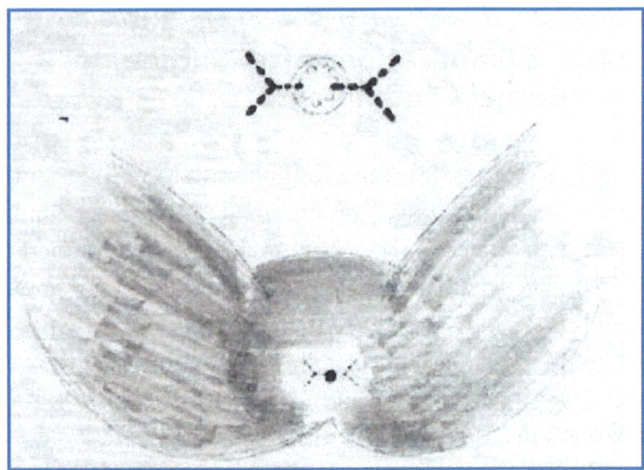

Fig. 7.3 Y-V bilateral incision for the treatment of anal stenosis

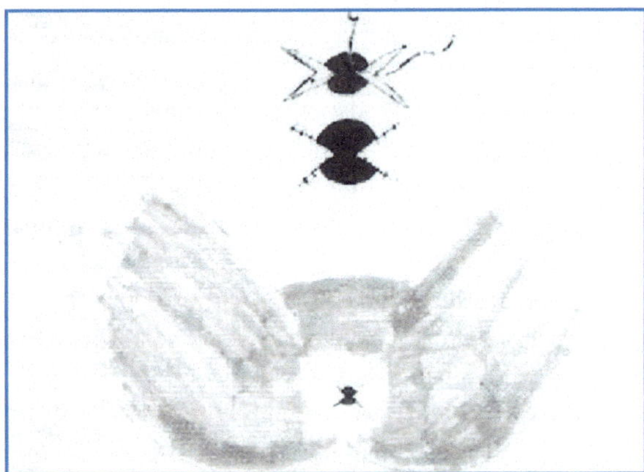

Fig. 7.4 The apex of both flaps is sutured within the anal canal, bilaterally, to reduce the tension on the sutures and consequently, the risk of dehiscence

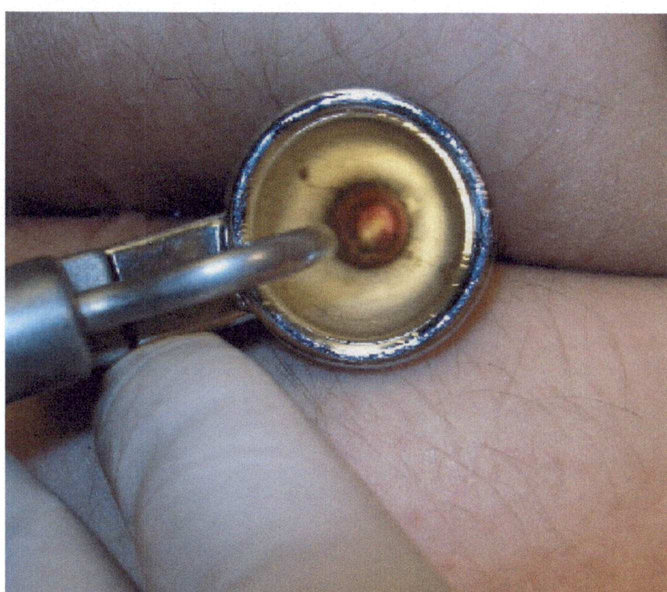

Fig. 7.5 Proctoscopy using an instrument similar to the otoscope to evaluate the rectum in patients with severe anal stenosis

preferred approach at our unit (Figs. 7.3, 7.4). When either a house or a diamond flap is performed, the use of post-anal skin should be avoided, as the vascular supply at the level of the posterior midline is less abundant than in other quadrants, reflecting the different anatomical arrangement, as shown by doppler studies. Therefore, there may be a greater risk of wound dehiscence in this area, which also is more prone to anal fissures.

Pfeifer et al. (1995), from the Cleveland Clinic in Florida, reported just one case of marginal flap ischemia out of 12 patients who underwent the house flap procedure, described in the "Live Surgery" section.

Instead, when flap anoplasty is performed to manage a Crohn's stricture, the results are less encouraging, both in terms of complications and recurrences (Linares et al., 1988). Either anocutaneous radial incisions or anal dilations may be carried out at the end of the anoplasty, aimed at preventing recurrent strictures. Anal stricturopasty is considered a good alternative when dealing with Crohn's strictures.

In case of severe anal strictures, a special anoscope, as thin as an otoscope, is required to evaluate the distal rectum. It is also useful to examine the perineal sinuses and narrowed inflamed rectal stumps, as it does not cause pain to the patient (Fig. 7.5).

A troublesome complication to treat is an ileoanal anastomosis that, following restorative proctocolectomy, has become either strictured or obliterated. Many years ago, we reported a difficult case that was successfully managed by means of an endoscopic trans-stomal and a surgical transanal rendez-vous (Pescatori et al., 1992) (Fig. 7.6).

For information on incontinence following a failed operation for anal stricture, the reader is referred to Chap. 9, which deals with fecal incontinence. Here, it suffices to say that sphincter reconstruction may be needed if the striated muscles are severely injured, whereas, in case of minor external sphincter lesions, sacral neuromodulation may be successful. If only the internal sphincter is disrupted, the injection of bulking agent may be the treatment of choice.

If the sphincters are intact, without extended perineal and anal fibrosis or scarring, biofeedback training should be attempted as the first-line therapy. The group of Bartolo (2004) reported satisfactory results using bowel retrograde irrigation with a plastic tube. Pizzetti et al. (2006) cured some of their patients with obstructed defecation using hydrocolon lavage, performed using a device that irrigated the bowel with warm water at constant temperature and flow. Both irrigation and hydrocolon lavage are safe procedures, as they are very unlikely to result in adverse events. When dealing with patients with strictured

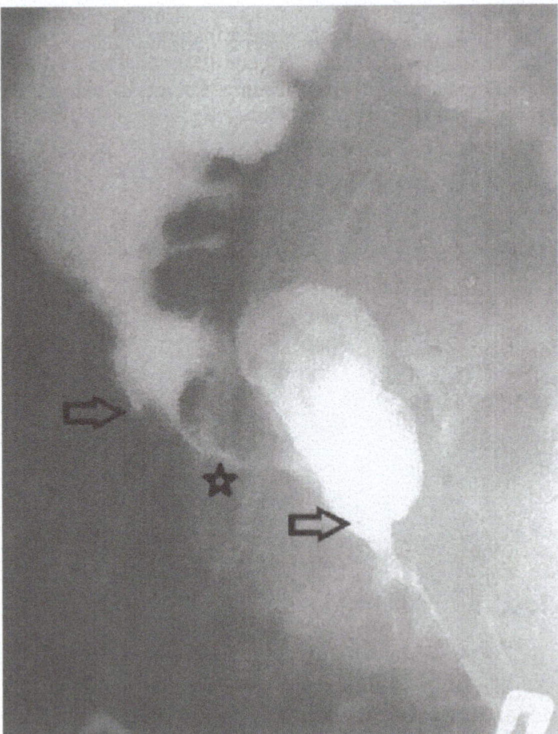

Fig. 7.6 a The pouchogram shows marked stenosis after ileoanal anastomosis dehiscence. The *upper arrow* indicates the ileal reservoir, the *lower arrow* the anal canal. The *star* shows the stenotic tract

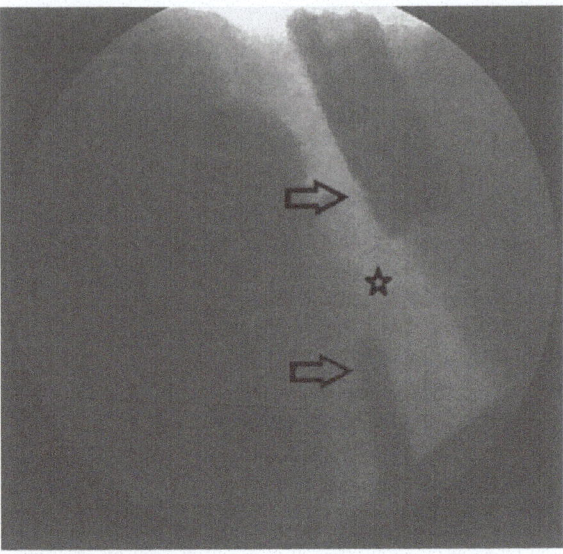

Fig. 7.6 b Abdominal X-ray: same symbols as in (a). A colonoscope is inserted into the reservoir through the diverting stoma and a Klemmer is inserted as a marker into the anal canal. Following the light path of the endoscope, a transanal section of the stenotic tract is performed together with a suture between the ileal mucosa and anal canal epithelium, thus restoring the intestinal continuity: the so-called rendez-vous-endoscopic surgery (from Pescatori et al., 1992)

anal canal, small irrigating probes are available to ensure the comfort of the patient. In case of severe recurrent problems that cannot be managed with other procedures, a terminal colostomy may be necessary, if accepted by the patient.

7.4 Complications After Surgery for Rectal Stricture

Rectal strictures may be low, middle, or high. For the management of low rectal strictures, those located just above the anorectal ring, the same procedures may be performed as previously reported for the surgical treatment of anal strictures. However, when dealing with either middle or high rectal stenosis, different techniques should be used, as the cutaneous advancement flap of an anoplasty cannot reach the middle or upper rectum.

Rectal strictures are usually the consequence of either an ischemia or the breakdown of a colorectal, coloanal or, less frequently, ileorectal or ileoanal anastomosis. The first option in such cases is a pneumatic balloon endoscopic dilation, but it may be followed by fissuration of the strictured bowel or significant bleeding. Less likely, and more dramatically, is the "Unforgettable Complication," reported and illustrated at the end of Chap. 8. If the latter complication occurs above the peritoneal reflection and is not promptly detected by the endoscopist, it may cause pelvic sepsis with frank peritonitis, potentially necessitating a diverting stoma. The clinical consequences will be less troublesome if the perforation occurs below the peritoneal reflection, where the rectum is covered by the levator ani. In this case, functional disturbances are more likely, due to the fibrosis created between the rectal ampulla and the rich nerve network above the puborectalis sling. The function of these nerves is to alert the CNS to a stimulus, such as the need to pass stool or a painful distention, triggered at the level of the pelvic floor

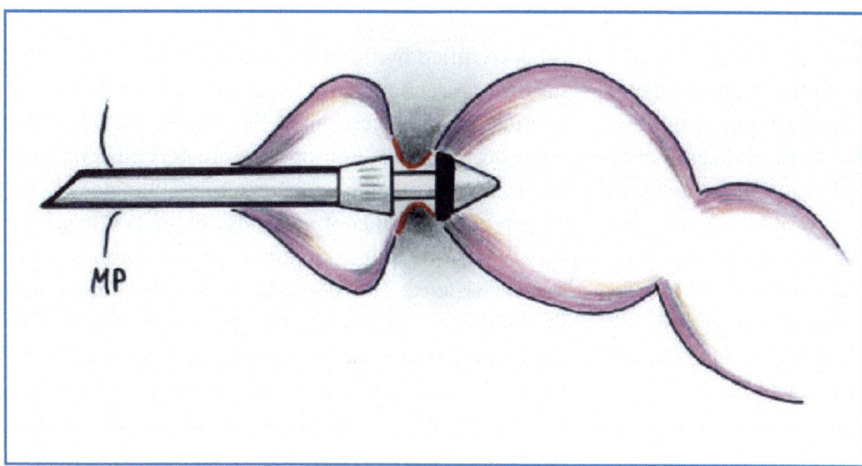

Fig. 7.7 Use of a circular stapler in the treatment of rectal stenosis

muscles and viscera. Since rectal sensation is paramount to the continence mechanism, if a fibrotic mass arising from a chronic infection is interposed between the somatic muscle funnel (the levator ani) and the visceral cylinder (the anorectum), the contact mediated by the mechanoreceptors and allowing awareness of the lower stimulus will be impaired and the mechanism of both anal continence and defecation will be affected. Basically, this is what happened to the patient with anterior resection syndrome, described in the Introduction of this chapter, whose fibrosis was the result of an anastomotic dehiscence of the low stapled suture.

However, the risk of peritonitis, retro-pneumoperitoneum, pneumomediastinum, pelvic sepsis, and the need of a re-intervention, possibly with a diverting stoma, will depend upon the site of the perforation.

Baatrup et al. (2010) successfully managed six patients in whom the rectal stricture was located 8 cm from the anal verge, without any complications. Dai et al. (2010) used a self expanding stent, under endoscopic and radiologic control, to dilate 14 rectal strictures located 6 cm above the anus, following colorectal anastomosis. One of the patients had a perianastomotic fistula. The authors reported four early and four late complications: proctitis (2), proctalgia (1), and stent dislocation (5).

The stricture may be resected either by a transanal manual excision or by using a circular stapler (Fig. 7.7). Rees et al. (2004) managed three rectal strictures using a stapler, two of them by means of a combined transanal and laparoscopic approach. Two of the three patients already had a diverting stoma and intestinal continuity was restored immediately after stricture excision in one patient.

7.5 "Live Surgery": The Prevention of Postoperative Complications After Anoplasty

This is the report of an operation I carried out on a 40-year-old man 7 years ago in Cuneo, a small town in northern Italy, at the request of my friend and colleague Diego Segre and the head of the department. The patient had undergone fulguration of a giant anal condylomata one year earlier, which was followed by scald, sepsis, and severe anal stricture. A diverting stoma was performed 2 months later, after several unsuccessful anal dilations, as the stricture was threatening to cause intestinal obstruction. Prior to commencing the operation, I appreciate that the stoma poses an advantage, because it greatly reduces the risk of local sepsis and wound dehiscence.

The patient is placed in the lithotomy position and I am able to feel the stricture, which is indeed severe and does not even allow introduction of the fifth finger into the anal canal. Fortunately, there are no residual or recurrent condylomata, at least neither anal nor perianal. After dilating the anus up to 16 mm with a Hegar dilator, I realize that the anal canal is fully disepithelialized over a length of 4 cm. Therefore an anoplasty is needed, with a large flap that is wide enough to cover the defect and effectively dilate the narrowed cylinder of the anal canal. I therefore prepare a pentagonal house flap with a 6-cm diameter, about the size of half a hand. While a flap of this size might seem too large to fill the 4 cm of disepithelialized tissue, this is not the case because it will slightly retract after the advancement upwards into the anal canal. When performing the skin incision, I keep the blade of the knife oblique rather than vertical, in order to harvest a flap with a good blood supply, with the base wider than the apex. This will minimize the risk of ischemia and subsequent suture dehiscence. For the same reason, I avoid diathermy to stop the minor bleeding of the flap's margins, preferring instead to compress the bleeding area using a gauze soaked with adrenaline. As the vascular supply of the flap is provided by the perforating vessels of the underskin, they should not be coagulated. An introflecting suture is then carried out using vicryl 3/0, taking a portion of underskin at a distance of 2-3 cm from the anus and anchoring it to the subcutis of the anal verge. After it is tied and cut short, the knot will disappear below the skin and the flap will start to advance towards the anal canal. Once completed, this deep suture layer will strongly anchor the flap and keep it in place even in case of a partial dehiscence of the superficial layer, which is more prone to local sepsis due to fecal contamination (but not in this patient who had a diverting stoma). During this maneuver, trauma to the flap is avoided using Kocher or Kelly forceps. Again, this minimizes the risk of suture breakdown and subsequent recurrence of the stricture.

The next step is to prepare the anal canal to be properly filled by the flap. This is achieved by gently inserting a retractor into the anal canal to perform a careful scissors excision of the fibrotic tissue of the stricture, without injuring the underlying internal sphincter and subcutaneous external sphincter, thereby preserving anal continence. Sometimes it is necessary to perform a distal internal sphincterotomy, if the muscle is tense and fibrotic. After determining that the base and margins of the endoanal defect are soft and vital, I suture the skin of the flap to the epithelium of the anal canal, still with asymmetrical stitches and using vicryl 3/0, with the goal of moving the flap upwards. The proximal limit of the anoplasty has to fall well inside the anal canal, to re-establish a new dentate line, and the lower rectal mucosa, or the epithelium of the upper anal canal, has to be strongly anchored to the cranial end of the flap. At the end of the suture, the upper half of the flap is positioned inside the anal canal, whereas the distal half is still in the perianal area. Therefore, the flap itself has been advanced at least 3 cm upwards and more than half of the previously strictured area has been filled with intact skin. The elasticity of the anal canal allows a digital exploration and the insertion of a proctoscope.

The stoma of the patient was closed after 2 months, and he was encouraged to perform sphincter exercises. After 7 years, he has not had a recurrence of the stricture or the condylomata and is fully continent. Figure 7.8 shows a cutaneous house-flap anoplasty carried out in a patient with fibrosis of the anal canal.

Fig. 7.8 a Male patient, 65 years old, with anal stricture due to multiple operations for anal fissures. The patient is in the lithotomy potition. A segment of fibrotic posterior anal canal has been excised. The defect has to be covered using a cutaneos flap

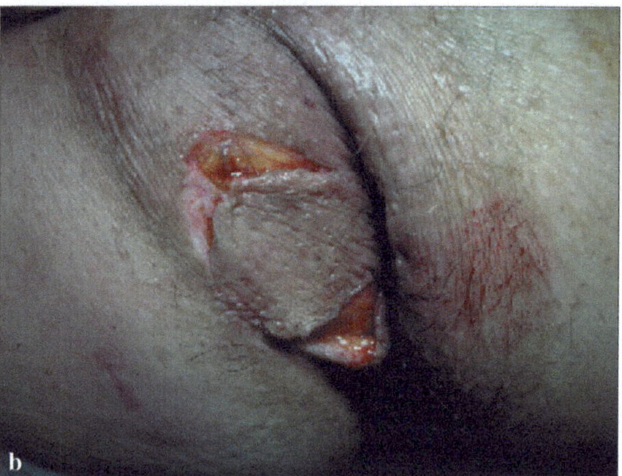

Fig. 7.8 b A "house" flap is harvested. The base of the flap is larger to ensure a good vascular supply. Diathermy is avoided to prevent flap's ischemia

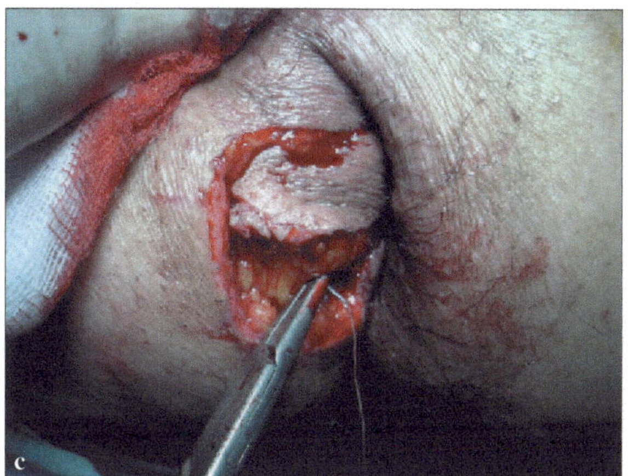

Fig. 7.8 c The flap is advanced towards the anal canal suturing its deep part to the subcutis by means of introflecting readsorbable stitches (Vicryl Rapid 2/0)

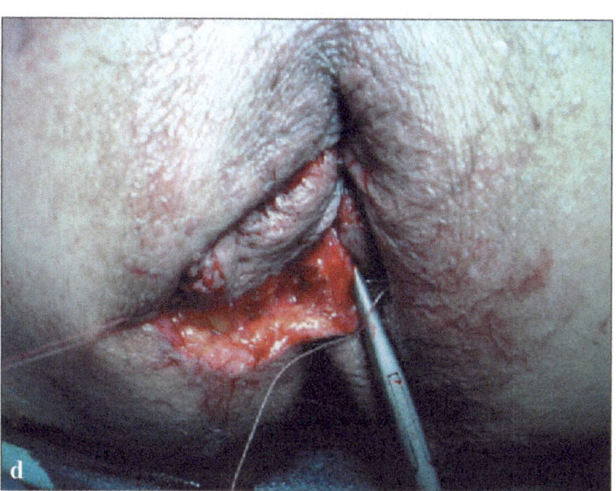

Fig. 7.8 d The stitches are positioned asimmetrically, aimed at advancing the flap towards the anal canal

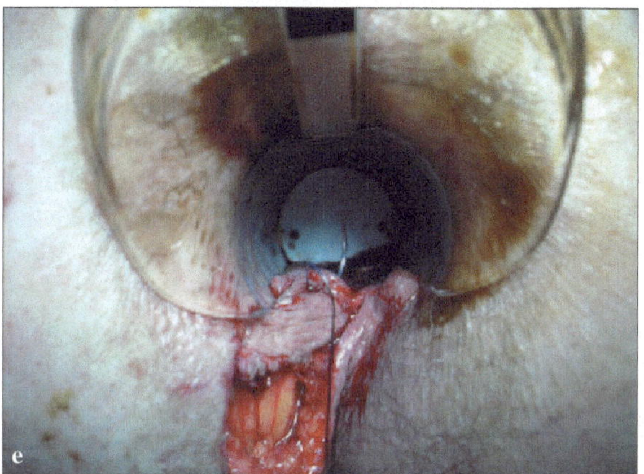

Fig. 7.8 e The upper part of the flap is stitched to the distal rectal mucosa, aimed at reconstructing the continuity of the anal canal, using Vicryl 3/0

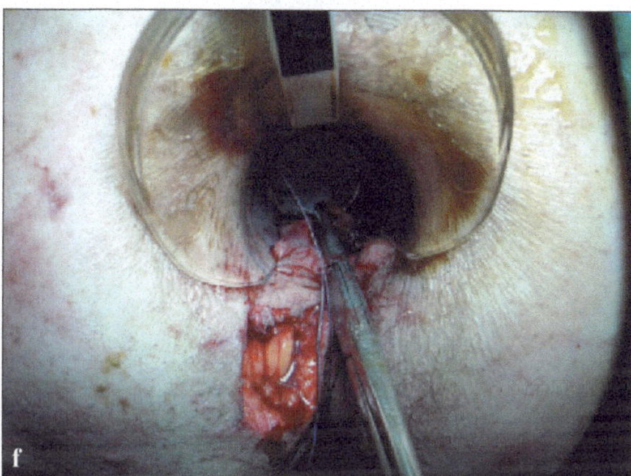

Fig. 7.8 f The suture is completed. A small bite of internal sphincter has been included

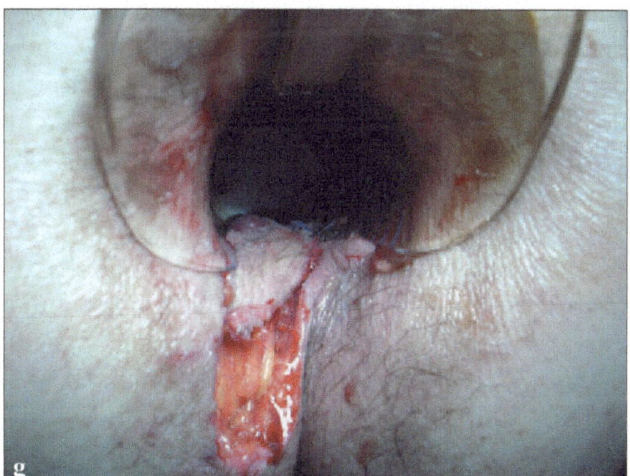

Fig. 7.8 g Once performed the endoanal suture, the flap is clearly displaced upwards

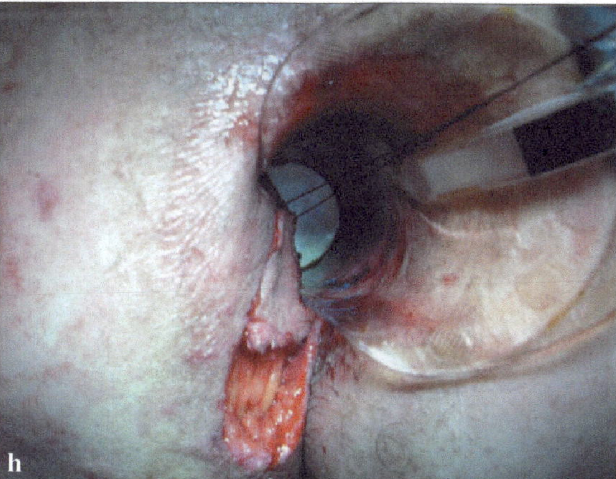

Fig. 7.8 h The lateral aspect of the flap is sutured to the distal part of the anal canal, just above the anal verge

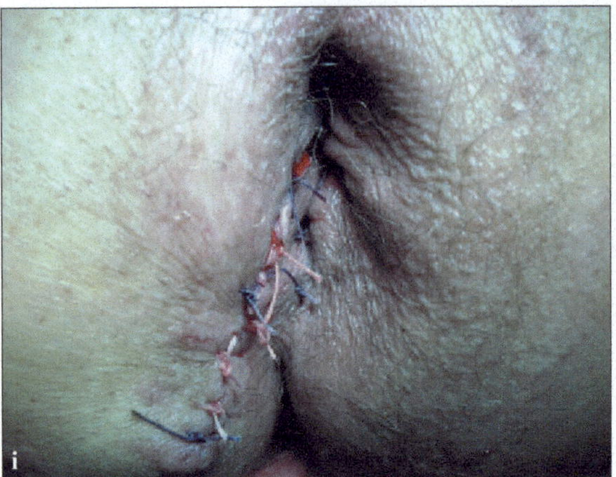

Fig. 7.8 i Finally, the residual defect at the donor site is sutured

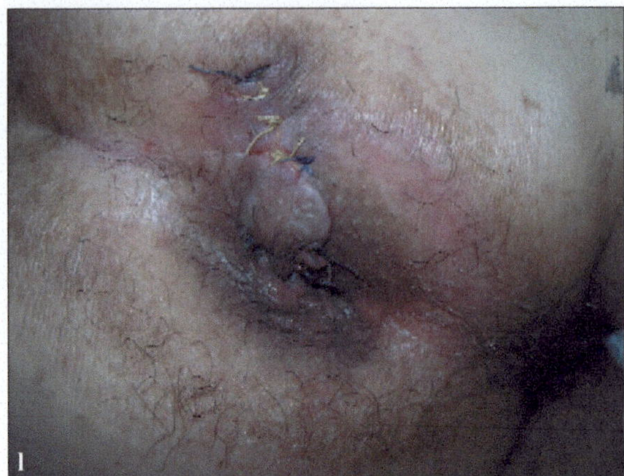

Fig. 7.8 l Patient in Sims position. The anoplasty wound is healed after 2 weeks. The patient is continent

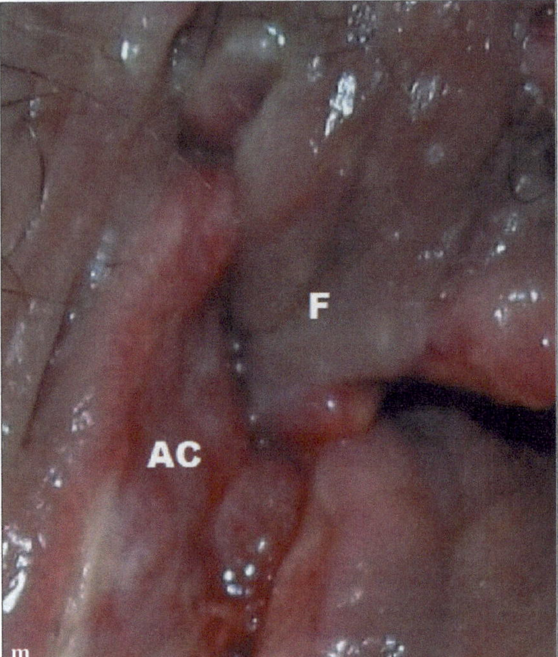

Fig. 7.8 m The endoanal portion of the anoplasty. *F*, Flap; *AC*, Anal Canal

7.6 A Trick of the Trade

This trick was already mentioned in Chap. 2, as I first used it to manage a patient who had a PPH, performed elsewhere, followed by inadvertent obliteration of the rectum (Pescatori, 2002). On that occasion, I was able to find the strictured lumen of the rectum, insert a 2-mm Hegar dilator and then a thin Foley catheter. The maneuver may be used in any severe rectal stricture, which has to be managed surgically, and renders the strictured area more accessible without stretching the anal sphincters with a retractor. After the Foley balloon has been inflated, the catheter is pulled and the strictured area is displaced downwards, almost outside the anus. While the surgical assistant keeps the catheter pulled out, radial incisions or other procedures aimed at correcting the stenosis may be easily performed, although attention must be paid not to puncture the balloon with either the scissors or diathermy.

7.7 An Unforgettable Complication

This occurred almost 20 years ago. The patient was a 37-year-old male from Sicily, who strongly denied that he was homosexual. He had four children and had undergone six operations for perianal condylomata. Unfortunately, the disease kept recurring. When I asked him to undress and lay down in the Sims position on the bed of my office, I could not believe what I saw. It is one thing is to see a disease pictured in a book, but another to have it in front of you. The perineum was fully covered by thick pinkish-white lozenges, with nodules and ulcers secreting pus and fluid. It was the first Buschke-Löwenstein tumor of my career! Of the three I have seen in 40 years, this very first one was certainly the worst (Fig. 7.9a).

The anus was strictured, almost hidden by condylomata. The perineum, at the edges of the rhomboid mass, was invaded by fistulous tracts secreting pus, up to the base of the scrotum and extending to the inguinal region, where several hard nodes were palpable. Two of them were biopsied and no malignant cells were found at histology. The disease is also called "verrucous cunniculans carcinoma", and I could well understand why: the fistulae had spread, forming tunnels filled with condylomata, like the tentacles of an octopus. Clearly, a seventh operation had to be performed, as the lesions were neither chemo- nor radiosensitive. I reviewed the literature and sought the opinion of an oncologist, based on the histology of the perineal lesions. There were no distant metastases, as shown by abdomino-pelvic ultrasound and chest X-ray. Nevertheless, Buschke-Löwenstein tumor is known to have local malignity. At rigid sigmoidoscopy, performed under anesthetics due to the narrowed anal canal, the lower rectum appeared to be invaded by condylomata.

The aim of surgery was twofold: 1) to remove the neoplasm and 2) to preserve anal continence. Unfortunately, the patient had strongly refused a colostomy; instead, I decided to carry out a two-stage operation, The first stage consisted of excision of the tumor, including the lower third of the rectum, via a perineal, transanal, and intersphincteric approach, leaving the rectal stump intubated and keeping the external sphincter intact. In the second stage, intestinal continuity would be restored by advancing skin flaps into the anal canal to prevent anorectal stricture, after the perineal wound had healed, keeping the patient constipated and under total parenteral nutrition for as long as needed. Fig. 7.9, taken from a paper by Abbas (2011) shows a similar case. Prior to surgery, we administered fluids, calories, and albumin to improve the patient's metabolic condition. The operation was carried out as illustrated at the end of this section. The tumoral condylomatous perineal lozenges were excised, without going too deep as the lesions were superficial, followed by excision of the strictured anus and anal canal together with the internal sphincter and the lower third of the rectum via an intersphincteric approach. Only a minimal part of the subcutaneous portion of the external sphincter was involved by condylomata and thus had to be removed. Finally, I sutured the distal end of the rectal stump to a large-size mushroom-shaped Depezzer tube, aimed at avoiding contamination of the perineal wound by fecal matter (Fig. 7.10). Everything went as planned and the patient was kept constipated with Loperamide while given nearly 2000 calories in the form of parenteral nutrition.

What do you think was the outcome of the operation?

Unfortunately, two adverse events occurred. First, healing of the perineal wound was slower than expected. Second, at examination under anesthesia, further condylomata were found at the level of the wounds, both anteriorly, invading the base of the urethra, and posteriorly, at the level of the sacral hollow. After 3 weeks, a CT scan showed condylomatous masses at the level of the femur's acetabulum and the presacral space. A surgical attempt was made to remove the anterior condylomata, but the urethra was slightly injured in the process, as it was also infiltrated by condylomata. The urethra was easily repaired and a Foley catheter was positioned. The posterior ano-coccygeal ligament was excised and the sacral cavity explored: the condylomatous mass had deeply invaded the area of the presacral veins such that an excision at that level was judged to be too dangerous. Sadly, the operation was interrupted and the patient's conditions progressively worsened, until he decided to return home to Sicily, where he died after 3 months.

It has been impossible to forget him or this case.

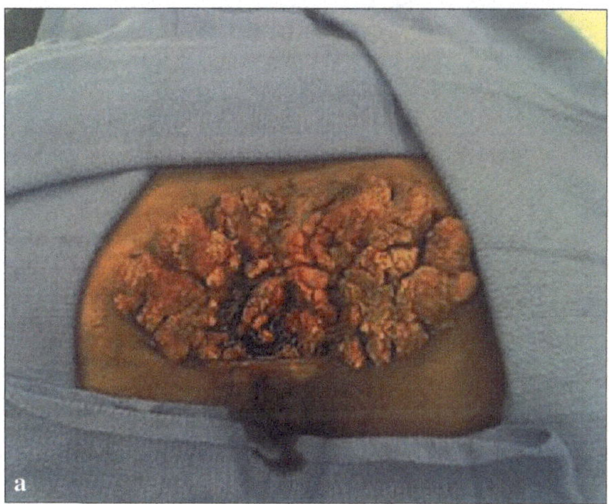

Fig. 7.9 a 37-year-old HIV-positive man with Buschke-Löwenstein tumor, a case similar to the one described in this section

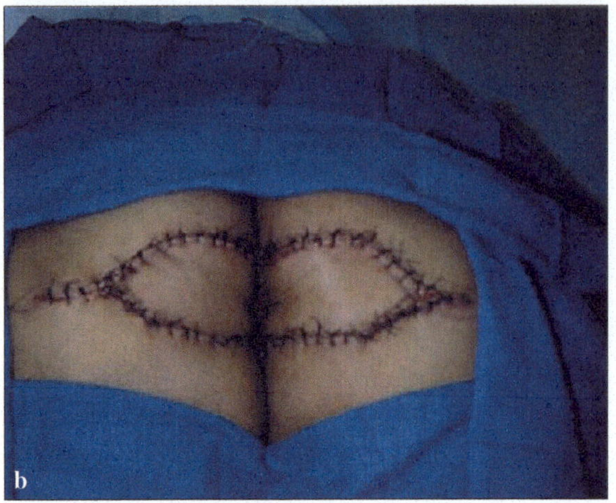

Fig. 7.9 b Excision with bilateral house flaps, an operation similar to the one we had planned for our patient

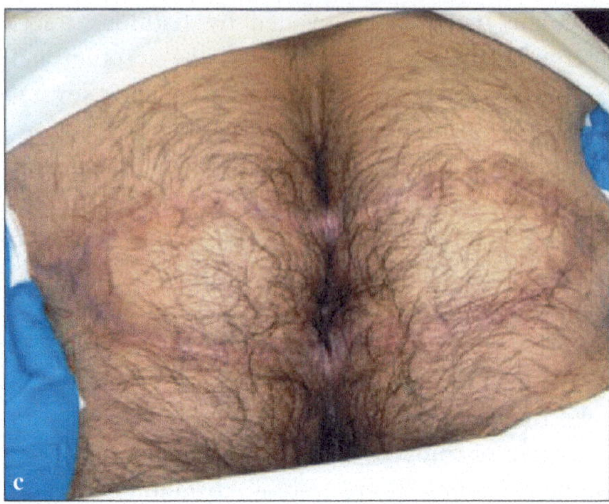

Fig. 7.9 c 2 months postoperatively (from Abbas, 2011)

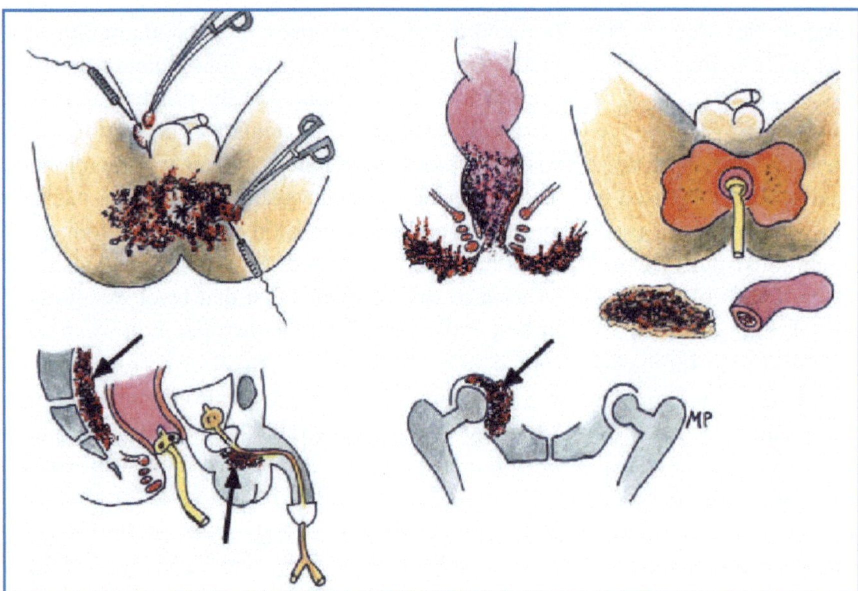

Fig. 7.10 Buschke-Löwenstein's tumor or condylomatosis cunniculata. The inguinal lymph nodes were biopsied and a macrobiopsy of the cancer obtained to confirm the diagnosis. The condylomatas are seen to invade the perineum, anal canal, and distal rectum. Perineal tumor and intersphincteric rectum excision was carried out as a first step. Unfortunately, in this patient, the condylomata invaded the presacral space, urethra, and acetabulum of the femur (*arrows*)

Summary

Scissors excision of a few anal or perianal condylomata is unlikely to be followed by significant complications. If diathermy excision is carried out, both early painful anal spasm and late bleeding may occur. Laser excision is carried out less frequently, as it is costly and may cause troublesome complications.

When dealing with giant condylomata or when they are located in the anal canal, there is the risk of anal stricture, which may be prevented by performing an anoplasty following condylomata excision. Wound healing is often delayed in immunodepressed patients.

Various types of anoplasty are used to manage anal strictures, the most common being cutaneous anoplasty, because a rectal mucosal flap will likely lead to an ectropion and thus to soiling. House, diamond, S, and V-Y anoplasties are more frequently carried out by specialists. The basic principles of plastic surgery should be followed to minimize the risk of suture dehiscence and recurrent stricture, including preservation of the vascular supply, avoidance of suture tension, and avoidance of traumas to the flap. Stretching or injury of the anal sphincters also should be avoided to prevent postoperative incontinence. Fecal contamination may cause local sepsis and subsequent suture breakdown, unless a diverting stoma is performed.

Rectal strictures are often due to the dehiscence of a colorectal anastomosis and may be managed endoscopically, either performing pneumatic dilation or inserting a stent. Stricture excision is another option, carried out by means a circular stapler but more often with a combined transanal and transabdominal open or laparoscopic approach, or even less invasively using the TEM procedure.

Suggested Readings

Abbas MA (2011) Wide local excision for the Buschke-Löwenstein tumor or circumferential carcinoma in situ. Tech Coloproctol 15:313-318

Aitola PT, Hiltunen KM, Matikainen MJ (1997) Y-V anoplasty combined with internal sphincterotomy for stenosis of the anal canal. Eur J Surg 163:839-842

Angelchik PD, Harms BA, Starling JR (1993) Repair of anal stricture and mucosal ectropion with Y-V or pedicle flap anoplasty. Am J Surg 166:55-59

Baatrup G, Svensen R, Ellensen VS (2010) Benign rectal strictures managed with transanal resection—a novel application for transanal endoscopic microsurgery. Colorectal Dis 12:144-146

Billingham RP, Lewis FG (1982) Laser versus electrical cautery in the treatment of condylomata acuminata of the anus. Surg Gynecol Obstet 155:865-867

Bonnichon P, Bellouard A, Richardson A et al (1988) Anal plasty after excision of giant condyloma acuminata. Presse Med 17:74-76

Brisinda G, Vanella S, Cadeddu F et al (2009) Surgical treatment of anal stenosis. World J Gastroenterol 15:1921-1928

Caplin DA, Kodner IJ (1986) Repair of anal stricture and mucosal ectropion by simple flap procedures. Dis Colon Rectum 29:92-94

Casadesus D, Villasana LE, Diaz H et al (2007) Treatment of anal stenosis: a 5-year review. ANZ J Surg 77:557-559

Christensen MA, Pitsch RM Jr, Cali RL et al (1992) "House" advancement pedicle flap for anal stenosis. Dis Colon Rectum 35:201-203

Consten EC, Slors FJ, Noten HJ et al (1995) Anorectal surgery in human immunodeficiency virus-infected patients. Clinical outcome in relation to immune status. Dis Colon Rectum 38:1169-1175

Crawshaw AP, Pigott L, Potter MA et al (2004) A retrospective evaluation of rectal irrigation in the treatment of disorders of faecal continence. Colorectal Dis 6:185-190

Dai Y, Chopra SS, Wysocki WM, Hünerbein M (2010) Treatment of benign colorectal strictures by temporary stenting with self-expanding stents. Int J Colorectal Dis 25:1475-1479

De Toma G, Cavallaro G, Bitonti A et al (2006) Surgical management of perianal giant condyloma acuminatum (Buschke-Löwenstein tumor). Report of three cases. Eur Surg Res 38:418-422

Dindo D, Nocito A, Schettle M et al (2011) What should we do about anal condyloma and anal intraepithelial neoplasia? Results of a survey. Colorect Dis 13:796-801

Duieb Z, Appu S, Hung K, Nguyen H (2010) Anal stenosis: use of an algorithm to provide a tension-free anoplasty. ANZ J Surg 80:337-340

Farid M, Youssef M, El Nakeeb A et al (2010) Comparative study of the house advancement flap, rhomboid flap, and Y-V anoplasty in treatment of anal stenosis: a prospective randomized study. Dis Colon Rectum 53:790-797

Gingold BS, Arvanitis M (1986) Y-V anoplasty for treatment of anal stricture. Surg Gynecol Obstet 162:241-242

Giordano P, Gravante G, Grondona P et al (2009) Simple cutaneous advancement flap anoplasty for resistant chronic anal fissure: a prospective study. World J Surg 33:1058-1063

González AR, de Oliveira O Jr, Verzaro R et al (1995) Anoplasty for stenosis and other anorectal defects. Am Surg 61:526-529

Guan YS, Sun L, Li X, Zheng XH (2004) Successful management of a benign anastomotic colonic stricture with self-expanding metallic stents: a case report. World J Gastroenterol 10:3534-3536

Habr-Gama A, Sobrado CW, de Araújo SE et al (2005) Surgical treatment of anal stenosis: assessment of 77 anoplasties. Clinics 60:17-20

Katdare MV, Ricciardi R (2010) Anal stenosis. Surg Clin North Am 90:137-145

Khawaja HT (1989) Podophyllin versus scissor excision in the treatment of perianal condylomata acuminata: a prospective study. Br J Surg 76:1067-1068

Klaristenfeld D, Israelit S, Beart RW et al (2008) Surgical excision of extensive anal condylomata not associated with risk of anal stenosis. Int J Colorectal Dis 23:853-856

Liberman H, Thorson AG (2000) How I do it. Anal stenosis. Am J Surg 179:325-329

Linares L, Moreira LF, Andrews H et al (1988) Natural history and treatment of anorectal strictures complicating Crohn's disease. Br J Surg 75:653-655

Maria G, Brisinda G, Civello IM (1998) Anoplasty for the treatment of anal stenosis. Am J Surg 175:158-160

Menteş BB, Yavuzer R, Cavuşo lu T et al (2001) Surgical treatment of anal stenosis following perineal shotgun injury. Plast Reconstr Surg 107:891-893

Mestrović T, Cavcić J, Martinac P et al (2003) Reconstruction of skin defects after radical excision of anorectal giant condyloma acuminatum: 6 cases. J Eur Acad Dermatol Venereol 17:541-545

Milsom JW, Mazier WP (1986) Classification and management of postsurgical anal stenosis. Surg Gynecol Obstet 163:60-64

Mistrangelo M, Mobiglia A, Cassoni P et al (2005) Verrucous carcinoma of the anus or Buschke-Löwenstein tumor of the anus: staging and treatment. Report of 3 cases. Suppl Tumori 4:S29-S30

Nadal SR, Manzione CR, Galvao VM et al (1998) Healing after anal fistulotomy: comparative study between HIV+ and HIV- patients. Dis Colon Rectum 41:177-179

Nickell WB, Woodward ER (1972) Advancement flaps for treatment of anal stricture. Arch Surg 104:223-224

Oh C, Zinberg J (1982) Anoplasty for anal stricture. Dis Colon Rectum 25:809-810

Pearl RK, Hooks VH 3rd, Abcarian H et al (1990) Island flap anoplasty for the treatment of anal stricture and mucosal ectropion. Dis Colon Rectum 33:581-583

Pescatori M (2002) Management of post-anopexy rectal stricture. Tech Coloproctol 6:125-126

Pescatori M, Maria G, Anastasio G (1992) Obliterated ileoanal anastomosis managed by intraoperative colonoscopy. Coloproctology 14: 86-88

Pfeifer J, Reissman P, Gonzales A et al (1995) "House" flap procedure for anal stenosis. Technique and results. Tech Coloproctol 3:62-65

Pidala MJ, Slezak FA, Porter JA (1994) Island flap anoplasty for anal canal stenosis and mucosal ectropion. Am Surg 60:194-196

Pizzetti D, Annibali R, Bufo A et al (2005) Colonic hydrotherapy for obstructed defecation. Colorectal Dis 7:107-108

Rakhmanine M, Rosen L, Khubchandani I et al (2002) Lateral mucosal advancement anoplasty for anal stricture. Br J Surg 89:1423-1424

Rees JR, Carney L, Gill TS, Dixon AR (2004) Management of recurrent anastomotic stricture and iatrogenic stenosis by circular stapler. Dis Colon Rectum 47:944-947

Rosen L (1988) Anoplasty. Surg Clin North Am 68:1441-1446

Sakai S, Yoshinaga R (1999) The prepuce flap in the reconstruction of male anal stenosis. Br J Plast Surg 52:660-662

Schlegel RD, Dehni N, Parc R et al (2001) Results of reoperations in colorectal anastomotic strictures. Dis Colon Rectum 44:1464-1468

Thompson JPS, Grace PH (1978) The treatment of perianal and anal condylomata: a new operative technique. Proc R Soc Med 71:180-185

Trombetta LJ, Place RJ (2001) Giant condyloma acuminatum of the anorectum: trends in epidemiology and management: report of a case and review of the literature. Dis Colon Rectum 44:1878-1886

Tsuchiya S, Sakuraba M, Asano T et al (2011) New application of the gluteal-fold flap for the treatment of anorectal stricture. Int J Colorectal Dis 7 epub ahead of print

Uribe N, Millan M, Flores J et al (2004) Excision and V-Y plasty reconstruction for giant condyloma acuminatum. Tech Coloproctol 8:99-101

8 Obstructed Defecation (OD) and Related Diseases

8.1 Introduction

Much has changed in the last three decades, since surgery for rectocele is no longer carried out by gynecologists alone and the term "obstructed defecation" is now well known even among non-specialists. Prior to 1980, only a few surgeons even considered the puborectalis muscle and very few radiologists had performed a defecography. Moreover, in this age of Internet medicine, you might receive a telephone call from a worried patient saying: "Doctor, please help me, I have a rectocele, I spend hours on the toilet and strain all the time!"

As far as rectal internal mucosal prolapse is concerned, its relationship with defecation and its endoscopic/radiologic grading were previously almost unknown. Solitary rectal ulcer syndrome was likely to be interpreted as a neoplasm or colitis, and psychologists were aware of "vaginismus" not "anismus." Thus, progress in knowledge and technology is most welcome, provided it does not result in surgical overtreatment. Indeed, surgery for obstructed defecation is rarely carried out at St. Mark's Hospital, to mention a well-known institution, as was the case 30 years ago.

Professor Phillips, Director of St. Mark's, in his Invited Commentary to the paper of Boccasanta et al. (2004) on the STARR procedure, wrote that for those who think that constipation is mainly a functional disease, to resect the rectum for constipation is like removing a lung from a patient with asthma. Professor Nicholls, at the Educational Meeting of the Italian Society of Colo-Rectal Surgery, held in Rome in 2008, reported that at St. Mark's almost no patients with constipation are treated surgically. At our unit, only 14% of patients with obstructed defecation (OD) undergo surgery (Pescatori et al., 2006). The rest are treated using conservative measures, with satisfactory outcome based on the following findings:

1. As reported in the literature, regardless of the operation, about half of the patients will have persisting or recurrent OD in the long term.
2. Any operation for OD is associated with the risk of postoperative complications. Some of them are severe, such as rectal ischemia following a Delorme procedure or pelvic sepsis after a STARR procedure (references will be quoted).
3. Any surgery for OD may be followed by the need for re-intervention, which is burdensome for the patients and for the hospital.
4. At our unit alternative measures are available as well as expert consultants who are able to treat functional associated disease, as described in the diagram of the "iceberg syndrome" (Fig. 8.1), which we follow when dealing with OD.
5. Conservative treatment is frequently offered to OD patients, such as psychotherapy, pelvic floor rehabilitation, high fiber diet, hydrocolon-lavage, yoga, and hypnosis, all of which have been reported in the literature as effective in over 50% of the patients.
6. Our liaison with industry is not so close that it forces us to use technological innovations instead of other, non-surgical procedures.
7. We are well aware of the financial limitations of public healthcare. In Italy, there are regions where the healthcare budget is low, hospitals are being closed, and doctors and nurses are being dismissed.
8. We know that surgery often restores anatomy but not function, as demonstrated by Vermeulen et al. (2005) and confirmed by Wexner (2005) in a series of patients operated on for rectocele and OD.
9. We are in favor of the holistic approach, which

takes into consideration the whole entity, psyche and body, and not just the affected organ.

10. We believe in the PNEI system, which considers the Psychological, Neurological, Endocrine and Immunological Systems, their relationships, and their feedback with both the large bowel and the pelvic floor. According to the PNEI system, surgery has a limited role in the management of these patients.

There are colleagues, with great expertise but more surgery-inclined, who follow different criteria. Here are three examples: In one year, Boccasanta et al. (2011) operated on 100 patients, out of 150 seen for OD, performing 50 STARR and 50 Transtar procedures. Within a 2-year period, Schwandner (2011) carried out 52 stapled rectal prolapsectomies in his patients with OD. We described this operation in 1997 (Pescatori et al., 1997, www.ucp-club.it/medici_articolo.asp) but have performed it in not more than 25 selected cases in 15 years. Ganio and Trompetto carried out about 150 internal Delormes in OD patients (personal communication), whereas we have performed this procedure in fewer than 10 patients. The long-term outcome of the procedures was not mentioned in any of these three studies (i.e. outcome at over 3 years after surgery). It should also be noted that, unfortunately, there are other colleagues, more often general than colorectal surgeons, who prefer to operate rather than to use conservative measures, even when surgery is not indicated.

The following case involves a 75-year-old woman who was seen in my outpatient clinic. She suffered from severe constipation and had experienced a mild TIA when straining at defecation. She had had three vaginal deliveries, her perianal sensation was impaired, the anal reflex was nearly absent bilaterally, and she had undergone hysterectomy. Therefore, she presumably had a pudendal neuropathy and rectal hyposensation. She was moderately depressed. Defecography showed a non-relaxing puborectalis muscle on straining, a small anterior rectocele, and a modest sigmoidocele. There was no sign of recto-rectal intussusception or rectal internal mucosal prolapse. Large bowel transit was markedly slow at a transit times study with radio-opaque markers. Based on these findings, I would have suggested conservative therapy, e.g., high residue diet, psyllium, bulking laxatives, biofeedback, and maybe hydrocolon lavage; perhaps, in case of failure, a mini-invasive surgical procedure, such as sacral neuromodulation. Instead, another surgeon had proposed a STARR as the first approach, which in my opinion would have been surgical overtreatment.

Here is another example, even more impressive: The patient was a 57-year-old multiparous woman who had undergone seven operations for OD in the last 3 years. Earlier, she had lost a baby; she was divorced, had troubles with her son, and lived alone, but her psychological pattern was never investigated. She complained that she had fragmented evacuation and had to strain, and that defecation was not possible without self-digitations. She also had a dolichosigmoid, but her intestinal transit times were normal. She previously underwent a PPH to excise a rectal internal mucosal prolapse, then an anterior levatorplasty to correct a rectocele, both performed by the same surgeon. Sacral neuromodulation and biofeedback training had also been attempted. Due to worsening symptoms, she underwent a laparoscopic sigmoidectomy. After an episode of intestinal obstruction, the sigmoidorectal anastomosis was dilated, but she still had constipation. A STARR was then carried out, but OD persisted. An enterocele was found by a radiologist, who thought that it was not the cause of symptoms; nevertheless, another surgeon carried out an obliteration of the pouch of Douglas, which was unsuccessful. Finally, the same surgeon constructed a diverting ileostomy. She had a poor quality of life with the stoma and complained of abdominal pain and urinary retention, which prompted her to see another surgeon, who suggested an anterior resection of the rectum.

I examined her in my office and performed both proctoscopy and endoanal/vaginal ultrasound (US), plus the "draw-the-family" psychological test (Miliacca et al., 2010). In addition, rectal capacity and sensation were measured using a latex balloon. She had a non-relaxing puborectalis muscle on straining, the rectal capacity was markedly decreased; she had a diversion proctitis, and was anxious and depressed. Her anal canal was short; she had a cystocele, an injured internal sphincter, a recto-rectal intussusception, and an internal rectal mucosal prolapse with a post-STARR (ear-pocket) rectal diverticulum. Thus, there were a number of functional and organic lesions typical of the "iceberg syndrome" (Fig. 8.1).

In my opinion, both sigmoidectomy and enterocele repair could well have been avoided in this patient. The levatorplasty and the STARR caused predictable damage. Moreover, an anterior resection most likely caused the fecal incontinence. Sadly, five of the above-mentioned operations had been performed by colorectal surgeons. My approach is to be more conservative, as are the colorectal surgeons at the Mayo Clinic, the Cleveland Clinic, and Minnesota University. This does not imply that I am overly cautious, as the ten above-listed criteria followed by all members of my unit may be considered a modern and wise approach to large bowel and pelvic floor diseases.

In any case, pragmatism is called for. If we are willing to carry out colorectal surgery effectively and safely, we should also be able to prevent and treat the postoperative complications, and, if at all possible, without re-intervention, which often is unsuccessful. This has certainly been our experience when dealing with re-intervention after a failed or complicated STARR procedure. The case reported at the end of this chapter, in "Two Unforgettable Complications", confirms this statement.

Two-thirds of patients with OD, most of them females, are anxious and/or depressed, as reported in a prospective study carried out at our unit (Pescatori et al., 2006). Since the 1980s, we have known that an altered psychological pattern is a negative predictor after colectomy and ileorectal anastomosis for severe chronic constipation (Yoshioka and Keighley). We published a series of 46 patients who had surgery for severe constipation (Coloproctology, 1993); 16 of them were operated upon for OD, seven of whom had an altered mental pattern, either anxiety or depression or hysteria, as shown by our psychologist. Nonetheless, after 20 years, only a few surgeons offer their constipated patients a psychological consultation prior to surgery.

We obtained similar findings in our patients who had transanal prolapsectomy for rectal internal mucosal prolapse and OD (Pescatori et al., 2006). After 3 years, nearly 80% of those with psychological distress prior to surgery were still constipated, compared with nearly 25% of those who had a normal psychological pattern. Of those who were re-operated on for persisting OD after failed STARR, nearly half had recurrent symptoms: all but one were either anxious or depressed prior to the re-intervention. Again, mental distress was a negative predictor in these patients (Pescatori and Zbar, 2009).

Therefore, we are in a minefield when dealing with complex patients, whose symptoms often have a psychosomatic etiology and require a holistic approach. The best way to avoid complications and failures in such patients is not to operate on

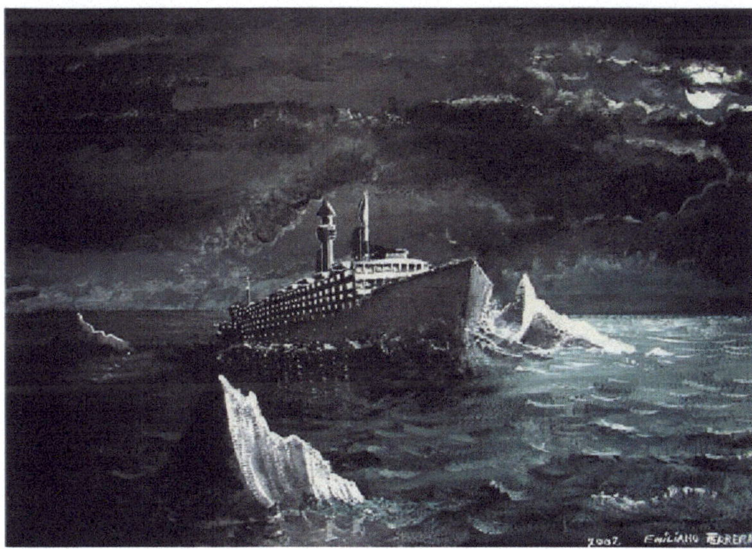

Fig. 8.1 a The "surgical ship" (equipped with stapler and scalpel) can be wrecked by the submerged rocks of an iceberg, i.e. occult functional and organic diseases such as anismus, rectal hypotension and enterocele (drawing by E. Ferrera)

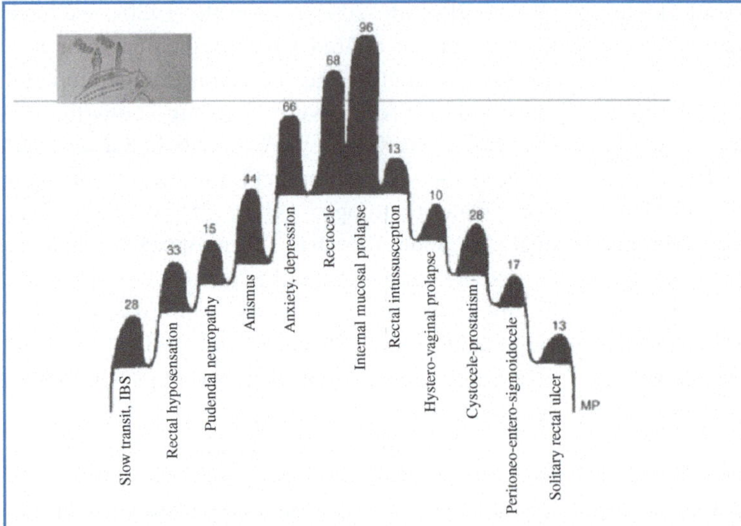

Fig. 8.1 b The hidden problems, often responsible for symptoms in patients with obstructed defecation, can be compared to the submerged, very dangerous portions of an iceberg (modified from Pescatori et al., 2006)

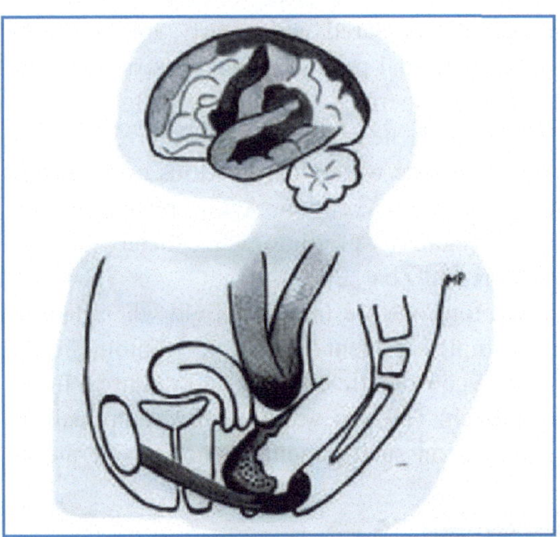

Fig. 8.2 Relationships between the psyche and morphofunctional alterations of the pelvis and perineum are typical in patients with obstructed defecation. These relationships are often undiscovered (also because surgeons are unlikely to look for them). *Bottom*: enterocele, internal mucosal prolapse of the rectum, and paradoxical contraction of the puborectalis muscle. Two-thirds of patients with obstructed defecation have an altered psychological pattern, which is also a negative predictive factor of surgery outcome

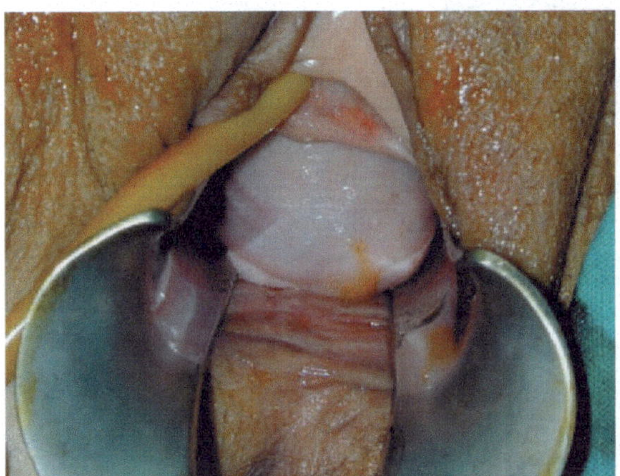

Fig. 8.3 a Bulky rectocele visible through the vagina

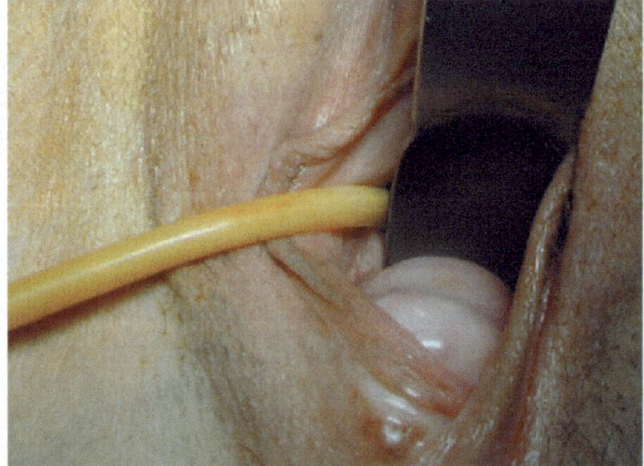

Fig. 8.3 b On inserting a retractor and asking the patient to push the doubled bulk of the rectocele is apparent. Above the rectocele (evident lesion) there is an enterocele (occult lesion)

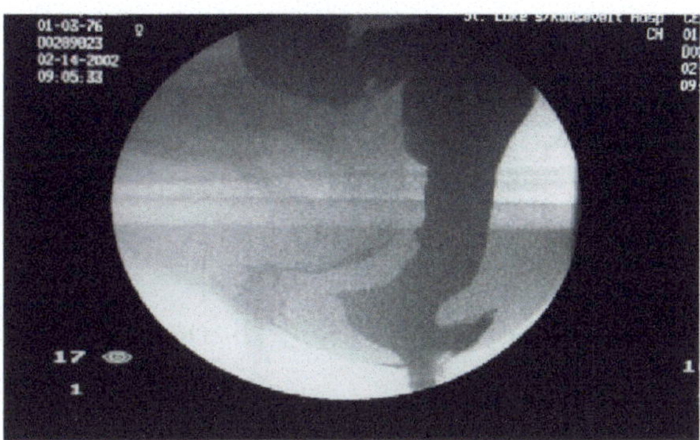

Fig. 8.3 c Defecography from the same patient shows the anterior rectocele and a certain grade of rectoanal intussusception. Consistent with the iceberg scheme, there are, apart from the evident disease (rectocele), two hidden lesions (enterocele and intussusception). Such lesions are revealed by instrumental maneuvers or other tests

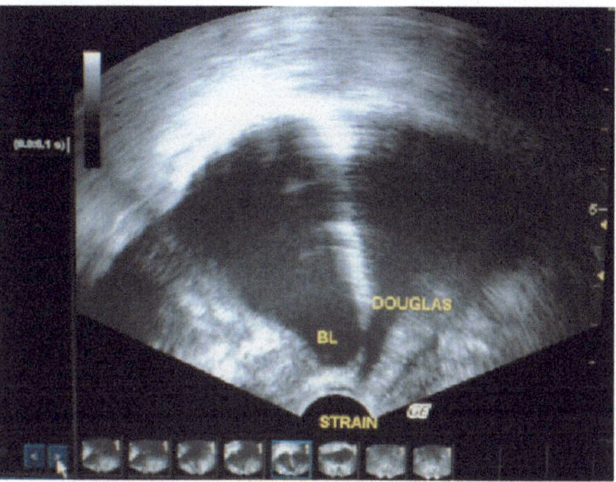

Fig. 8.3 d Dynamic perineal ultrasonography in a patient with an enterocele. On straining, the pouch of Douglas moves downwards between the vagina and anal canal

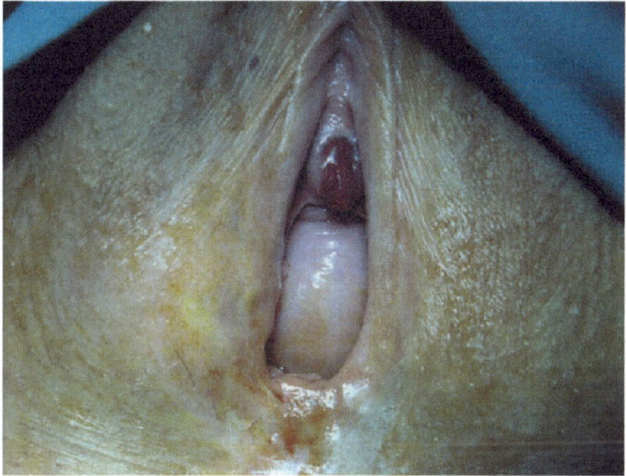

Fig. 8.3 e Urethrocele and cystocele: urologic problems such as these are frequent in patients with OD

them at all. However, surgery might be useful in a minority, perhaps 10-20%, and some of these patients will insist on surgery. This has been my experience in a few cases, which are presented further on, together with the literature's view on postoperative complications after surgery for OD.

I should first mention that I refer to OD as the "iceberg syndrome," since much of what afflicts these patients is difficult to see and may ultimately "sink the surgical ship." The largely visible aspects, i.e. rectocele and mucosal prolapse, which are usually the targets of surgery, are more likely to be the effects rather than the causes of excessive and prolonged straining. Only in the advanced stage of these diseases they may become non-causes, with the main obstacle being occult functional disorders, not curable by surgical means.

Figure 8.1b serves as a reminder to me of the difficulties in dealing with patients with OD and I hope that you also find it instructive.

8.2 Our Relevant Complications Following Surgery for Obstructed Defecation

Table 8.1 lists the relevant postoperative complications, i.e., those requiring re-admission, re-operation, or a prolonged stay in the hospital, which occurred in patients who were operated on for OD at our unit in the last few decades. The data are based on a paper we published in 2009 (Pescatori et al.), which included a meta-analysis of the literature.

It should be noted that all of our patients who were re-operated upon for recto-rectal intussusception suffered from either anxiety, depression, or both, as discussed in the Introduction to this chapter. One case of temporary mild hemospermia after manual transanal excision of second-degree rectal internal mucosal prolapse occurred recently and is not listed in Table 8.1. In this patient, I used a slightly different technique: diathermy of the prolapsed mucosa clamped with Kelly forceps. The mucosal stump was then sutured over the Kelly. A

Table 8.1 Complications and re-interventions after surgery for OD in 183 patients operated on via the transanal or transperineal route, from a total of 283 patients surgically managed for OD at our unit between 1988 and 2007

Diagnosis	Technique	(n)	Complication	(n)	Treatment	(n)	Outcome
Rectocele	Block	(49)	R-V granuloma Ischemic colitis	(1) (1)	Excision & stoma L. hemicolectomy		OD I
Rectocele	Sarles	(27)	Pelvic sepsis Rectal stricture Incontinence	(1) (2) (1)	Diverting stoma Dilation Bulking agents	 (2) 	C I I
Rectocele	Levatorplasty	(20)	Perineal sepsis	(2)	Drainage	(2)	OD, C
Rectocele	R-V mesh	(1)		0			
Recto-rectal intussusception	Delorme	(8)	Suture dehiscence Rectal stricture	(1) (1)	TPN Dilation		I C
Recto-anal intussusception	Manual mucosectomy	(13)	Rectal stricture Bleeding	(2) (2)	Dilation Suture		C C
Recto-anal intussusception	Stapled mucosectomy	(23)	Bleeding Rectal stricture	(1) (2)	Suture Dilatation	PPH (1) (1)	C G
Recto-anal intussusception	Cauterization plication	(4)	Bleeding	(1)	Suture		OD
Recto-anal intussusception	STARR	(1)	Bleeding	(1)	Suture		OD
Rectal internal mucosal prolapse	Manual mucosectomy Obliterative suture	(13) (3)	Bleeding	(3) 0	Tamponade		C
Solitary rectal ulcer syndrome	Manual mucosectomy	(7)		0			
Solitary rectal ulcer syndrome	Altemeier	(1)		0			
Rectocele after STARR	Cauterization-plication	(1)		0			
Rectocele after STARR	Levatorplasty	(2)		0			
Proctalgia after STARR	Agrapphectomy-anoplasty	(2)		0			
Mucosal prolapse and R-V fistula after STARR	Levatorplasty	(1)	Dehiscence-bleeding		Diverting stoma		OD
Recto-rectal Intussusception after STARR	Sarles	(5)	Dehiscence Pelvic sepsis	(1) (1)	Re-suture Stoma		Lost to follow-up Lost to follow-up

C, cured; *F-U*, follow-up; *I*, improved; *OD*, persistence of obstructed defecation; *RVF*, recto-vaginal fistula; *TPN*, total parenteral nutrition.

small area of fibrosis very close to the intact prostate capsule was detected at prostatic US carried out postoperatively, as shown in Figure 8.4. Hemospermia lasted only 4 days following prolapsectomy. Clearly, a small local surgical trauma had occurred.

However, just five out of 26 patients with relevant postoperative complications had severe problems, as shown in Table 8.1, which reports a specialist's experience. Surgeons not trained in surgery of the anorectum and pelvic floor might have more complications, as suggested by Binda et al. (2005).

Rectal bleeding, suture dehiscence, and anorectal stricture were the most frequent complications. Bleeding may be controlled by means of a Foley catheter balloon, as reported in patients with posthemorrhoidectomy bleeding, but the procedure

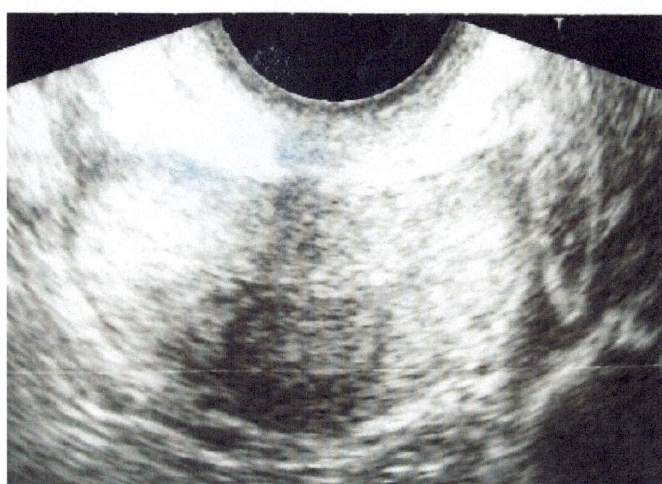

Fig. 8.4 Transitory hemospermia after endoanal excision of a rectal internal mucosal prolapse in patient with obstructed defecation. The hyperechogenic area of the anorectum, adjacent to the prostatic capsule, is suggestive of postoperative fibrosis and small local trauma. Hemospermia continued for a few days and then spontaneously subsided

does not work in most cases, as the source of hemorrhage is in the lower rectum and not in the upper anal canal or at the level of the anorectal ring, i.e., higher than after hemorrhoidectomy. Suturing of the bleeding area is often required, as happened in five out of six cases.

Suture dehiscence may also occur, either circumferential, as in case of internal Delorme, or linear, as after Block and mucosal stripping, or double, as following STARR. Suture breakdown affecting more than 25% of the circular or curved suture is likely to be followed by a significant rectal stricture.

8.3 Postoperative Complications After Internal Delorme

The most troublesome complication is a wide anastomotic breakdown following an internal Delorme in a patient with a clinical history of straining at stools and with weak anal sphincters who is operated upon for either recto-rectal or recto-anal intussuception. In this case, the rectal mucosa may be displaced 3-4 cm upwards, and a significant stricture may be found at digital exploration with a small denuded rectal cylinder.

The patient may complain of fecal incontinence, proctalgia, tenesmus, urgency, and OD due to the stricture, and may present with rectal bleeding. I have seen three such patients, one male and two females. Dilation was carried out in all cases, but was effective only in one. Re-suturing was attempted twice with no success, due to the excessive tension. A diverting sigmoidostomy was needed in one patient who developed pelvic sepsis following an anterior Delorme; the stoma was subsequently closed in another hospital.

This is the reason why I have performed not more than ten internal Delormes in three decades. Other surgeons used to carry out this procedure more frequently, as reported in the Introduction. While an internal Delorme may be anatomically successful, a report of long-term functional results is still lacking (Fig. 8.5).

Let me report how to deal with postoperative perianastomotic sepsis, a not infrequent, apparently trivial, but somewhat occult and intriguing mild complication, which followed my last internal Delorme. If not adequately and timely managed, it was likely to cause a pelvic abscess with severe clinical consequences. This 43 year-old constipated primiparous female developed symptoms of obstructed defecation three years after prolonged straining, suggested by her gynecologist following her delivery, aimed at facilitating evacuation. She then developed a recto-rectal and recto-anal intussusceptions with wide rectocele, all seen at defecography, facilitated by the delivery itself, the weight loss and the repeated straining at stool.

She had a Delorme-Rehn procedure performed at our unit, with mechanical preparation and antiobiotic prophylaxis, Metronidazole and Kefalosporine. She also suffered from spastic colon and internal

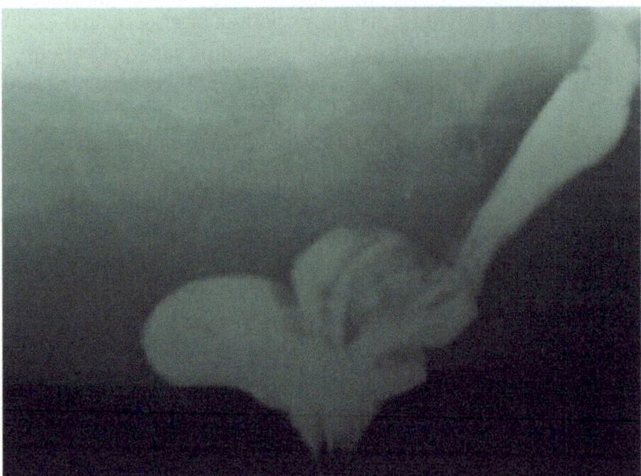

Fig. 8.5 a Defecography from a patient with obstructed defecation due to rectocele and rectal intussusception

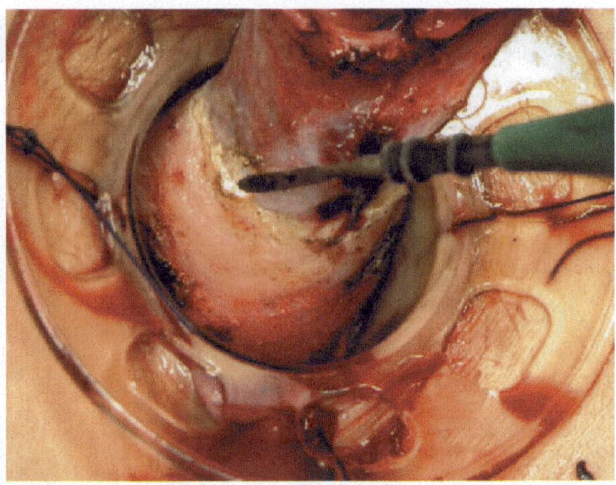

Fig. 8.5 b Internal Delorme's operation: transanal prolapsectomy

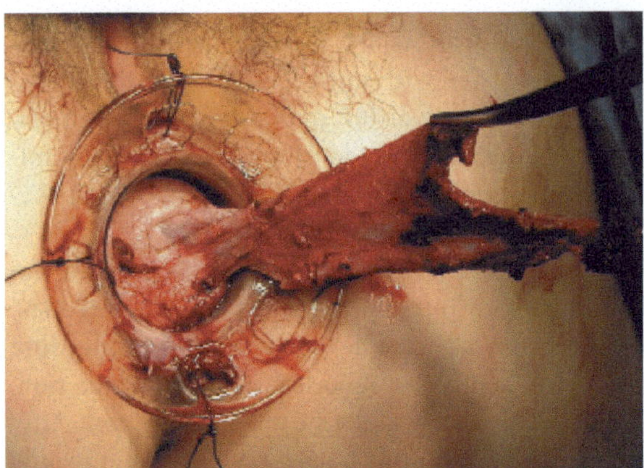

Fig. 8.5 c The mucosal excision is completed; the whitish rectal muscle fibers are seen

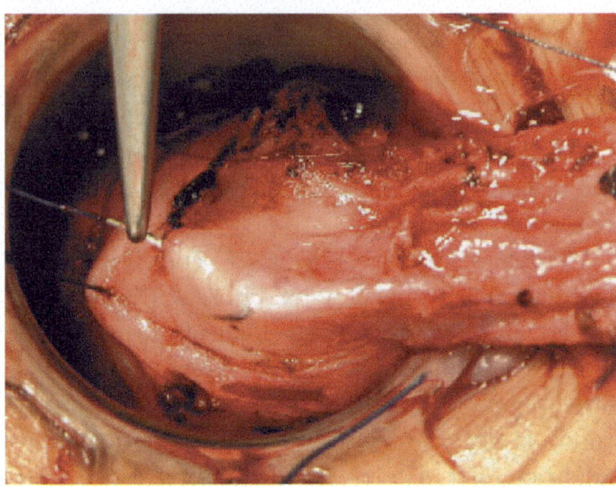

Fig. 8.5 d Plication of the muscle layer

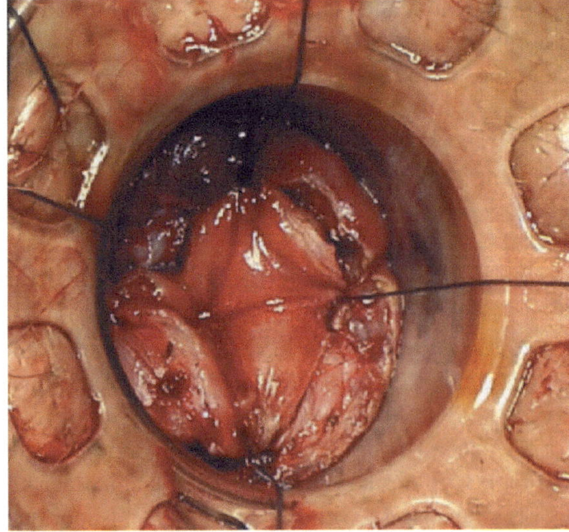

Fig. 8.5 e First suture stitches between rectum and anal canal

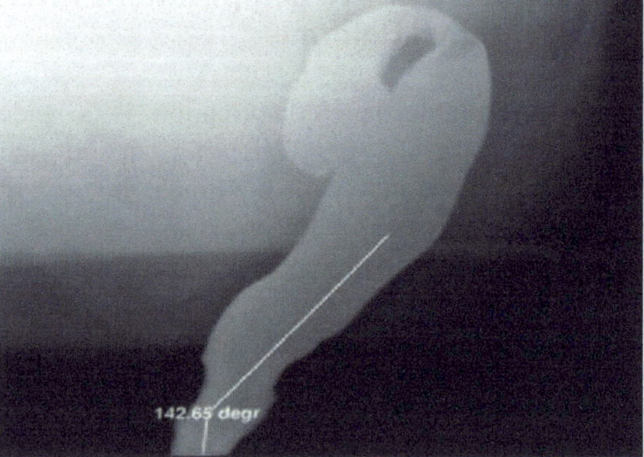

Fig. 8.5 f Postoperative defecography shows the correction of the previous defects. Bleeding, dehiscence, and stenosis are reported following this operation. Anal incontinence can occur because the rectal reservoir is reduced. Postoperative complications are not frequent (from Trompetto et al., 2006)

sphincter hypertonia, possibly due to frequent gymnic exercises. From a psychological point of view, she was rather anxious, strongly fighted against her parents during childhood, and suffered for both the loss of the husband and the mother, when she was over thirty. Then she had a baby with a fiancée, who left them before the delivery. Therefore, as any case of obstructed defecation seen bearing in mind the iceberg diagram, she had, apart the prolapse and the rectocele, several occult both muscular and psychological disorders. The operation went well and was followed by an eventful early postoperative course. Figures 8.6 and 8.7 show the dynamics of her subse-

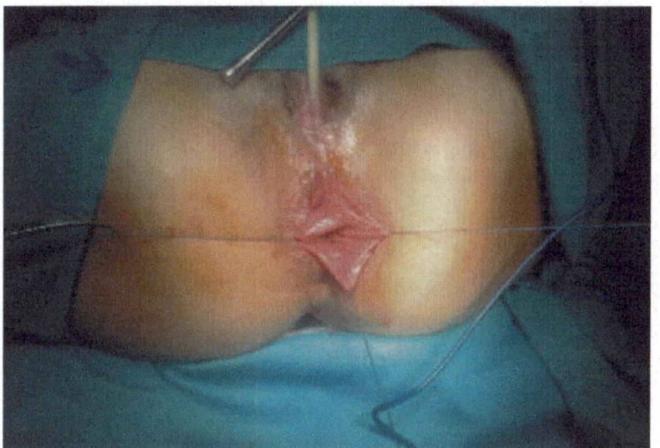

Fig. 8.6 a The patient, a 43 year-old female, had a Delorme procedure with anterior levatorplasty for obstructed defecation related to recto-rectal, recto-anal intussusception and rectocele. The patient is in the lithotomy position and the rectal mucosal prolapse is shown in the first picture

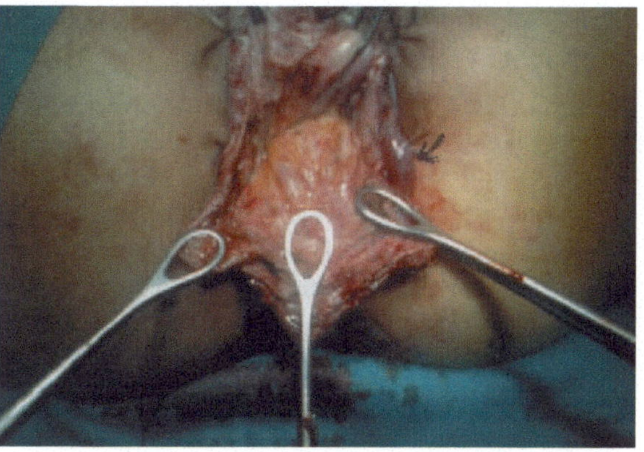

Fig. 8.6 b Transanal rectal prolapsectomy. The whitish rectal muscle is grasped with forceps in the upper part of the figure

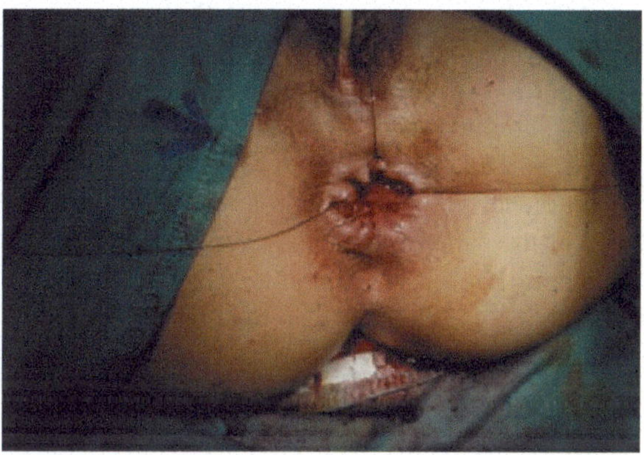

Fig. 8.6 c Recto-anal anastomosis. The suture is almost completed

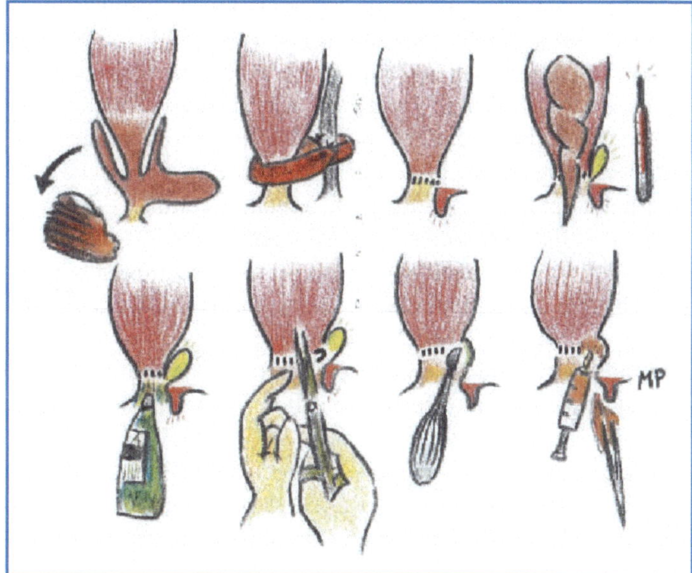

Fig. 8.7 Etiology and management of perianastomotic sepsis in the same patient of Fig. 8.6. *Top figures, from left to right*: the originally diseased rectum with intussusception and wide rectocele; transanal rectal prolapsectomy, recto-anal anastomosis and anterior levatorplasty; early detection of an edematous and painful skin tag, with an intact anastomosis, on postoperative day 3; when the patient evacuated he had fever (38°C), vomiting and rectal pain. *Bottom figures, from left to right*: an anterior supra-anastomotic abscess was then suspected and palpated on digital exploration, calcium-antagonist ointment with local analgesic (Antrolin, Bracco) was used to relax the hypertonic internal sphincter and reduce pain; the corresponding stitch was removed by cutting it on the guide of the finger; once the stitch was released, the infected fluid came out of the pocket, which was then gently curetted; irrigation with Betadine followed by the positioning of a gauze into the pocket. The endoanal wound healed after two weeks

quent complications. The steps are underlined in details in the captions.

Everything ended well, but, if not dealt with on time at the patient's bedside in postoperative day 6, the mild complication would have turned to a more severe one, requiring a formal re-operation.

The management of post-dehiscence rectal strictures was described in Chap. 7. Among other procedures, a TEM rectoplasty may be carried out.

In the book Rectal Prolapse, edited by Altomare and Pucciani and published by Springer-Verlag Italy in 2008, Ganio and Giani reported the postoperative complications occurring in 53 cases of internal Delorme. Anastomotic dehiscences were seen in 9.4% of the patients, more than one-third of whom required re-operation for rectal stricture. A case of hematoma of the rectovaginal septum was also reported. Half of the patients complained of fecal urgency 2 weeks after surgery. This symptom was still present in 7.5% after 1 month but disappeared after 6 months. Instead, fecal urgency was still present after 3 years in one-third of the patients who had undergone a STARR procedure (Boccasanta et al., 2011), presumably because the double-stapled rectotomy affected the compliance of the rectal reservoir more severely than did the Delorme. STARR, by excising two segments of the rectal wall, is likely to damage the local innervation and affect the adaptation reflex that allows postponement of the need to pass stool.

Table 8.2 Transanal and transperineal surgical procedures used for the management of rectocele and rectal internal mucosal prolapse

Transanal route
1. Obliterative suture of the rectocele and the mucosal prolapse, according to Block (Fig. 8.8)
2. Anterior mucosectomy and rectal muscle plication, according to Sarles (Fig. 8.9)
3. Rectocele repair according to Khubchandani
4. Rectocele repair according to Sullivan
5. Rectal mucosectomy and muscle plication according to Delorme-Rehn
6. Rectal circular stapled mucosectomy or PPH
7. Double stapled rectal resection or STARR
8. Rectocele and mucosal prolapse resection using an endoGIA
Transperineal route
1. Anterior levatorplasty
2. Rectocele repair with the interposition of a non-reabsorbable mesh (polypropylene)
3. Rectocele repair with the interposition of a reabsorbable mesh (Permacol or Surgisis)
4. Rectocele repair with fascia lata interposition
5. Resection and plasty with Goretex interposition
6. Resection and plasty with Permacol interposition (trans-perineal EXPRESS)

8.4 Anal Incontinence Following Surgery for Rectocele and Rectal Internal Mucosal Prolapse

The most frequently used surgical procedures for the management of rectocele and rectal internal mucosal prolapse, which affects the majority of patients with rectocele, are listed in Table 8.2.

For further details, the reader is referred to the review by Zbar et al. (2003).

We retrospectively reviewed and published our experience with rectocele repair (Ayabaca et al., 2006). Postoperative new-onset anal incontinence occurred in 5% of the patients after Block, Sarles, and anterior levatorplasty procedures.

Different findings were reported by others, e.g., Boccasanta et al. (2006), with two out of ten patients complaining of anal incontinence and fecal urgency after STARR carried out for OD. Among the possible causes, we might consider damage to the sphincters, stretched by both the stapler and the 36 mm wide CAD. However, this is not convincing, as a larger device is introduced transanally in other procedures, e.g., in TEM, and, as reported in Chap. 6, this procedure is unlikely to be followed by fecal incontinence. Instead, the main cause of post-STARR incontinence and urgency is more likely to be a reduction of the rectal reservoir, due to the rectal resection, with a partial impairment of its storage function.

As mentioned in the previous section, a similar complication may occur following an internal Delorme, which is more appropriate for the management of recto-rectal or recto-anal intussusception than of rectocele and may cause postoperative incontinence in 29% to 33% of the patients after 36 and 43 months, respectively (Berman et al., 1990, Liberman et al., 2000). However, it should be noted that some of these patients suffered from anal incontinence prior to surgery, as most were

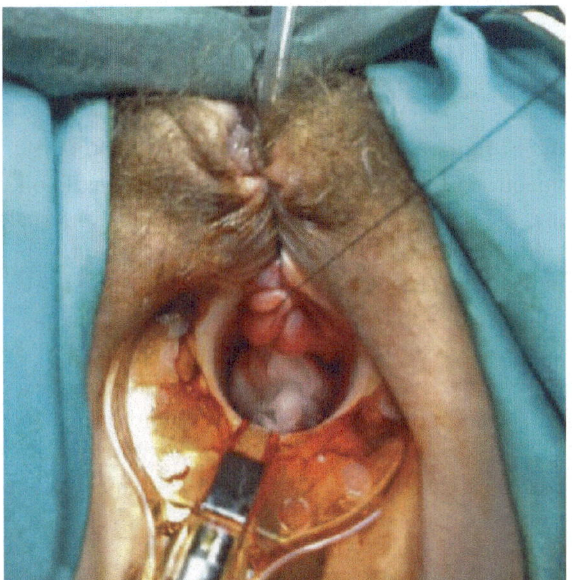

Fig. 8.8 Obstructed defecation surgery: Block's operation. The patient is in the lithotomy position. Final stage of transanal suturing of a rectocele and concomitant internal mucosal rectal prolapse. Out of about 60 such operations, the author had two important complications, of which one was surgically related: an ischemic colitis that required a left colectomy, and a granuloma of the rectovaginal septum that caused severe proctalgia and was surgically removed. Less than 5% of these patients have new onset anal incontinence following rectocele repair at our unit

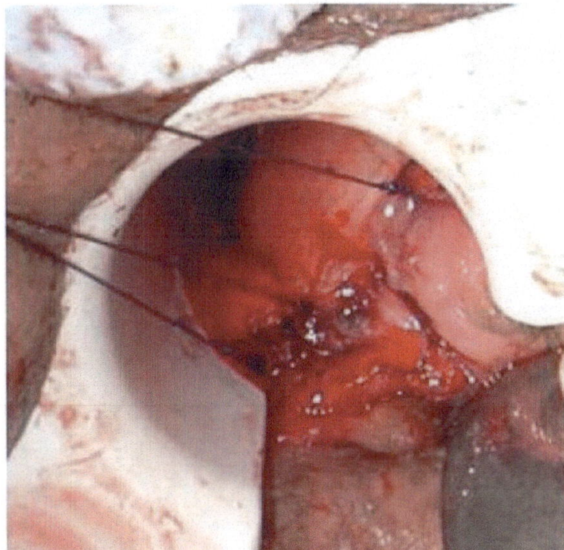

Fig. 8.9 Sarles's rectocele repair, a type of anterior hemi-Delorme. The patient is in the lithotomy position after anterior prolapsectomy and rectal muscle plication. Suturing between the middle rectum and anal canal

multiparous females with perineal descent, worsened by chronic straining.

Using a tailored approach in our patients, the rate of postoperative anal incontinence 3 years after manual and stapled prolapsectomy for OD and rectal intussusception with or without rectocele was only 10.6%.

Besides the rates cited in the papers of Boccasanta (2004, 2011), rates of fecal incontinence after STARR of 3 and 19% were reported in the 2008 review of Pescatori and Gagliardi. Better results have been achieved using the Transtar with the new Contour stapler, as new-onset incontinence was only 5% (Lenisa et al., 2009). A somewhat worse result was reported in another study, comparing STARR and Transtar: 20% using the former, 15% with the latter (Wadhawan et al., 2010).

8.5 The Prevention of Postoperative Incontinence

It is better not to operate on patients at risk for anal incontinence, i.e., elderly multiparous women, as they are likely to have both rectal hyposensation, easily detectable by simply inflating a latex balloon and recording the sensory thresholds, and pudendal neuropathy, which is more difficult to diagnose, as a more sophisticated EMG study measuring the nerve terminal motor latency is required. Both the damaged rectum, which does not allow sensation of the need to pass stool, and the damaged nerve, which does not allow squeezing of the sphincters, are responsible for anal incontinence. Moreover, nearly all the procedures mentioned thus far (some more, such as the STARR, some less, such as the Delorme) reduce the volume of the rectal reservoir and require sphincter dilation, more prolonged in the case of internal Delorme. The type of anal dilator used may make the difference: Schouten and coworkers reported incontinence in their patients after prolonged use of the Parks retractor. Seow-Choen's group found lesions of the internal sphincter at anal US after using the CAD of the PPH (as described in Chap. 2). The internal sphincter may also be damaged by inadvertently dividing some of the fibers of its upper portion when either a Delorme or a Sarles mucosectomy, which starts just above the dentate line, is performed.

Moreover, when performing a mucosectomy (Delorme) or a rectotomy (STARR), we alter the shape of the rectum, from an "hourglass", partially obstructed by the internal folding due to the intussusception but still elastic and with intact intrinsic nerves, to a more rigid and less compliant "tube". This might well cause urgency and loss of feces, as the integrity of the rectal reservoir is important for anal continence.

Therefore, these operations may be less appropriate in patients with anxiety and irritable bowel syndrome, who have increased smooth muscle tone and rectal sensation, as reported by Schwandner (2011) in a paper on the "conversion rate" of PPH and STARR. A tight anus may contraindicate an anal stapling procedure.

8.6 The Treatment of Postoperative Incontinence

According to Spyrou and De Nardi (2005), the injection of bulking agents may be effective if soiling is due to a localized lesion of the internal sphincter (Fig. 8.10). A sphincteroplasty may be indicated in case of more extended damage of the sphincters, which is unlikely to occur after a perineal operation for OD.

When the cause of incontinence is altered rectal sensation, transanal electrostimulation may be helpful, provided that retained staples are not emerging through the rectal mucosa, which might cause local burning due to the stimulating

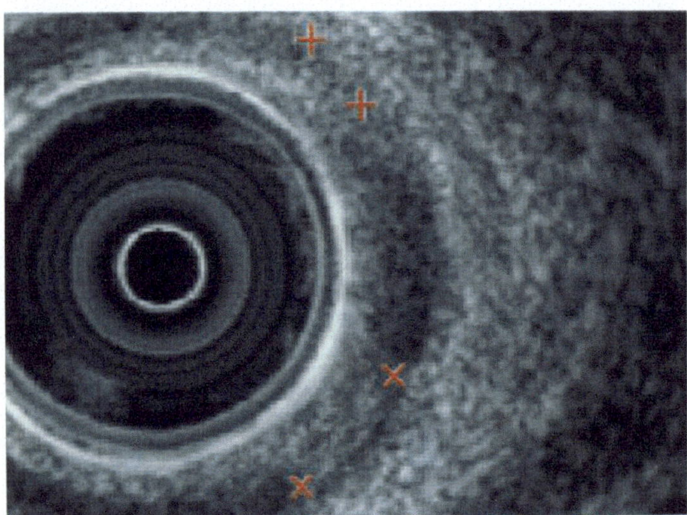

Fig. 8.10 a Partial anal incontinence after STARR because of internal sphincter lesions. Transanal ultrasonography shows two interruptions of the hypoechogenic ring. The patient is in the left lateral position

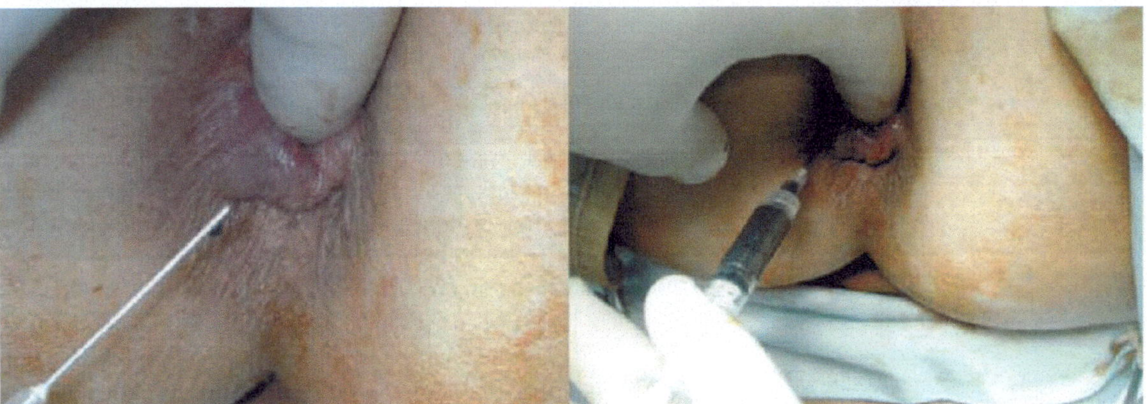

Fig. 8.10 b A needle was perianally inserted to inject a bulking agent (Durasphere) to treat incontinence (from Spyrou and De Nardi, 2005)

endoanal probe. Sacral neuromodulation may also work.

Biofeedback may be carried out in patients with sphincter weakness (Lacima et al., 2010), but the endoanal probe may cause discomfort or pain in case of rectal granulomata. Alternatively, transcutaneous electrostimulation of the posterior tibial nerve may be used (Eléouet et al., 2010).

8.7 Postoperative Complications After STARR and Transtar

Complications occurred in 30% of the 122 patients who underwent these procedures at the Colorectal Clinic of Orlando (Bahna et al., 2010). They merit a separate section in this chapter because some were unusual, since this is a relatively new technique. However, it is first necessary to briefly mention the relationship between the recurrence of OD after STARR and both the learning curve and follow-up.

De Bahna's group had a 50% recurrence rate in their early cases and 9-20% in their later cases. Madbouly et al. (2010) reported a 6% recurrence rate at 18 months, 22% at 36 months, and 35% at 42 months. As mentioned in the Introduction, patients with this disease typically worsen over time, regardless of the surgical technique used to treat them. This may be because of hidden causes, probably not addressed by the operation, which affect the patient's clinical condition and are part of the so called "iceberg syndrome."

Transtar, as its name implies, was developed from STARR and involves a new suturing device, the Contour stapler (Ethicon Endosurgery), instead of the stapler used in PPH. This should be a sign of progress, and the procedure does in fact allow more gradual, more controlled, and less "blind" resection. Nevertheless, severe complications after Contour Transtar have been reported, for instance a very large retrorectal hematoma that required a re-intervention (Gelos et al., 2010). However, the occurrence of postoperative complications is, to some extent, unavoidable.

Some recent trials (like that of Shorthouse's group; Wadhawan et al., 2010) did not show any significant improvements of Transtar compared to STARR. In particular, in 27 patients these British authors observed major rectal bleeding after Transtar due to stapler malfunction. Significant rectal bleeding was also described by Dodi et al. (2003) after STARR.

In the Shorthouse study, only one patient had urinary retention after STARR while 11% had postoperative pain. Defecation urgency was reported by 44% (this is important as it is linked to defects in the rectal reservoir, as mentioned earlier). The percentage of postoperative anal incontinence was notable: 15% new-onset incontinence after Transtar and 20% after STARR.

Moving on to Italian authors and STARR, a multicenter SICCR study by Gagliardi et al. (2008) reported a few cases of postoperative rectovaginal fistulae, a complication also observed by Bassi et al (2006), by us (Pescatori et al., 2006), and by Naldini (2011). Let's find out why.

When operating on a patient with rectocele, especially a large rectocele, one observes that anteriorly, above the anorectal ring, the musculature of the rectum gradually becomes thinner until it disappears (this is clearly visible in a Sarles-type or anterior hemi-Delorme procedure). There is a significant displacement of the muscles, which are pushed to each side by the rectocele in the center. In this stretch of the rectum, which can be several centimeters long, the distance between the rectal mucosa and the vaginal mucosa is minimal, so that the trauma, compression, and ischemia resulting from dissection and suturing can provoke damage (Fig. 8.11). This often becomes evident not immediately but further along, in the postoperative period, and results in tissue loss and formation of a fistula between the rectum and the vagina. If the procedure is performed manually, these structures are readily visible and damage to them easily avoided. With a stapler, without direct vision of the area being dissected and sutured, the risks are higher.

Sciaudone et al. (2008) reported the formation of a rectal diverticulum after STARR that had to be removed via transanal resection.

There are also life-threatening complications necessitating major re-operations, usually including stoma construction. These complications can also occur after other operations.

In a patient treated with a Sarles procedure, I had to construct a sigmoidostomy, which was later closed, because of pelvic sepsis. Another case of pelvis sepsis, which was unfortunately fatal, was

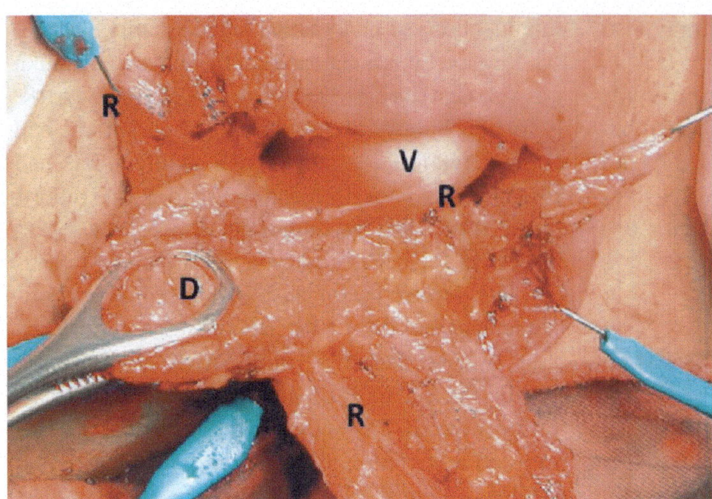

Fig. 8.11 The photo was taken during a Sarles's procedure for rectocele and rectal internal mucosal prolapse in a patient with obstructed defecation. It shows the high-risk area between rectum (*R*), vagina (*V*), and pouch of Douglas (*D*), which may contain an elytrocele and an enterocele. In patients with severe rectocele, the muscularis propria of the distal rectum can be anteriorly displaced and the rectal lumen shifted very near to the vagina. Without direct vision of the sutures, as occurs using the endoanal stapler in a STARR operation, recto-vaginal fistulae may occur (modified from Pescatori et al., 2006)

reported by Gagliardi et al after STARR (2007). Stolfi et al. (2009), described a case of retroperitoneal sepsis with pneumomediastinum after a STARR procedure. Treatment consisted of retroperitoneal drainage and a sigmoidostomy. Complications after STARR and the data regarding their frequency were described by Pescatori and Gagliardi in a review article (2008).

Considering these severe complications, it is difficult to agree with Lehur (in Altomare and Pucciani, 2008), that "STARR is a technically safe and minimally invasive procedure". Surgeons who perform the procedure and patients who are treated with it must be well aware of the risks involved. Web sites (e.g., www.emorroidiestipsi.com) that deny the existence of complications after STARR are not helpful. Indeed, the procedure is actually potentially dangerous, therefore the company that produces the Contour stapler used in Transtar trains and certifies surgeons at its center in Germany. A consensus paper on STARR (Corman et al., 2006) was published, in which well-known specialists established the indications and contraindications for the procedure, and concluded by stating that STARR should only be performed by colorectal surgeons. While these efforts were highly praiseworthy, this recommendation is not always followed.

Schwandner (2011) reported that in 5% of patients undergoing STARR and 11% undergoing Transtar, it was necessary to convert to a manual technique because of proctitis, fistula, or the impossibility of introducing the instrument, due to the conformation of the perineum. Another of the expert recommendations in the consensus paper was that STARR should not be performed in a patient with a large enterocele because the prolapsed pouch of Douglas together with a loop of the ileum might end up in the stapler. In fact, as Carriero et al. suggested (2010), if an enterocele is present a combined transanal and laparoscopic approach should be used. Instead, according to Reibetanz et al. (2011), enterocele is not a contraindication to STARR.

The European STARR Registry is an interesting initiative that has been excellently organized and has published various reports. According to the report presented by two coordinators of the Coloproctology Units of the Italian Society of Colo-Rectal Surgery involved in the Registry, at the Annual Meeting (Chianciano Terme, Italy), in May 2008, a financial contribution is provided to surgeons of the Registry who perform STARR procedures, based on the number of patients who are treated and followed. It would be wonderful if the same thing was done in Italy by public institutions, but instead cuts are being made in funding for research.

To return to the theme of this book, the complications described in the most recent multicenter study on Transtar (Lenisa et al., 2009) are presented below.

Seventy-five patients were studied. In one out of ten, there were intraoperative complications, such as partial dehiscence of a rectal anastomosis which

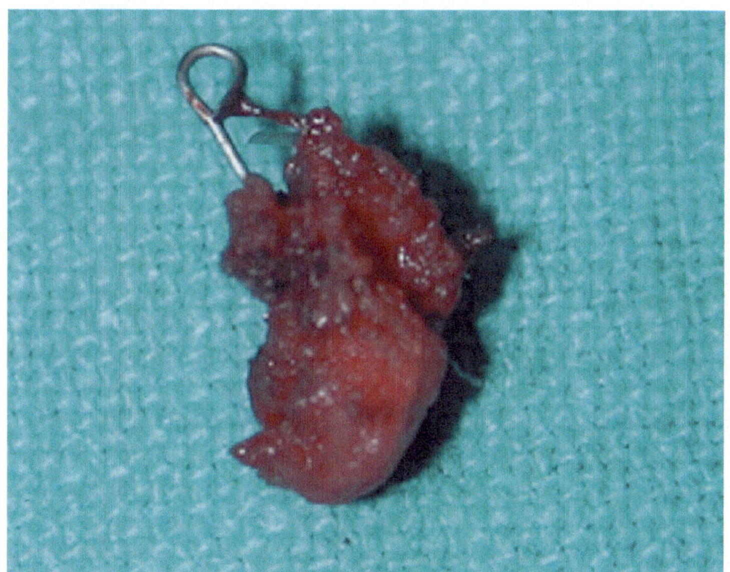

Fig. 8.12 Puborectalis muscle fragment in a woman who was re-operated on after STARR because of severe chronic proctalgia. The staple on the muscle is the possible cause of the pain, because of the permanent stimulus of the nerve endings (from De Nardi et al., 2007)

required manual suturing. This is reminiscent of an article by Arroyo et al. (2008), in another multicenter study, but involving traditional STARR. The authors reported a 50% incidence rate of intraoperative hemorrhage. This was not problematic, simply requiring a little more time to perform manual suturing, as in the case of Lenisa et al. (2009).

An English multicenter study by Knight et al. on PPH for hemorrhoids also reported that supplementary suturing was required, in half of the cases in fact. Still, it is better that suturing be done during the procedure than after surgery when the patient has severe rectal bleeding.

The most important thing to consider is that postoperative hemorrhage after Transtar is not as frequent. According to Lenisa et al. (2009), the incidence of postoperative bleeding is 5.4%. While not exactly a small number, it is acceptable. The staples can end up on the highly innervated puborectalis muscle, as demonstrated by De Nardi et al. (2007) (Fig. 8.12), which leads us to reflect on one of the main problems patients have after STARR: chronic proctalgia.

Severe chronic proctalgia can have a very negative effect on the quality of life. It affects two out of 10 patients, according to Boccasanta et al. (2004), and one out of 10 according to the data on over 1000 cases from the European Registry, presented recently at the ASCRS congress in the USA (Stuto et al., 2007).

Returning to the 2009 study of Lenisa et al. (2009) on the Transtar procedure. One would assume that if the manufacturers produced a new instrument, it was because the procedure needed to be improved. But what about severe chronic pain after Transtar? Has it been reduced? It seems so. One year after undergoing a Transtar procedure, 2% of patients have chronic pain. Only 5% complain of diminishing anal continence; fecal urgency was reported by 13% of patients. In a study of over 1000 STARR patients cited above, the number was twice as high.

So, in contrast to the claims of Wadhawan et al.'s (2010) trial, the results of Lenisa et al. (2009) indicate that Transtar is associated with fewer complications than STARR. Nonetheless, at the end of the article there was a conflict of interest declaration stating that the authors are consultants of Ethicon Endosurgery. I do not refer to this in order to cast doubt on the credibility of the results or to bring up the controversial topic of conflict of interest and the literature on innovations, but for a different reason, to focus on chronic pain.

Out of the over 1000 patients from the European STARR Registry, 9% had chronic pain whereas this complication occurred in only 2% of the 75 patients in the Transtar study conducted by the "consultants". That's a much lower number. Is it due to the different technique? Perhaps. However, apart from the technique, there is an important difference between the studies that may have influenced the results. The patients who suffered less pain were operated on only by surgeons with extensive experience in transanal stapling, as is certainly the case for the "consultants" of the company that manufactures the staplers. The patients who complained of more severe pain were those who were operated on also by surgeons without much experience with the technique. This is why it is essential that these procedures are performed by specialists and not by general surgeons.

A final note on Transtar: the costs. Six Contour cartridges are needed for each procedure. That means a total of at least 1560 Euros. Does it make sense to spend so much money before we know for sure that this technique is superior to the others?

At this point in the chapter, we have extensively discussed the complications after STARR, less about how to prevent them, and even less about how to treat them. The latter topic is now addressed.

In a multicenter SICCR study conducted by Gagliardi et al. (2008), the authors reported an 8% incidence of re-operations because of complications. Recently (2010), Jongen et al., from Germany, presented at the ASCRS their analysis of 53 STARR procedures for OD. Re-operations (15%), problems with anal continence (27%), and incomplete defecation (44%) reduced patient satisfaction. Meurette et al. (2010) had similar results: a 16% incidence of re-operations and a 32% incidence of persistent constipation requiring laxatives. In 2009, Andrew Zbar and I published an article entitled "Reinterventions after STARR," (Int J Colorect Dis 2009).

In the past 8 years, about 100 patients suffering from complications after PPH or STARR carried out elsewhere have come to my outpatient clinic. One out of three patients had re-operations, which ranged from simple procedures, i.e. the removal of staples that caused persistent pain or bleeding, to an Altemeier procedure (Fig. 8.12). So far I have re-operated on 16 patients after STARR, including a woman with severe postoperative bleeding.

About half of the patients who must be re-operated on have either no improvement or worsening symptoms. Most of the latter patients were operated on the first time for the wrong indications (for instance, constipation due to irritable bowel syndrome) and, even more importantly, were suffering from anxiety or depression. This is noteworthy since the literature describes an altered psychological pattern as one of the negative predictive factors in patients with OD.

Among the complications after STARR, the most difficult to treat, in my experience, is chronic proctalgia with no clearly defined organic cause. Even if an organic cause is found, it is almost certain that there are at least two functional causes that cannot be managed with surgery ("iceberg syndrome", Fig. 8.1).

Re-operation on a patient who has proctalgia after STARR (Figs. 8.13 and 8.14) should be care-

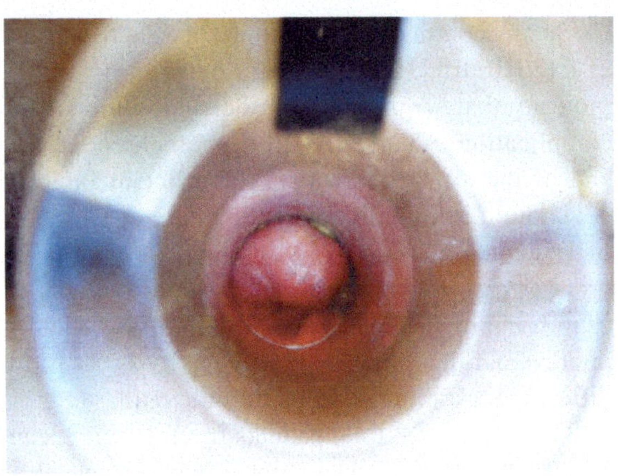

Fig. 8.13 a Obstructed defecation and chronic proctalgia after STARR. Two years postoperatively, the patient had a recurrence of rectal internal mucosal prolapse, very evident at proctoscopy

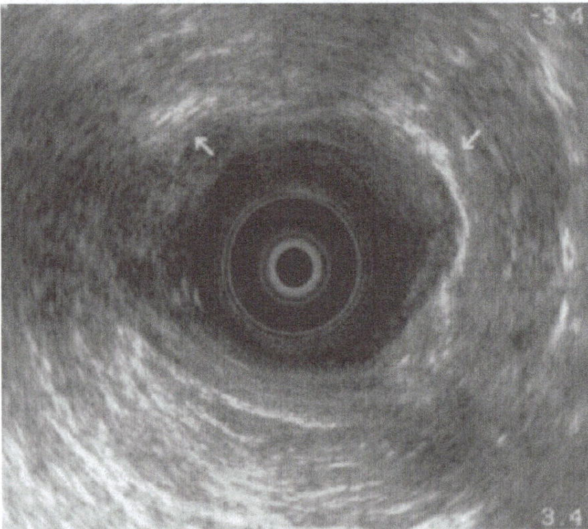

Fig. 8.13 b Transanal ultrasonography with rotating probe shows many retained staples (*arrows*). These were probably the causes of the patient's pain, which became important during defecation

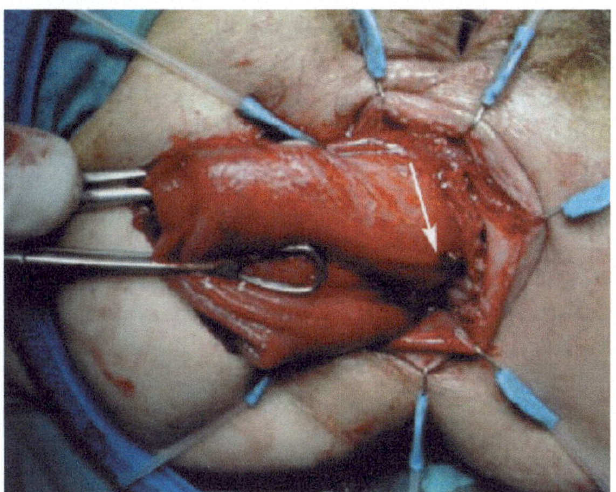

Fig. 8.14 a Beginning of Altemeier's operation in a patient with proctalgia and rectal procidentia after STARR. Staples on the levator ani (*arrow*)

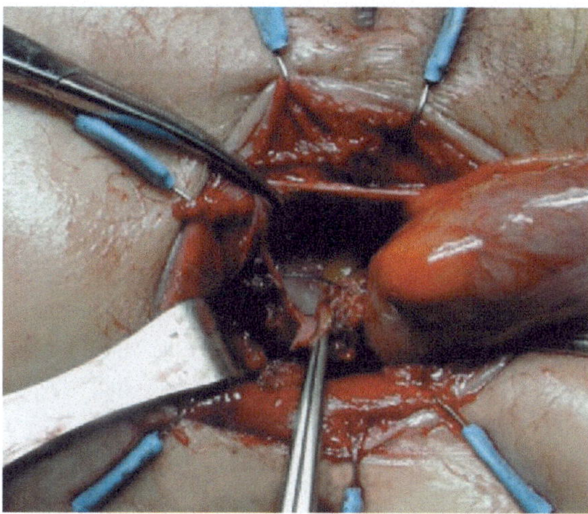

Fig. 8.14 b Partial excision and repair of the pouch of Douglas (elytrocele)

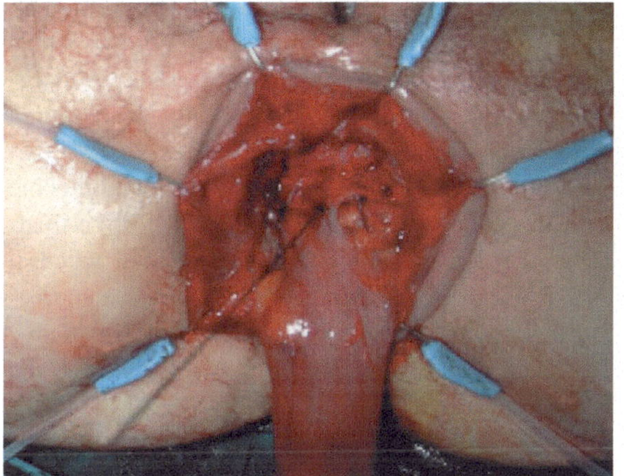

Fig. 8.14 c Suture between the Douglas and sigmoid

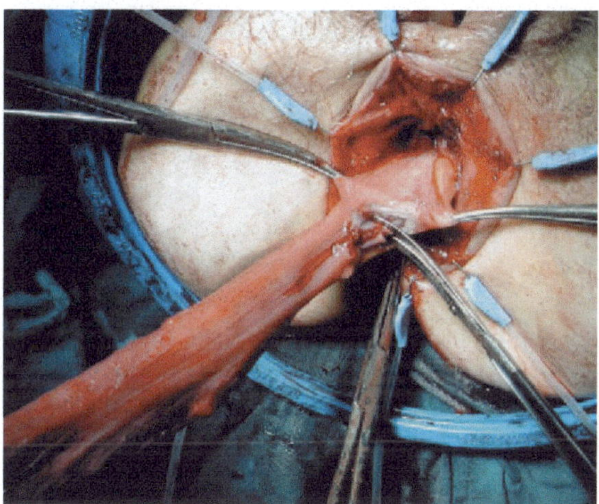

Fig. 8.14 d Prolapsed bowel resection

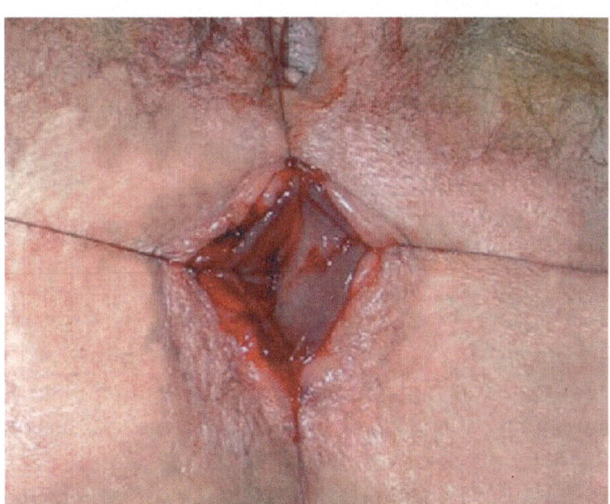

Fig. 8.14 e Colo-anal anastomosis

fully considered, especially if he/she suffers from a psychological disorder. Since it might be the case that the patient is nervous because of the pain rather than having pain because of being nervous, he or she should be sent to a competent psychologist who can perform an evaluation and clear up any doubts, scoring both trait and state anxiety.

In addition, before assuming that a patient's symptoms are due to retained staples that must be removed (this is very likely, as the device fires 52 staples) try using conservative treatment such as gabapentin, injections of analgesics or cortisone, psychotherapy, hypnosis, acupuncture, tranquilizers, hot sitz baths, even reassuring talks. Yes, hot water and reassurance can truly help against proc-

Table 8.3 Postoperative complications after STARR

Complication	Frequency (%)	Author and Year
Severe rectal bleeding	11	Gagliardi, 2007
	4.4	Stuto, 2007
	3.1	Lehur, 2008
	4	Boccasanta, 2011
Requiring re-intervention	2.7	Arroyo, 2007
	3,3	Scarcliff, 2010
Anorectal stricture	3	Pechlivanides, 2010
	3.6	Ellis, 2007
	1.2	Stuto, 2007
	1.5	Lehur, 2008
Requiring re-intervention	3.3	Scarcliff, 2010
Anorectal and/or pelvic pain	20	Boccasanta, 2004
	9.5	Stuto, 2007
	11	Gagliardi, 2007
	13	Meurette, 2011
Fecal urgency	22	Nicolas, 2004
	23	Stuto, 2007
	44	Wadhavan, 2010
	34	Boccasanta, 2011
Anal incontinence	14	Nicolas, 2004
	3	Boccasanta, 2004
	16	Pechlivanides, 2007
	27	Jongen, 2010

talgia, as discussed by Jeyarayah et al. (2010). According to Petersen et al. (2011), already quoted in Chapter 2, agrapphectomy is unlikely to be successful when dealing with patients who complain of chronic proctalgia following STARR.

We end this section with Table 8.3, on the complications after STARR.

The data on rectorrhagia, defecation urgency, proctalgia, and incontinence after STARR are not very positive and they explain the search for a new instrument and a modified procedure (Transtar). According to Boccasanta et al. (2011), Transtar causes less fecal urgency (14% vs.34%), although the technique is associated with certain major complications (e.g., a 2% incidence of vaginal lesions).

8.8 Other Operations for Rectocele Using a Transanal Stapler

Basically there are two: PPH and resection with EndoGIA. Although there are very few reports on these procedures, two criticisms must be raised. First, the efficacy of an operation that does not reinforce the rectovaginal septum must be questioned, as this is the major anatomical defect in case of rectocele. Second, the use of transanal stapling in these patients with OD raises concern, as they are likely to have perineal and pelvic descent due to chronic straining; thus, a relatively "blind" procedure, without direct observation of the anatomical structures, might cause a concomitant peritoneo-, colpo-, and enterocele. However, since objective data are more important than theoretical concerns, let us review the literature on this topic.

8.8.1 Circular Stapler

Regadas et al. (2005) described an interesting procedure, i.e., a combination of diathermy excision and stapling using a PPH device. They operated on eight women and had only one postoperative complication, a perianal hematoma that required re-intervention. Neither incontinence nor dyspareunia was reported using this technique.

Mathur et al. (2004) reported a positive outcome with the same procedure we described for the treatment of internal and small external rectal mucosal prolapse causing OD, i.e., circular stapled mucosectomy (Pescatori et al., 1997). They used a double purse-string and were careful to avoid vaginal tears, but did not provide any data on the size of the rectoceles and barium entrapment at preoperative defecography. Moreover, the follow-up was short and postoperative defecographies were not performed.

As for the above-mentioned risk of vaginal lesions following transanal stapling, Angelone et al. (2006), McDonald et al., Bassi et al. (2006), Gagliardi et al. (2008), and Naldini (2011) reported 12 cases of rectovaginal fistulae following either PPH or STARR.

8.8.2 Linear Stapler

The rectal internal mucosal prolapse is excised according to a combined manual and stapling procedure, using an endoGIA, with a suture placed anteriorly, at the level of the rectal muscle, as in the Block operation. D'Avolio et al. (2005) performed this procedure in 15 women, in whom the following postoperative operations were reported: urinary retention (one patient), mild prolonged rectal bleeding (six), fecal urgency and proctitis (five), moderate proctalgia (three).

8.9 Postoperative Complications After Rectocele Repair Using Prosthetic Meshes

The meshes used in these cases are slowly reabsorbable, either synthetic or biological. Their advantage is that they stay "in situ" until there is connective tissue growth. Therefore, they create an effective barrier between the rectum and the vagina to prevent rectocele recurrence. By contrast, the potential disadvantages of non-reabsorbable meshes are infections and sepsis, although Azanjac did not report either one in a small series of six patients (1999). Mercer-Jones, in 2004, reported two cases of sepsis in 24 patients operated on using a polypropylene mesh.

If a transanal procedure with either mucosectomy or rectotomy is performed, there is a risk of stretching the anal sphincters and both affecting rectal compliance, which might cause fecal incontinence. If either transvaginal or perineal repair is carried out, e.g., anterior levatorplasty, postoperative dyspareunia might occur. Such complications are likely to be prevented by positioning a slowly reabsorbable mesh to reinforce the rectovaginal septum.

Milito, Cadeddu and coworkers presented their series at the last Biennial Meeting of the Eurasian Colorectal Technologies Association (Turin, 2011, abstract published in Techniques in Coloproctology, 2011). They reported encouraging results and estimated a cost of about 400 Euros per mesh per patient. To avoid this expensive procedure, rather than a mesh one might use the fascia lata harvested from the thigh, as reported by Ismail Shafik at the Biennial Meeting of the Mediterranean Society of Coloproctology (Rome, 2008).

Mercer-Jones et al. (2007) used a slowly reabsorbable porcine collagene mesh in operating on 10 females with rectocele and reported the following complications: perineal hematomas (two patients), which they suggested preventing by means of a Redivac suction drain; dyspareunia (two) and erosion of the skin due to the mesh (one). The latter complication was managed by simply cutting off the sharp angle of the prosthesis.

De la Postilla et al. (2010), after having excised the rectocele and the mucosal prolapse transanally by an endoGIA, sutured a reabsorbable Goretex Seamguard mesh to the staple line to reinforce the rectovaginal septum. The procedure was rather costly, due to both the stapler and the prosthesis, but was followed by no complication in ten patients, except for two who still complained of fecal urgency after one year.

The trans-perineal EXPRESS procedure was reported by Williams et al. (2005), who used a Permacol mesh to treat both rectocele and mucosal prolapse in 17 patients with OD. These authors had one case of postoperative sepsis at the level of the rectovaginal septum, which unfortunately, required a diverting stoma—subsequently closed. There were also three cases of temporary proctalgia.

Ellis (2010) operated on two groups of females with rectocele. The first (88 patients) underwent manual rectocele repair, while in the second (32) a Cook Surgisis slowly reabsorbable synthetic mesh was used. Functional results were similar, with six cases of urinary retention occurring in both groups but those operated on with the mesh had fewer postoperative complications: 16% (abscesses, dehiscences and one rectovaginal fistula) in the first group, 6% (dehiscences and sepsis) in the second. Dr. Ellis is a Cook consultant.

Attention must be paid when reading or listening to the positive outcome of a costly innovation. Years ago, the results of a novel technological procedure (not meshes) were presented at a congress. A colleague who had submitted his cases to the multicentric study was sitting beside me in the audience, when a slide was presented reporting no postoperative bleeding at all after the novel procedure. He was surprised and disappointed, since two of his submitted cases involved severe hemorrhage. This demonstrates that, sometimes, not all complications are properly reported.

As regards the use of meshes in the management of patients with rectocele and OD, the conclusion is that these procedures are more costly, but are likely to be associated with fewer complications than in manual operations.

8.10 Complications After Surgery for Anismus or a Non-relaxing Puborectalis Muscle

As reported by Devroede (2004), anismus may represent multiorgan failure associated with uro-

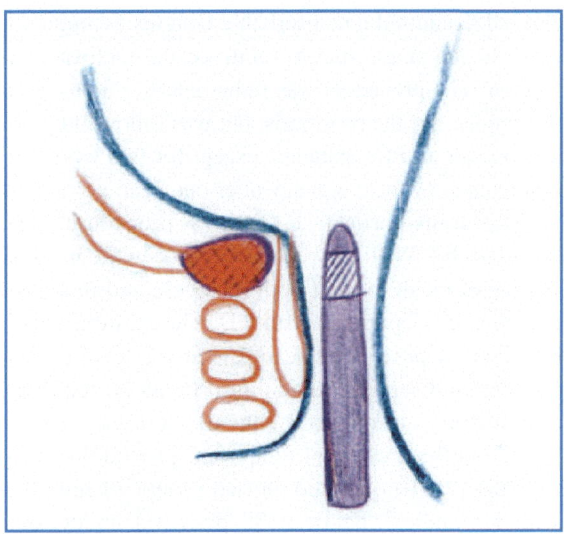

Fig. 8.15 a The ultrasound probe is inserted into the anus, with the rotating head close to the puborectalis muscle

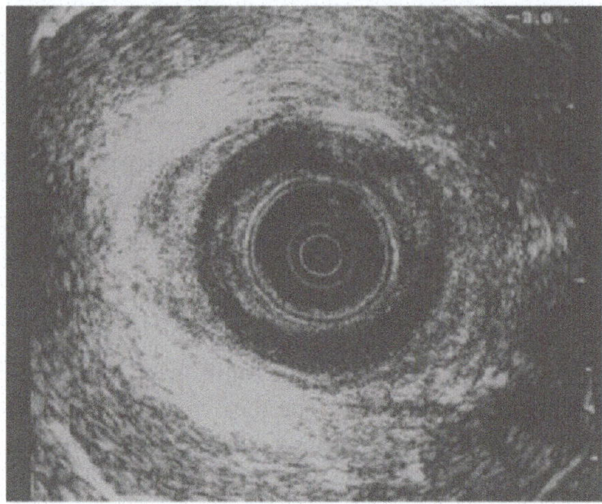

Fig. 8.15 b Transanal ultrasonography with rotating probe in a woman with obstructed defecation because of abdominopelvic dyskinesia or anismus. The patient is in the Sims position

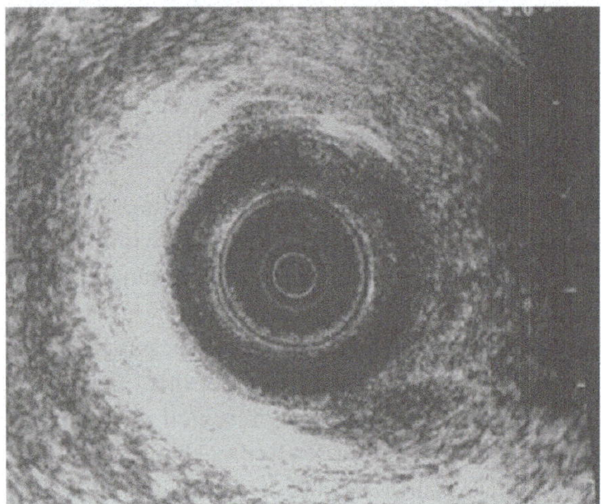

Fig. 8.15 c When the patient strains at defecation, the hyperechogenic puborectalis sling does not relax but contracts. The distance between the external margin of the hypoechogenic ring (internal sphincter) and the internal margin of the hyperechogenic sling (puborectalis muscle), rather than increasing, is reduced (from Dodi et al., 2003)

logical, gastroenterological, and mental disturbances. One-third of the females with OD and pelvic-perineal discomfort, if properly questioned, report a history of sexual traumas in their childhood or adolescence. Ghislain Devroede, from Sherwood, Canada, is a "psychosomatic surgeon," and I would recommend his wonderful chapter on the psychopathological aspects of chronic constipation in the book "Constipation," edited by Wexner and Bartolo (1997).

In these patients, OD is due to a lack of relaxation or to a paradoxical contraction of the puborectalis muscle on straining, which might be detected either at digital exploration or anal manometry, defecography, or transanal US (Fig. 8.15). Sphincter needle-EMG may also be helpful but is rarely used because it causes discomfort to the patient.

Botox injection, yoga, transanal electrostimulation, and psychotherapy have also been reported to yield encouraging results, according to the literature. Another approach is biofeedback. In the last 2 years, we have been using a novel procedure, psycho-echo-biofeedback, which is a combination of psychologically guided relaxation techniques and vaginal ultrasound. The technique is indicated in patients with anxiety and/or depression and allows them to visualize and facilitate the opening of the puborectalis muscle on straining.

In the early 1980s, at St. Mark's, I observed cases of anismus treated with the Wasserman procedure, i.e., posterior division of the puborectalis muscle, an operation likely to be followed by fecal incontinence.

Recently, Farid et al. (2009) described a similar procedure, involving partial bilateral division of the puborectalis muscle, which caused mild anal incontinence in three out of 15 patients and cured anis-

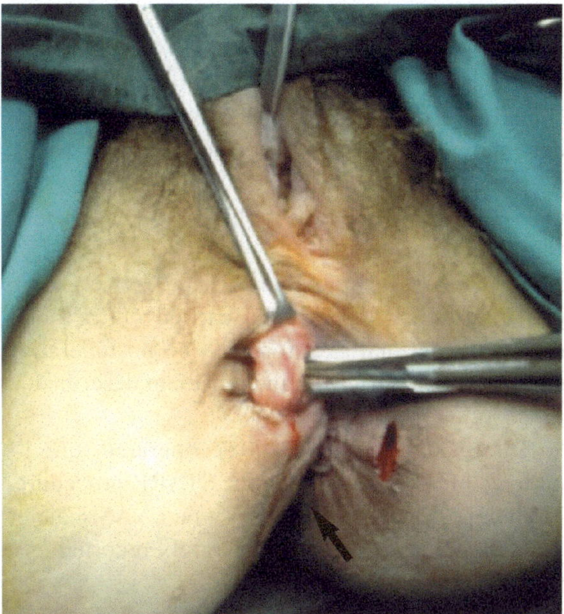

Fig. 8.16 a Obstructed defecation surgery in a young woman with anismus, treated by biofeedback without success. The patient is in the lithotomy position. Modified Farid's operation. Through two small perianal incisions, lateral branches of the puborectalis muscle are visible

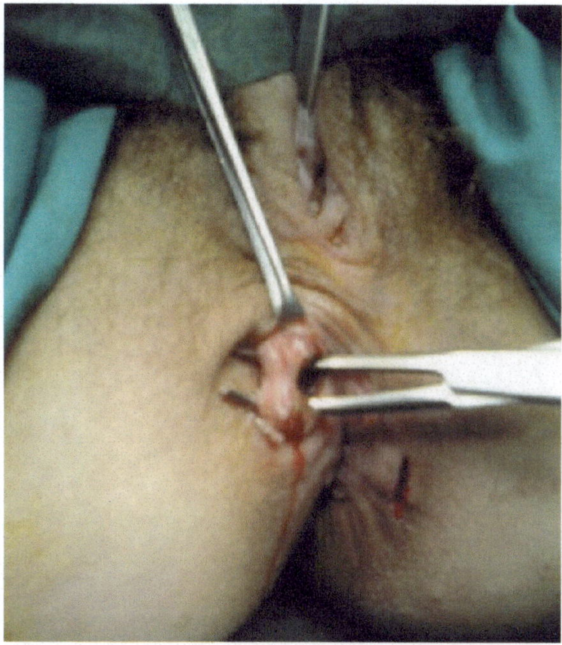

Fig. 8.16 b The semi-internal aspect of the muscle is divided. Cutaneous wounds are left open, to reduce the risk of local sepsis. The partial (half) and lateral sections of the muscle reduce the risk of anal incontinence

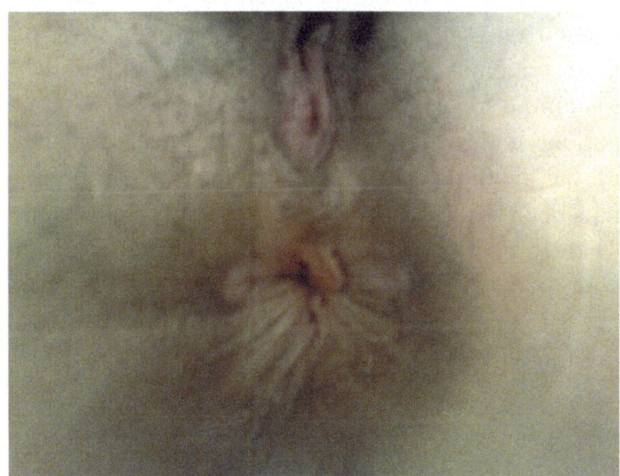

Fig. 8.16 c One month later, only a small scar is detectable at the sites of the surgical perianal incisions

mus in the majority (66%). Local sepsis at the site of the sutured perianal surgical wounds was seen in ten patients. We slightly modified the technique by leaving open the small perianal wounds. There was no sepsis or incontinence; relief from OD in the short term was achieved in the first three patients, who had not responded to a biofeedback training course (Fig. 8.16). Larger series with longer follow-up are needed to confirm both the safety and the efficacy of this novel minimally-invasive procedure.

8.11 Operating on a Patient with Solitary Rectal Ulcer Syndrome (SRUS) and Obstructed Defecation

SRUS may be occasionally localized to the sigmoid and is likely to be due to: fecal stasis, rectal intussusception, chronic ischemia, or excessive straining (Ignjatovic et al., 2010, Yagnik, 2011).

The first case I encountered in my career was in the late 1970s. A 36-year-old woman complained of rectal bleeding and OD. A 3 cm in diameter, partially ulcerated polpyoid lesion at the level of the mid-rectum, suggestive of a neoplasm, was detected at endoscopy. Small conventional surface biopsies indicated adenocarcinoma. However, I was not convinced, due to the relatively young age of the woman, the presence of a concomitant internal mucosal prolapse, and the fact that the patient was fit and well-nourished, without any family history of cancer. Therefore, I carried out a macrobiopsy, i.e., a transanal nearly total excision of the lesion, with the

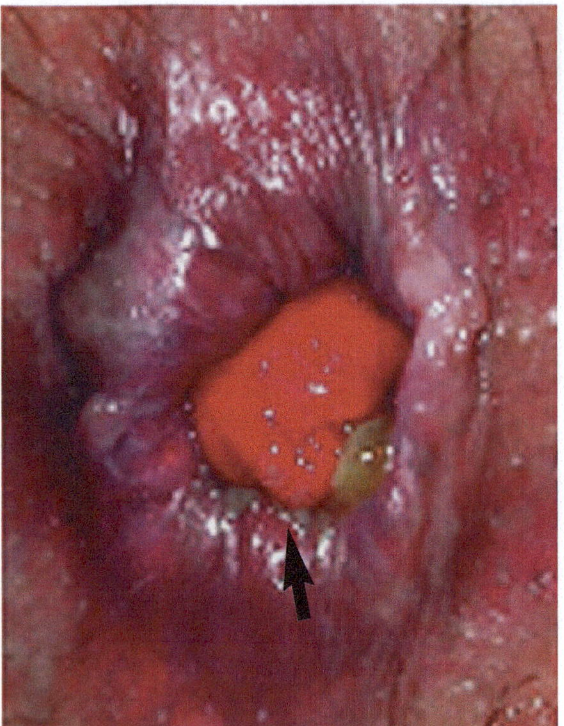

Fig. 8.17 Patient with obstructed defecation and rectal solitary ulcer syndrome. A small rectal mucosal prolapse is observed on straining, with whitish pseudopolypoid lesions (*arrow*)

patient under anesthesia and mailed the whole specimen to Dr. Basil Morson, pathologist at St. Mark's. His definitive diagnosis was "pseudopolypoid solitary rectal ulcer syndrome." The postoperative course of the patient was uneventful.

Since then, I have seen and treated 40 SRUS patients, most with small lesions, in the 33 years at my unit (Fig. 8.17). Fifteen of them were operated on due to persistent bleeding, rectal procidentia, or rectal intussusception/internal mucosal prolapse causing OD. An Altemeier procedure was carried out in one patient, with no postoperative complications. Three patients had a sacral mesh rectopexy. One of them, a young male, complained of temporary loss of ejaculation, presumably due to a periprosthetic fibrosis traumatizing the hypogastric nerves. A transanal manual rectal mucosectomy was performed in the other nine patients, one of whom had local sepsis and had been operated on in 1987. Finally, I carried out a rectal cauterization/plication, i.e., the El Sibai/Shafik procedure, a kind of anterior hemi/Delorme, in a female patient who had to be re-operated on for rectal bleeding. The operation is described in Chap. 10.

Tseng et al. (2004) operated on 19 patients who had SRUS causing massive rectal bleeding. All needed to be transfused and admitted to the ICU. Bleeding was stopped either with endoscopic coagulation (four cases), ethanol injection (one), transanal suturing (three), or balloon tamponade (11). Eight patients had re-bleeding that needed transanal suturing.

In one case of polypoid SRUS, Privitera et al. (2010), at the Mayo Clinic, carried out a three-quadrant transanal excision with no postoperative complications, as we did in the patient described at the beginning of this section.

Boccasanta et al. (2008) operated on 14 patients in two years, using the STARR procedure. Median postoperative pain was 4 on a VAS scale of 1-10. In other series, pain was rarely reported as a significant complication.

Over a period of more than 10 years, Torres et al. (2007) reported severe proctalgia in one out of 16 patients operated on for SRUS. Among other complications, there were two cases of rectal bleeding, which required re-intervention, and three cases of sexual dysfunctions (all after abdominal procedures). It should be noted that these authors carried out a transanal operation only in 20% of their patients. Most procedures were either rectosigmoid resections or sacral rectopexies. One patient underwent an abdominoperineal excision of the rectum, presumably because a carcinoma had been either diagnosed or strongly suspected. Therefore, we may conclude that the most feared complication in a patient with SRUS is a permanent stoma; thus, attention should be paid to making the correct diagnosis.

8.12 Two Unforgettable Complications

8.12.1 Case Number One

It was 1986 and I had just started to operate on patients with rectocele. I was rather interventionist, as, I'm afraid, are many colleagues nowadays when dealing with a disease that, to some extent, may be better considered as a "physiologic" finding. Almost all multiparous women over age 50 and with a history of chronic straining at stools present with a rectocele. The literature is very clear in stating that rectocele is not the main causes of defecatory disorders. In addition, it is well-recognized that two-thirds of these patients, as reported in the literature, are anxious and/or depressed and their obstructed defecation is more likely to be psychosomatic rather than an organic alteration. But, at that time, this was not clear to me. Moreover, I was strongly interested in increasing my surgical experience by operating on as many patients as possible.

I had learned the Block procedure, i.e., obliterative transanal suture of rectocele and rectal internal mucosal prolapse, in Ravenna, Italy, not at St. Mark's Hospital in the UK, where I had trained, since at that institution there had been almost no case of obstructed defecation requiring surgical treatment. The Block procedure is minimally invasive, as it does not require any excision, only a running suture aimed at rendering the superficial layers of the rectum ischemic and fibrotic at the level of both the prolapse and the rectocele. The only potential risk is to enter the vagina, although to this day I have never made this error, after operating on about 60 patients using this technique. The advantage of the operation is that it is unlikely to be followed by either anal incontinence, as the sphincter stretch is mild and short, or postoperative bleeding, as no open surgical wound is left.

The patient was a 75-year-old woman, whose mother was recently deceased. Apart from the anxiety, clearly related to the loss of her mother, and the fractioned evacuation and frequent straining, her main complaint was proctalgia. But I could not find any organic or functional cause at proctoscopy and manometry, not even a non-relaxing puborectalis muscle or a significant rectal internal mucosal prolapse, i.e., reaching the dentate line on straining. Therefore, I decided to carry out an evaluation, with the patient under anesthesia: no anomaly was found upon a careful 10-minute exploration of the rectum and the anal canal. Namely, there was no evidence of chronic abscess, which might well have caused pain. Nothing at all. The only finding was an anterior rectocele, 3-4 cm in diameter, more evident on sedation. Therefore, I decided to carry out a Block procedure.

The operation lasted less than 20 minutes and the early postoperative course was uneventful. On postoperative day two, the patient had her first evacuation and there was some dark blood in the stool. I was not surprised, since she had had an endorectal suture, but during the night she continued to pass bloody stool. As the rectal bleeding persisted and the patient was becoming tachycardic and pale, intravenous fluid therapy was started. Then, after rectal irrigation with saline, a Foley catheter was inserted through the anus and the balloon inflated in the lower rectum to tamponade the bleeding area, which I thought was at the site of the surgical wound. This maneuver is almost always successful in case of post-hemorrhoidectomy bleeding. However, it did not work and the patient kept bleeding through the catheter.

What is your hypothesis on the cause of bleeding after a minimally invasive rectocele repair in an elderly patient with preoperative proctalgia?

We performed an urgent colonoscopy. Unexpectedly, the rectum was normal and there was no bleeding from the surgical wound. The lower sigmoid also was normal, but, at the level of the upper sigmoid and the ascending colon, there were many bleeding ulcers surrounded by dystrophic mucosa. Therefore, the diagnosis of postoperative ischemic colitis was made, possibly caused by the anesthesia-related hypotension, in a patient with insufficient mesenteric vascular supply due to advanced age.

After 3 days, as bleeding continued, a left hemicolectomy was carried out. The postoperative course was uneventful and the patient was discharged after a week.

I searched the literature when writing this book and found a paper by Medina et al. (2004), in which left colon resection was described in 12 out of 18 patients who developed acute ischemic colitis.

After one year, my patient no longer had a rectocele, but she still complained of obstructed defecation and proctalgia and still had not gotten over her mother's death.

8.12.2 Case Number Two

This patient was also a woman and while she had not lost any relatives, she was extremely anxious. She was 28 years old and was accompanied by her parents when she visited my office. "My problem", she said, "is that despite several operations I spend hours on the toilet trying to defecate but never empty my

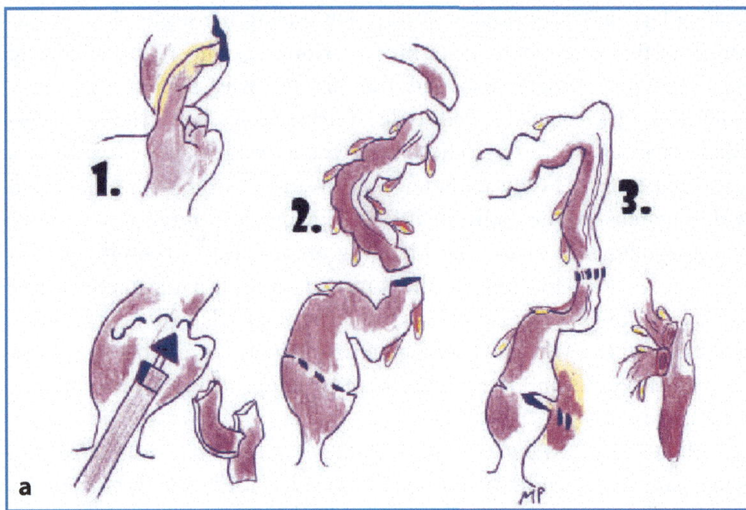

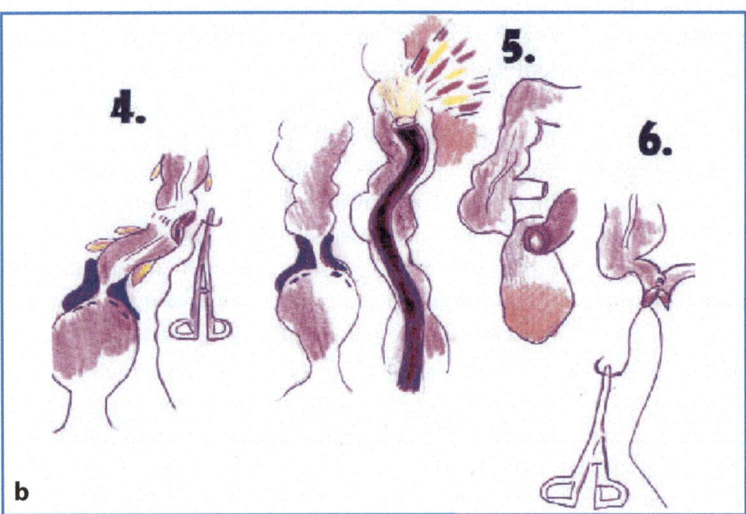

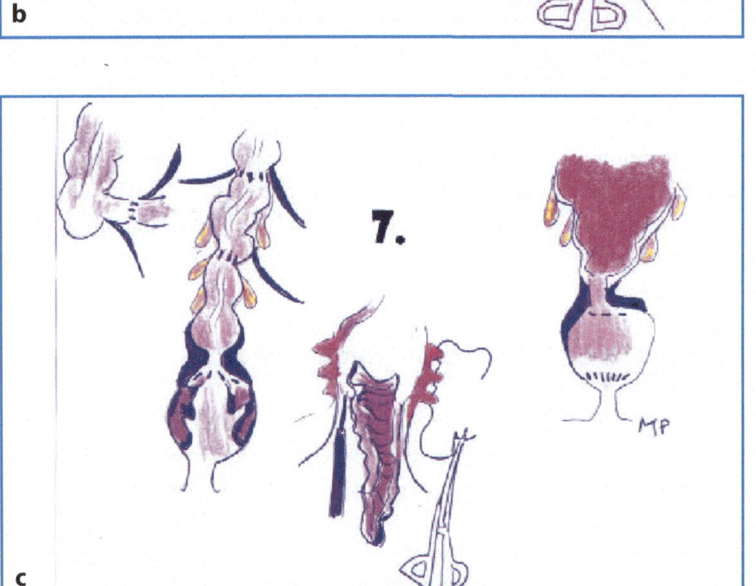

Fig. 8.18 a-c Operations performed in a 28-year-old woman after STARR and laparoscopic sigmoid resection because of chronic constipation, dolichocolon; and rectal internal mucosal prolapse. **a** The diagnosis was made by rectal exploration (*1*), the first double operation (*2*) and postoperative complication (*3*): rectal suture dehiscence after STARR with peritonitis, which required a diverting stoma. **b** Stoma closure (*4*) and, the second complication, perforation during colonoscopy, followed by an urgent loop ileostomy (*5*), and then its closure (*6*). In the "operation-free" periods, the patient suffered from worsening symptoms: abdominal pain and constipation. **c** The last operation, performed before the patient came to us: Delorme-Rehn's internal prolapsectomy for recurrence of a rectal internal prolapse and rectal stenosis. The operation was unsuccessful, necessitating dilatations under local anesthesia to treat recurrence of the stenosis (images from the Italian Society of Colo-Rectal Surgery, website: www.siccr.org)

bowel. I have a dolichosigmoid and suffered from anorexia". She was indeed as thin as a rake.

Unlike the patient in the previous case, who was examined in the mid 1980s, nowadays, there is transanal ultrasound and MRI; we are knowledgeable about psychosomatics and can take advantage of highly technological surgery. That's why the patient had previously undergone a STARR procedure, supposedly "the new deal" for the management of obstructed defecation.

She had seen a surgeon, who convinced her to undergo STARR, saying: "You have an internal prolapse of the rectum that must be excised, otherwise it will come out and become as big as a melon." This is what the patient reported to me, while her parents nodded in confirmation.

Once the STARR was completed, the surgeon, still in operating green, told the parents that he was afraid their daughter would continue to be constipated unless the dolichosigmoid was adequately treated with a bowel resection, which might be safely carried out by a laparoscopic surgeon. Obviously, the parents agreed and the second part of the operation took place. (Note: no intestinal transit time study had been performed.)

On postoperative day five, the patient had fever and abdominal pain, but the surgeon reassured her. After two days she was frankly peritonitic and the parents moved her to another hospital, where a low rectal suture breakdown was found and a diverting stoma performed.

Two months later, the stoma was closed, but she was still constipated and had to strain to defecate. A rectal stricture was found and a course of dilations were scheduled, but the girl called the first surgeon, who strongly advised her to refuse dilations and instead return to his hospital for a colonoscopy. Unfortunately, an intestinal perforation occurred during endoscopy and she required an emergency ileostomy.

After closure of the second stoma, she still complained of obstructed defecation plus crampy abdominal pain, probably due to adhesions. She became increasingly depressed, because she realized that her condition had worsened after four operations. Her parents took her to a third surgeon, who performed a rectal prolapsectomy to correct a recto-rectal intussusception, which he believed was the main cause for her symptoms (Fig. 8.18).

Following the internal Delorme, the patient complained of the same symptoms and came to my clinic.

What is your hypothesis about this difficult case? In summary: STARR and laparoscopic sigmoid resection, rectal suture breakdown, two diverting stomas closed, internal Delorme, continued obstructed defecation. What would you expect to find at this stage?

Examination of the abdomen revealed surgical scars and a palpable painful mass suggesting a spastic colon. Digital exploration was performed and a severe stricture was felt at about 7 cm from the anal verge. The pediatric proctoscope revealed a fibrotic stricture of the lower rectum, with two retained staples partly anchored to the mucosa, which were easily removed. A rectal dilation was performed under local anesthesia by means of Hegar dilators up to 18 mm and then continued gently using my fingers.

I gave the patient an anal dilator, instructing her to use it at home twice a day, and recommended that she return after a week for a second dilation, which I performed in the theatre with the patient under sedation and local anesthesia. Two more retained staples were removed, at the site of the stricture, above a rectal granuloma. At the end, a normal proctoscope, 23 cm in size, could be inserted in the rectum beyond the stricture, albeit with some difficulty.

The patient never came back for the third and probably last dilation under anesthesia. Maybe she was tired of suffering or skeptical about the dilations. This was unfortunate because I was certain that more dilations, and possibly even a rectal resection with a coloanal anastomosis, would have been needed to solve her problem.

This case started with a STARR procedure, carried out for what was likely to have been a psychogenic irritable bowel syndrome.

Summary

The most frequent complications after transanal and transperineal surgery for obstructed defecation are rectal bleeding and local sepsis with suture dehiscence and consequent rectal stricture.

Hemorrhage may require an emergency re-intervention with suture of the bleeding area, while pelvic sepsis may require a diverting stoma, usually a sigmoidostomy.

Local infection is less frequent when a slowly reabsorbable, either synthetic or biological mesh is used for rectocele repair. Stricture may require rectal dilations under anesthesia; less frequently, an anoplasty is needed.

Some patients may present with anal incontinence, pre-existing rather than of new onset. It is likely to occur after transanal procedures, due to intraoperative sphincter stretching and, more often, to a reduced compliance of the rectal reservoir following both internal Delorme and STARR. It may be managed with the injection of bulking agents or with pelvic floor rehabilitation.

Dyspareunia may occur after anterior levatorplasty, but severe chronic proctalgia is more debilitating and, when present, is likely to affect the quality of life. Painful defecation may occur in up to 20% of the patients who have undergone a STARR procedure and might be related to chronic stimulation of the levator ani and puborectalis muscle neural network by the fibrosis around the staples. Transtar is still costly but carries less risk of proctalgia and fecal urgency. Both procedures should be performed by colorectal surgeons trained in trans-anal stapling.

Agrapphectomy is unlikely to relieve rectal and pelvic pain. Re-interventions after either a complicated or a failed STARR have a poor outcome in patients with anxiety and/or depression.

The "iceberg diagram" is based on the concept that obstructed defecation is caused more often by occult functional disorders than by rectocele and rectal internal mucosal prolapse. It is helpful in selecting patients suitable for surgical management and for minimizing the risk of postoperative complications possibly arising from a concomitant anismus or an enterocele.

Suggested Readings

Alabiso ME, Grassi R, Fioroni C, Marano I (2008) Iatrogenic rectal diverticulum in patients treated with transanal stapled techniques. Radiol Med 113:887-894

Altomare DF, Pucciani F (eds) (2008) Rectal prolapse - diagnosis and clinical management. Springer Verlag

Ambe P, Köhler L, Janghorban-Esfahani B, Meyer A (2010) Double-stapled transanal rectotomy (STARR procedure) for obstructed defecation syndrome seems to have a low degree of acceptance amongst older surgeons. Int J Colorectal Dis 25:915

Angelone G, Giardiello C, Prota C (2006) Stapled hemorrhoidopexy. Complications and 2-year follow-up. Chir Ital 58:753–760

Arroyo A, González-Argenté FX, García-Domingo M et al (2008) Prospective multicentre clinical trial of stapled transanal rectal resection for obstructive defaecation syndrome. Br J Surg 95:1521-1527

Arroyo A, Pérez-Vicente F, Serrano P et al (2007) Evaluation of the stapled transanal rectal resection technique with two staplers in the treatment of obstructive defecation syndrome. J Am Coll Surg 204:56-63

Ayabaca SM, Zbar AP, Pescatori M (2006) Anal continence after rectocele repair. Dis Colon Rectum 45:63-69

Bassi R, Rademacher J, Savoia A (2006) Rectovaginal fistula after STARR procedure complicated by haematoma of the posterior vaginal wall: report of a case. Tech Coloproctol 10:361-363

Beco J (2008) Interest of retro-anal levator plate myorrhaphy in selected cases of descending perineum syndrome with positive anti-sagging test. BMC Surg 8:13

Berman IR, Harris MS, Rabeler MB (1990) Delorme's transrectal excision for internal rectal prolapse. Patient selection, technique, and three-year follow-up. Dis Colon Rectum 33:573-580

Binda GA, Pescatori M, Romano G (2005) The dark side of double-stapled transanal rectal resection. Dis Colon Rectum 48:1830-1831

Boccasanta P, Venturi M, Barbieri S, Roviaro G (2006) Impact of new technologies on the clinical and functional outcome of Altemeier's procedure: a randomized controlled trial. Dis Colon Rectum 49:652-660

Boccasanta P, Venturi M, Calabrò G et al (2008) Stapled transanal rectal resection in solitary rectal ulcer associated with prolapse of the rectum: a prospective study. Dis Colon Rectum 51:348-354

Boccasanta P, Venturi M, Roviaro G (2007) Stapled transanal rectal resection versus stapled anopexy in the cure of hemorrhoids associated with rectal prolapse. A randomized controlled trial. Int J Colorectal Dis 22:245-251

Boccasanta P, Venturi M, Roviaro G (2011) What is the benefit of a new stapler device in the surgical treatment of obstructed defecation? Three-year outcomes from a randomized controlled trial. Dis Colon Rectum 54:77-84

Boccasanta P, Venturi M, Salamina G et al (2004) New trends in the surgical treatment of outlet obstruction. Clinical and functional results of two novel stapled techniques from a randomized controlled trial. Int J Colorectal Dis 19:359-369

Boccasanta P, Venturi M, Stuto A et al (2004) Stapled transanal rectal resection for outlet obstruction: a prospective, multicenter trial. Dis Colon Rectum 47:1285-1296; discussion 1296-1297

Bouchoucha M, Devroede G, Arsac M (2004) Anismus: a marker of multi-site functional disorders? Int J Colorectal Dis 19:374-379

Carriero A, Picchio M, Martellucci J et al (2010) Laparoscopic correction of enterocele associated to stapled transanal rec-

tal resection for obstructed defecation syndrome. Int J Colorectal Dis 25:381-387
Church JM (2003) The application of percutaneous endoscopic colostomy to the management of obstructed defecation (commented summary). Tech Coloproctol 7:121
Corman ML, Carriero A, Hager T et al (2006) Consensus conference on the stapled transanal rectal resection (STARR) for disordered defaecation. Colorectal Dis 8:98-101
D'Avolio M, Ferrara A, Chimenti C (2005) Transanal rectocele repair using EndoGIA: short-term results of a prospective study. Tech Coloproctol 9:108-114
de la Portilla F, Rada R, Vega J et al (2010) Transanal rectocele repair using linear stapler and bioabsorbable staple line reinforcement material: short-term results of a prospective study. Dis Colon Rectum 53:88-92
De Nardi P, Bottini C, Faticanti Scucchi L, Palazzi A, Pescatori M (2007) Proctalgia in a patient with staples retained in the puborectalis muscle after STARR operation. Tech Coloproctol 11:353-356
Dodi G, Pietroletti R, Milito G, Binda G, Pescatori M (2003) Bleeding, incontinence, pain and constipation after STARR transanal double stapling rectotomy for obstructed defecation. Tech Coloproctol 7:148-153
Eléouet M, Siproudhis L, Guillou N, Le Couedic J, Bouguen G, Bretagne JF (2010) Chronic posterior tibial nerve transcutaneous electrical nerve stimulation (TENS) to treat fecal incontinence (FI). Int J Colorectal Dis 25:1127-1132
Ellis CN (2004) Anterior levatorplasty for the treatment of chronic anal fissures in females with a rectocele: a randomized, controlled trial. Dis Colon Rectum 47:1170-1173
Ellis CN (2007) Stapled transanal rectal resection (STARR) for rectocele. J Gastrointest Surg 11:153-154
Ellis CN (2010) Outcomes after the repair of rectoceles with transperineal insertion of a bioprosthetic graft. Dis Colon Rectum 53:213-218
Farid M, Youssef T, Mahdy T et al (2009) Comparative study between botulinum toxin injection and partial division of puborectalis for treating anismus. Int J Colorectal Dis 24:327-334
Farouk R, Bhardwaj R, Phillips RKS (2009) Stapled transanal resection of the rectum (STARR) for the obstructed defaecation syndrome. Ann R Coll Surg Engl 91:287-291
Frascio M, Stabilini C, Ricci B et al (2008) Stapled transanal rectal resection for outlet obstruction syndrome: results and follow-up. World J Surg 32:1110-1115
Gagliardi G, Pescatori M, Altomare DF et al Italian Society of Colo-Rectal Surgery (SICCR) (2008) Results, outcome predictors, and complications after stapled transanal rectal resection for obstructed defecation. Dis Colon Rectum 51:186-195; discussion 195
Gelos M, Frommhold K, Mann B (2010) Severe mesorectal bleeding after stapled transanal rectal resection (STARR-operation) using the 'Contour Transtar curved cutter stapler'. Colorectal Dis 12:265-266
Goede A, Glancy D, Carter H et al (2011) Medium term results of stapled transanal rectal resection (STARR) for obstructed defecation and symptomatic rectal-anal intussusception. Colorectal Dis 13:1052-1057
Grassi R, Romano S, Micera O, Fioroni C, Boller B (2005) Radiographic findings of post-operative double stapled trans anal rectal resection (STARR) in patient with obstructed defecation syndrome (ODS). Eur J Radiol 53:410-416
Guarnieri A, Cesaretti M, Tirone A et al (2008) Stapled transanal rectal resection (STARR) in the treatment of rectocele: personal experience. Chir Ital 60:243-248
Habr-Gama A, e Sous AH Jr, Roveló JM et al (2003) Stapled hemorrhoidectomy: initial experience of a Latin American group. J Gastrointest Surg 7:809-813
Hammond KL, Ellis CN (2010) Outcomes after transanal repair of rectoceles. Dis Colon Rectum 53:83-87
Harmston C, Jones OM, Cunningham C, Lindsey I (2010) Comment on: Stapled transanal resection of the rectum (STARR) for obstructed defaecation syndrome. Ann R Coll Surg Engl 92:85-86
Ignjatovic A, Saunders BP, Harbin L, Clark S (2010) Solitary 'rectal' ulcer syndrome in the sigmoid colon. Colorectal Dis 12:1163-1164
Isbert C, Reibetanz J, Jayne DG, Kim M, Germer CT, Boenicke L (2010) Comparative study of Contour Transtar and STARR procedure for the treatment of obstructed defecation syndrome (ODS)—feasibility, morbidity and early functional results. Colorectal Dis 12:901-908
Jayne DG, Schwandner O, Stuto A (2009) Stapled transanal rectal resection for obstructed defecation syndrome: one-year results of the European STARR Registry. Dis Colon Rectum 52:1205-12012; discussion 1212-1214
Jeyarajah S, Chow A, Ziprin P, Tilney H, Purkayastha S (2010) Proctalgia fugax, an evidence-based management pathway. Int J Colorectal Dis 25:1037-1046
Kessler M, Joos AK, Bussen D (2008) Rare complication after STARR operation. Chirurg 79:580-583
Lacima G, Pera M, Valls-Solé J, González-Argenté X, Puig-Clota M, Espuña M (2006) Electrophysiologic studies and clinical findings in females with combined fecal and urinary incontinence: a prospective study. Dis Colon Rectum 49:353-359
Lang RA, Buhmann S, Lautenschlager C et al (2010) Stapled transanal rectal resection for symptomatic intussusception: morphological and functional outcome. Surg Endosc 24:1969-1975
Lenisa L, Schwandner O, Stuto A et al (2009) STARR with Contour Transtar: prospective multicentre European study. Colorectal Dis 11:821-827
Liberman H, Hughes C, Dippolito A (2000) Evaluation and outcome of the Delorme procedure in the treatment of rectal outlet obstruction. Dis Colon Rectum 43:188-192
Lovatsis D, Drutz HP (2002) Safety and efficacy of sacrospinous vault suspension. Int Urogynecol J Pelvic Floor Dysfunct 13:308-313
Madbouly KM, Abbas KS, Hussein AM (2010) Disappointing long-term outcomes after stapled transanal rectal resection for obstructed defecation. World J Surg 34:2191-2196
Mathur P, Ng KH, Seow-Choen F (2004) Stapled mucosectomy for rectocele repair: a preliminary report. Dis Colon Rectum 47:1978-1980; discussion 1980-1981
McDonald PJ, Bona R, Cohen CR (2004) Rectovaginal fistula after stapled haemorrhoidopexy. Colorectal Dis 6:64-65
Medina C, Vilaseca J, Videla S, Fabra R, Armengol-Miro JR, Malagelada JR (2004) Outcome of patients with ischemic colitis: review of fifty-three cases. Dis Colon Rectum 47:180-184
Mercer-Jones MA, Sprowson A, Varma JS (2004) Outcome after transperineal mesh repair of rectocele: a case series. Dis Colon Rectum 47:864-868

Meurette G, Wong M, Frampas E, Regenet N, Lehur PA (2010) Anatomical and functional results after stapled transanal rectal resection (STARR) for obstructed defaecation syndrome. Colorectal Dis 21 in press

Mongardini M, Pappalardo G (2003) The use of Floseal in the prevention and treatment of intra- and post-operative hemorrhage in the surgical treatment of hemorrhoids and colporectocele. Preliminary results. G Chir 24:377-381

Morio O, Meurette G, Desfourneaux V et al (2005) Anorectal physiology in solitary ulcer syndrome: a case-matched series. Dis Colon Rectum 48:1917-1922

Naldini G (2011) Serious unconventional complications of surgery with stapler for haemorrhoidal prolapse and obstructed defecation due to rectocele and rectal intussusception. Colorectal Dis 13:323-327

Ommer A, Albrecht K, Wenger F, Walz MK (2006) Stapled transanal rectal resection (STARR): a new option in the treatment of obstructive defecation syndrome. Langenbecks Arch Surg 391:32-37

Patel CB, Ragupathi M, Bhoot NH, Pickron TB, Haas EM (2011) Patient satisfaction and symptomatic outcomes following stapled transanal rectal resection for obstructed defecation syndrome. J Surg Res 165:e15-e21

Pechlivanides G, Tsiaoussis J, Athanasakis E et al (2007) Stapled transanal rectal resection (STARR) to reverse the anatomic disorders of pelvic floor dyssynergia. World J Surg 31:1329-1335

Pescatori M (2011) STARR and the older surgeon: what makes the difference? Int J Colorectal Dis. 2011 in press

Pescatori M, Aigner F (2007) Stapled transanal rectal mucosectomy ten years after. Tech Coloproctol 11:1-6

Pescatori M, Boffi F, Russo A, Zbar AP (2006) Complications and recurrence after excision of rectal internal mucosal prolapse for obstructed defaecation. Int J Colorectal Dis 21:160-165

Pescatori M, Dodi G, Salafia C, Zbar AP (2005) Rectovaginal fistula after double-stapled transanal rectotomy (STARR) for obstructed defaecation. Int J Colorectal Dis 20:83-85

Pescatori M, Favetta U, Dedola S, Orsini S (1997) Transanal stapled excision of rectal mucosa prolapse. Tech Coloproctol 1:96-98

Pescatori M, Gagliardi G (2008) Postoperative complications after procedure for prolapsed hemorrhoids (PPH) and stapled transanal rectal resection (STARR) procedures. Tech Coloproctol 12:7-19

Pescatori M, Milito G, Fiorino M, Cadeddu F (2009) Complications and reinterventions after surgery for obstructed defecation. Int J Colorectal Dis 24:951-959

Pescatori M, Quondamcarlo C (1999) Prevention of intraoperative complications during stapled excision of rectal mucosal prolapse. Tech Coloproctol 3:103-104

Pescatori M, Spyrou M, Pulvirenti d'Urso A (2006) A prospective evaluation of occult disorders in obstructed defecation using the 'iceberg diagram'. Colorectal Dis 8:785-789

Pescatori M, Zbar AP (2009) Reinterventions after complicated or failed STARR procedure. Int J Colorectal Dis 24:87-96

Privitera A, Smyrk TC, Dozois EJ (2010) Three-quadrant mucosal excision for solitary rectal ulcer syndrome. Tech Coloproctol 14:187-188

Ram E, Alper D, Atar E et al (2010) Stapled transanal rectal resection: a new surgical treatment for obstructed defecation syndrome. Isr Med Assoc J 12:74-77

Regadas FS, Regadas SM, Rodrigues LV et al (2005) New devices for stapled rectal mucosectomy: a multicenter experience. Tech Coloproctol 9:243-246

Regadas FS, Regadas SM, Rodrigues LV et al (2005) Transanal repair of rectocele and full rectal mucosectomy with one circular stapler: a novel surgical technique. Tech Coloproctol 9:63-66

Reibetanz J, Boenicke L, Kim M et al (2011) Enterocele is not a contraindication to stapled transanal surgery for outlet obstruction: an analysis of 170 patients. Colorect Dis 13:e131-e136

Renzi A, Talento P, Giardiello C, Angelone G, Izzo D, Di Sarno G (2008) Stapled trans-anal rectal resection (STARR) by a new dedicated device for the surgical treatment of obstructed defaecation syndrome caused by rectal intussusception and rectocele: early results of a multicenter prospective study. Int J Colorectal Dis 23:999-1005

Rosen A (2010) Obstructed defecation syndrome: diagnosis and therapeutic options, with special focus on the STARR procedure. Isr Med Assoc J 12:104-106

Scarcliff SD, Parker M (2010) Efficacy of stapled transanal rectal resection (STARR) for the treatment of obstructive defecation syndrome. Dis Colon Rectum 53:591

Scarcliff SD, Parker M, Birmingham AL (2010) The American Society of Colon and Rectal Surgeons annual meeting May 15–19, 2010. Minneapolis, Minnesota. Poster: efficacy of stapled transanal rectal resection for the treatment of obstructive defecation syndrome

Schiano di Visconte M, Piccin A, Di Bella R et al (2006) Cost-revenue analysis in the surgical treatment of the obstructed defecation syndrome. Chir Ital 58:743-752

Schwandner O (2011) Conversion in transanal stapling techniques for haemorrhoids and anorectal prolapse. Colorectal Dis 13:87-93

Schwandner O, Fürst A (2008) Actual role of stapled transanal rectal resection (STARR) for obstructed defecation syndrome. Zentralbl Chir 133:116-122

Schwandner O, Fürst A, German STARR Registry Study Group (2010) Assessing the safety, effectiveness, and quality of life after the STARR procedure for obstructed defecation: results of the German STARR registry. Langenbecks Arch Surg 395:505-513

Schwandner O, Stuto A, Jayne D et al (2008) Decision-making algorithm for the STARR procedure in obstructed defecation syndrome: position statement of the group of STARR Pioneers. Surg Innov 15:105-109

Sciaudone G, Di Stazio C, Guadagni I, Selvaggi F (2008) Rectal diverticulum: a new complication of STARR procedure for obstructed defecation. Tech Coloproctol 12:61-63

Smart NJ, Mercer-Jones MA (2007) Functional outcome after transperineal rectocele repair with porcine dermal collagen implant. Dis Colon Rectum 50:1422-1427

Song K-H, Lee D-S, Shin J-K et al (2011) Clinical outcomes of stapled transanal rectal resection (STARR) for obstructed defecation syndrome (ODS): a single institution experience in South Korea. Int J Colorectal Dis 26:693:698

Spyrou M, De Nardi P (2005) Fecal incontinence after stapled transanal rectotomy managed with Durasphere injection. Tech Coloproctol 9:87

Stolfi VM, Micossi C, Sileri P, Venza M, Gaspari A (2009) Retroperitoneal sepsis with mediastinal and subcutaneous emphysema complicating stapled transanal rectal resection (STARR). Tech Coloproctol 13:69-71

Torres C, Khaikin M, Bracho J et al (2007) Solitary rectal ulcer syndrome: clinical findings, surgical treatment, and outcomes. Int J Colorectal Dis 22:1389-1393

Trompetto M, Clerico G, Realis Luc A, Marino F, Giani I, Ganio E (2006) Transanal Delorme procedure for treatment of rectocele associated with rectal intussusception. Tech Coloproctol 10:389

Tseng CA, Chen LT, Tsai KB et al (2004) Acute hemorrhagic rectal ulcer syndrome: a new clinical entity? Report of 19 cases and review of the literature. Dis Colon Rectum 47:895-903; discussion 903-905

Vermeulen J, Lange JF, Sikkenk AC, van der Harst E (2005) Anterolateral rectopexy for correction of rectoceles leads to good anatomical but poor functional results. Tech Coloproctol 9:35-41; discussion 41

Wadhawan H, Shorthouse AJ, Brown SR (2010) Surgery for obstructed defaecation: does the use of the Contour device (Trans-STARR) improve results? Colorectal Dis 12:885-890

Williams NS, Dvorkin LS, Giordano P et al (2005) EXternal Pelvic REctal SuSpension (Express procedure) for rectal intussusception, with and without rectocele repair. Br J Surg 92:598-604

Yagnik V (2011) Solitary 'rectal' ulcer syndrome in the sigmoid colon. Colorectal Dis 13:344

Zbar AP, Lienemann A, Fritsch H, Beer-Gabel M, Pescatori M (2003) Rectocele: pathogenesis and surgical management. Int J Colorectal Dis18:369-384

Zehler O, Vashist YK, Bogoevski D et al (2010) Quo vadis STARR? A prospective long-term follow-up of stapled transanal rectal resection for obstructed defecation syndrome. J Gastrointest Surg 14:1349-1354

Zhang B, Ding JH, Yin SH, Zhang M, Zhao K (2010) Stapled transanal rectal resection for obstructed defecation syndrome associated with rectocele and rectal intussusception. World J Gastroenterol 16:2542-2548

Zhao K, Ding JH, Song WL, Zhu J, Yin SH, Tang HY (2009) Application of stapled transanal rectum resection in the treatment of obstructed defecation syndrome. Zhonghua Wai Ke Za Zhi 47:1846-1848

Fecal Incontinence

9

9.1 Introduction

Between 1972, when I graduated, and 1981, when I went to St. Mark's Hospital, in London, for a fellowship, I saw only two patients with fecal incontinence. At St. Mark's, I was taught how to manage this disease; since 1983, I have seen and treated more than 1000 such patients.

The number of incontinent patients is no doubt an underestimate, because most of these patients are ashamed and do not admit to the problem unless properly and insistently questioned by their physician.

Patients with fecal incontinence should undergo a "functional" perineal examination and digital exploration, aimed at detecting perineal descent and assessing anal sphincter tone and contraction. The means to carry out anal manometry and transanal/vaginal rotating probe ultrasound (US) and/or transperineal dynamic US examinations should be available in the proctologist's office. If fecal incontinence is determined, it is initially treated using conservative measures, the main one being pelvic floor rehabilitation.

In fact, very few patients with fecal incontinence need to be treated surgically, less than 15% according to the Annual Report of the SICCR Coloproctology Units (UCP Club), published yearly by Bruni and Occelli and even less, about 1%, according to Bartolo, as reported in a consensus paper by Baeten et al. in 2007. Surgical treatment has the disadvantage that some of the procedures used to treat fecal incontinence are likely to be followed by complications, such as suture dehiscence, local sepsis, and other adverse events, e.g., pacemaker dysfunction or prosthesis displacement. This is the case with dynamic graciloplasty and artificial bowel sphincter, two procedures, discussed below, whose use has recently declined.

Some innovations have proven to be effective, e.g., sacral neuromodulation and, to a minor extent, bulking agents, but sphincter reconstruction and plication may still be helpful in selected cases. Both classical and novel procedures may be followed by complications and the specialist has to be prepared to prevent and to manage them. Moreover, while new technologies are important, as in the treatment of obstructed defecation, when dealing with incontinent patients a holistic approach is needed (Chatoor et al., 2007).

In the following, instead of providing a commented list of postoperative complications, as done in the previous chapter, I use the "live surgery" method as the basis for a discussion of how to prevent them—an approach that the reader may find more appealing.

9.2 Complications During and After Post-anal and Total Pelvic Floor Repair: "Live Surgery"

Recently, a consensus conference chaired by Norman Williams (Baeten et al., 2007), confirmed that Parks' post-anal repair technique continues to have a place in the surgical management of incontinent patients. Elderly patients without severe sphincter dystrophy and those unable to use sophisticated therapeutic devices are the most suitable cases. Mackey et al. (2010) reported an 80% success rate in the long-term in patients with neurogenic incontinence who were selected on the basis of preoperative anorectal physiology tests. This is likely to be a rather optimistic view, as, among our patients, not more than half show significant improvement, also following postoperative sphincter rehabilitation, and only a quarter are fully continent in the medium term. However,

M. Pescatori, *Prevention and Treatment of Complications in Proctological Surgery*,

regardless of the success rate, the Parks procedure is still used, which necessitates a review of its potential complications. So let us now proceed to the operating theatre.

First, a few words about the preoperative preparation. As noted in the Introduction, intraoperatively, rectal perforation occasionally occurs. It even happened to the surgeon who invented the procedure and used it to operate on more than 150 patients. In case of perforation, it is essential to avoid fecal spillage, with contamination of the retrorectal spaces; therefore, mechanical preparation of the patient, with the rectum emptied, should be carried out prior to surgery. In case of iatrogenic lesion, the defect should be sutured, or, if it is large and there has been significant fecal contamination, a diverting sigmoidostomy might be needed. Antibiotic prophylaxis should also be performed, aimed at minimizing the risk of local sepsis. We use metronidazole and last-generation kephalosporins.

Our patient is in the lithotomy position, but the jack-knife position may also be used. A spinal anesthesia may be preferred, possibly implemented with sedation using i.v. Diprivan, as most patients are elderly and fragile and the operation lasts less than one hour. General anesthesia carries the advantage that the surgeon may better appreciate sphincter tone, but I prefer the spinal approach, as it provides full analgesia for several hours after surgery, which is useful in patients with potentially painful muscle sutures. If general anesthesia is performed, it is better to inject Naropine, a long-lasting local anesthetic, at the end of the operation and to ask the anesthetist to insert an i.v. elastomer with either morphine or Ketorolac and gastric protective drugs, bearing in mind that a prolonged use of morphine may increase sigmoid segmental contractions and delay first evacuation.

After making a post-anal "V"-shaped incision, we are faced with the first potential complication: damage of either the sphincter or the anal canal. Specifically, although we have to identify the intersphincteric plane, the incision must correspond with the subcutaneous part of the external sphincter in order to keep the surgical wound at least 4 cm behind the anus, less prone to fecal contamination and local sepsis. Therefore, the correct plane has to be identified between the lower edges of the external sphincter, which has to be left posteriorly, and those of the internal sphincter, located anteriorly. To differentiate between the two muscles, we can seldom rely upon their color, unlike in patients undergoing surgery for anal fissure after the intersphincteric groove has been identified. The difference is that elderly neurogenically incontinent females have pale denervated striated sphincters. A simple trick is to touch the muscles with diathermy: the external sphincter usually reacts with a circumferential contraction. As soon as the intersphincteric plane is entered, it should be kept in mind that the internal sphincter is thin in these patients, especially in its upper part, corresponding to the upper anal canal. Therefore, attention must be paid to avoid injury of the anal canal; otherwise, the defect will have to be closed with a fine extraluminal absorbable running suture.

Continuing the dissection higher up, not more than 3-4 cm from the anal verge, as the anal canal is short in these incontinent, often female patients, we reach the posterior part of the puborectalis muscle, which is gently pulled downwards with a Mathieu retractor (Fig. 9.1). The upper part of the intersphincteric plane is then entered bilaterally, by blunt scissors dissection or using a small swab, until the entire puborectalis sling is separated from the inner visceral muscle up to the anorectal ring.

At this point, the dissection can be ended if a "limited" post-anal repair is performed, in case the anal canal, which is an important factor for anal continence, does not need to be markedly lengthened, or if an anterior levatorplasty is planned.

Alternatively, if the dissection has to be continued upwards to carry out a formal Parks post-anal repair, the Waldeyer fascia, a whitish fibrotic tissue, is divided to identify the pubococcygeus and ileococcygeus muscles, which subsequently will be plicated. Yellow spots indicating the posterior distal mesorectum will appear and a careful dissection between the levator plane and the rectal smooth muscle is subsequently carried out in the posterior hemicircumference, avoiding inadvertent rectal injuries. This plane is embryologically avascular; therefore, if bleeding appears, it means that we entered at the wrong plane, cutting some of the striated muscle fibers. At the end of this maneuver, the lower rectum will be freed and lifted up with a Morris retractor. It is better not to use a Mathieu retractor at this stage, as its distal hooks might cause injury to the rectum.

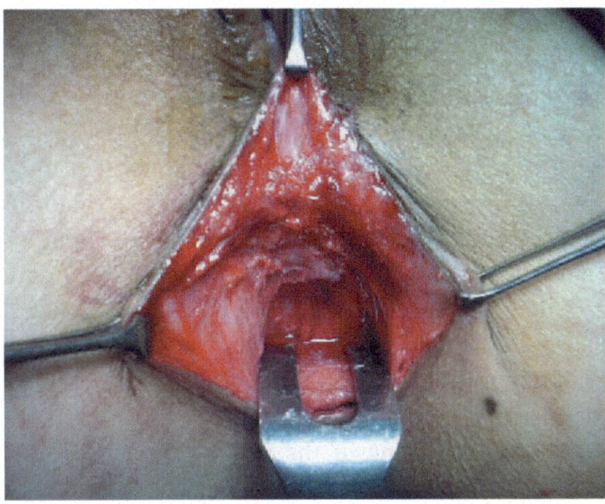

Fig. 9.1 a Parks' plication of the posterior pelvic floor for the treatment of neuropathic fecal incontinence. A Mathieu retractor pulls below the deep part of the external sphincter. Above: the anal canal

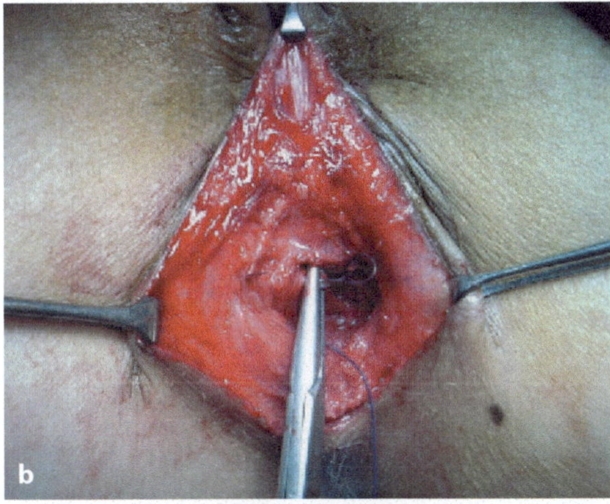

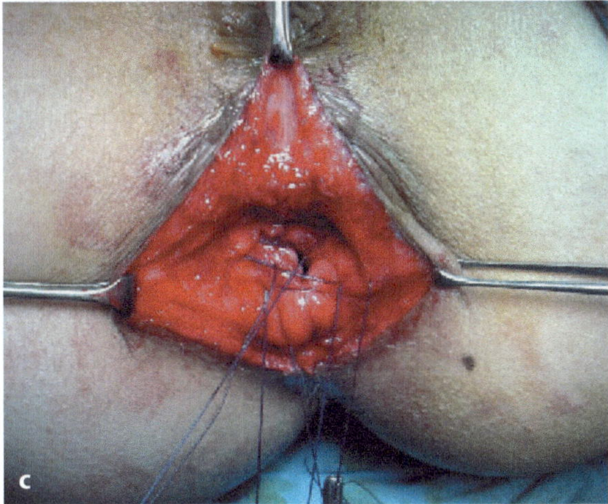

Fig. 9.1 b, c Plication of the puborectalis muscle. **b** Initial; **c** Final plication of the puborectalis muscle

The dissection is complete and the levator muscle is plicated bilaterally with non-absorbable sutures, which are not completely tightened to prevent laceration of the muscle fibers. A kind of suspending net should be created behind the rectum, aimed at elongating the anal canal and narrowing the anorectal angle. Care should be taken not to incorporate segments of the rectal wall in the plicating suture, to prevent endoluminal migration of the prolene stitches—an error that I made twice in my early experience. Slowly absorbable suture may be used when plicating the puborectalis muscle, a few centimeters below the levator ani, as at this level the knots may be tightened. The plicated muscle of the two sides will be in contact with each other, and the subsequent fibrosis will favor the adhesion of the tissues at the plication site. Both the deep and the superficial part of the external sphincter are plicated posteriorly using Vicryl Rapid, avoiding a tight knot as it is likely to cause postoperative pain. After careful hemostasis, a Penrose drain may be left in the retrorectal space; however, in most cases I do not leave any drainage.

I prefer not to suture the underskin so as not to close all of the spaces, which could favor the growth of anaerobic microorganisms. It is better not to carry out a complete horizontal closure of the skin incision, to reduce the risk of fecal and bacterial contamination and to avoid stretching of the wound, which might leave a gaping anus. The "V" incision is then partially closed with cross-shaped suturing and the very distal edge of the skin flap excised, to less than 1 cm, as it is otherwise likely to become necrotic and infected.

At the final digital exploration, we should feel a tightened anus and an elongated anal canal, with a narrowed anorectal angle, both of which mean that the operation has been anatomically successful.

Mackey et al. (2010), working with Lubowski who trained with Sir Alan Parks, reported a 10% rate of postoperative complications in 57 patients, most females, who underwent post-anal repair. There was one deep venous thrombosis, two hemorrhoidal thromboses, one fecal impaction, one case of severe nausea and vomiting, and one of urinary retention. Thus, at least in the hands of those authors, post-anal repair is a very safe procedure. By contrast, in my early experience, some of my patients had local sepsis, described in the section

"Unforgettable complications". The risk of infection may be minimized using several intraoperative maneuvers, as discussed below.

Should we decide to perform a total pelvic floor repair, a wide curved incision, anteriorly convex, is made between the anus and the vagina (most of these patients are females), followed by plication of both the external sphincter and the lateral branches of the puborectalis muscle with U-shaped stitches, which are unlikely to lacerate the muscles, using slowly absorbable sutures and, again, without completely closing the skin but instead leaving a cross-shaped wound. During the anterior dissection, care should be taken to prevent injuries of the posterior wall of the vagina. In case of minor bleeding, rather than using diathermy, it is often advisable to wait until natural coagulation takes place, facilitated by compression with a swab soaked in adrenaline.

Before going on to the complications that may occur following other operations, I present the procedures currently available for the management of anal incontinence. They are listed in Table 9.1 and consist of manual operations as well as procedures based on technological devices, e.g. prostheses, thus underlining the important role of industry in the progress of therapy.

I have used nine of the above-reported procedures, the most recent being tibial nerve electrostimulation and the most frequent being post-anal

Table 9.1 Main operations for the management of incontinent patients. Authors who either invented the procedure or published the largest series are listed in chronological order

Intervention	First author	Year
Manual operations		
Gluteoplasty	Chetwood	2002
	Devesa	1992
Sphincter reconstruction	Lockart- Mummery	1923
	Blaisdell	1942
Graciloplasty	Pickrell	1952
Post-anal repair	Parks	1975
Anoplasty and "re-routing"	Nixon	1984
Puborectalis-external sphincteroplasty	Christiansen	1987
Gracilo-smooth muscle-plasty	Pescatori	1990
Total pelvic floor repair	Keighley	1991
Procedures with prosthesis or other devices		
Dacron ring	Labrow	1980
Magnetic ring	Schier	1986
	Lehur	2010
Silicone-Marlex ring	Devesa	2011
Artificial sphincter	Corman	1983
	Christiansen	1987
	Wong	2002
Dynamic graciloplasty	Baeten	1988
	Williams	1991
Injection of bulking agents	Shafik	1993
	Tjandra	2004
Sacral neuromodulation	Matzel	1995
Radiofrequency	Takahashi	2002
Tibial nerve electrostimulation	Shafik	2003
Polyester puborectalis sling	Yamaha	2003
Acupuncture	Scaglia	2009

and total pelvic floor repair and sphincter reconstruction. I abandoned graciloplasty due to the large number of adverse events. I do not use gluteoplasty due to its frequent complications, or the artificial sphincter procedure due to its high cost and frequent failures.

9.3 Anterior Levatorplasty

Rather than "levatorplasty," a more accurate description is plasty of the puborectalis, which is the muscle involved in the procedure, as the puborectalis muscle is not part of the levator ani, according to a recent publication (Guo et al., 2010).

The postoperative complications include pain, which may be due to the muscular sutures, especially if they have been markedly tightened, since the anal sphincters are highly innervated. Dyspareunia may also occur whereas rectovaginal fistulae are uncommon. There may be bleeding, possibly from the posterior vaginal wall. Local sepsis and suture dehiscence rarely require parenteral feeding or stoma formation.

9.4 Sphincter Reconstruction

This procedure is required in case of moderate or severe incontinence following trauma to the anal sphincters, due either to an accident or as a byproduct of an operation, e.g., sphincter division during a fistulotomy, or to a vaginal delivery with or without an episiotomy. Significant continence disorders are more likely the result of an external sphincter lesion, with the goal of surgery being to reconstruct the continuity of the sphincter ring.

According to a recent study carried out at our unit, involving over 1,000 patients and based on a prospective database (Bondurri et al., 2011), fecal incontinence due to traumatic lesions of the anal sphincters and to congenital malformations have a significantly worse score (> 4) in the 0-6 grading system of Pescatori et al. (1992) than incontinence related to other etiologies.

If the patient with a diverting stoma comes to our attention, sphincter reconstruction is unlikely to be followed by local sepsis and suture dehiscence, as there is no risk of fecal contamination. The stoma will be closed after the surgical wounds have healed.

The most frequently used operation is the overlapping procedure (Fig. 9.2), carried out without excision of the fibrotic ends of the divided muscle, which is thought to ensure a stronger suture. However, excessive scarring itself may make overlap impossible (Moscovitz et al., 2002). Unlike in patients who undergo post-anal repair, those who require sphincter reconstruction after trauma do not have neuropathic dystrophic sphincters; therefore, postoperative incontinence is less frequent, ranging between 20 and 30% over the medium term in most series. Nevertheless, Evans et al. (2006) reported that only 21% of their patients were fully continent in the long term, although, according to the same authors, after 4 years another 32% had flatus incontinence only. Therefore, more than half of the patients in this series had either good or satisfactory continence over the long term following sphincter reconstruction.

Watson et al. (2005) reported only four minor complications in 17 cases (one hematoma, two superficial dehiscences, and one local sepsis), but a deterioration of anal continence 5 years after surgery, even if the sphincteroplasty seemed to be intact at anal US. Again, as noted in the previous chapter, according to Vermeulen et al. (2005), restoration of the normal anatomy after rectocele repair did not lead to a restoration of normal function. Similar findings were reported by Osterberg et al. (2000), Pinta et al. (2003) and Barisic et al. (2006).

To minimize the risk of a progressive deterioration of anal continence with time, Ferreira et al. (2010) reinforced the sphincter reconstruction with a Permacol mesh, the same as used for rectocele and, more rarely, for rectovaginal fistulae. Use of the mesh did not increase the rate of postoperative complications, whereas continence in the short term was improved compared with sphincter reconstruction without use of the mesh.

To minimize the risk of suture dehiscence, it is better not to isolate the divided sphincter endings for more than 2.5 cm, thus maintaining a good vascular supply, and to avoid the use of diathermy. Also, extension of the lateral dissection risks damaging the nerve supply to the sphincters at the level

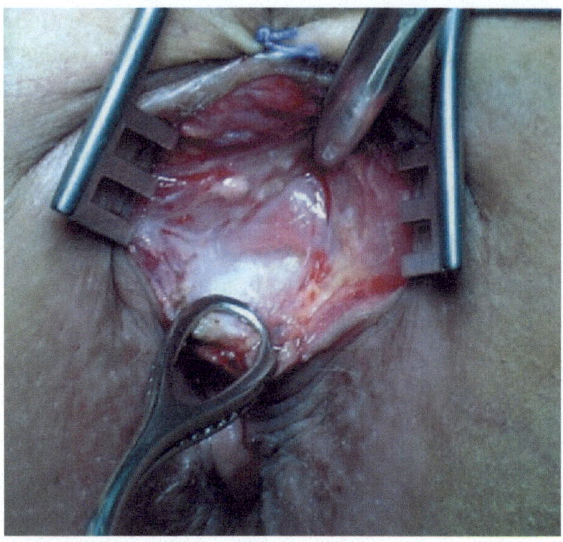

Fig. 9.2 a Sphincter reconstruction in the treatment of fecal incontinence after local excision of anal cancer. A postoperative and post-radiotherapy fibrosis is present

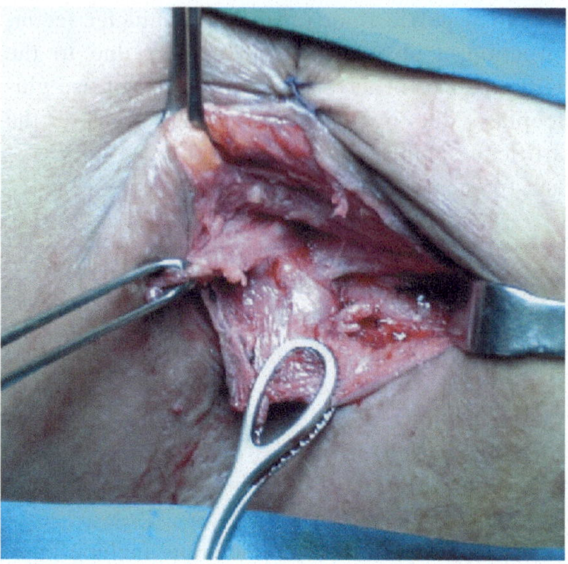

Fig. 9.2 b External sphincter ends, sectioned in the previous operation, are identified and prepared. It is important that they not be devascularized

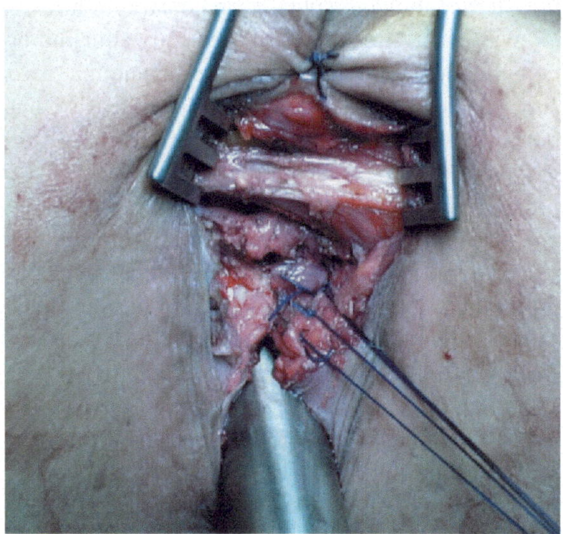

Fig. 9.2 c Reconstruction using the overlapping procedure. Some authors report good functional results using direct suturing. Patient in the lithotomy position

of the Alcock canal and injuring the nerves crossing the ischiorectal space laterally and posteriorly.

As far as the type of suture, according to Oberwalder et al. (2008), direct suture of the divided ends of the sphincters does not improve functional results compared with the overlapping procedure. Zorcolo, Covotta, and Bartolo (2005) reported their experience based on 84 patients in 8 years: a 26% rate of wound sepsis and dehiscence, which in my patients operated on by post-anal repair has occurred more frequently. In their group, a diverting stoma was required in a patient with suture breakdown. To minimize the risk of local sepsis, they recommended leaving the wound partially open and drained with a Penrose.

Postoperative bleeding is rare and may be caused by the erosion of a vessel at the site of the plasty due to local infection. Therefore, antibiotic prophylaxis is recommended to minimize the risk of hemorrhage. In case of more complex muscle reconstruction, with wide tissue dissection, a diverting sigmoidostomy or, in some cases, a course of total parenteral nutrition may be indicated to prevent fecal contamination of the wound. Bowel motions may be delayed using constipating agents; however, afterwards, the evacuation of hard feces with excessive straining might damage the sphincteroplasty. Therefore, standard sphincter reconstruction does not need to be followed by any dietary restrictions. Instead, a high-fiber diet might be helpful to keep the stool soft and non-traumatizing. Self-digitation should be avoided, to prevent suture disruption.

This reminds me of an impressive case involving one of our patients, whose sphincter reconstruction failed due to the failure to consider a holistic approach. This 35-year-old woman, suffering from severe fecal incontinence due to a congenital anomaly, came to our unit approximately 15 years ago. She lived with her relatives, who were attentively taking care of her. Since she had a fiancée and was planning to marry, she felt that her disabling disease had to be cured. After an appropriate preoperative work-up, a sphincteroplasty was planned and then carried out, in which the continuity of the muscle ring was re-established around the anal canal. The postoperative course was uneventful and the patient was discharged with the recommendation to eat a high-fiber diet and to drink plenty of water to keep the stool soft, and to avoid enemas and self-digitation. A course of pelvic floor exercises was also prescribed, as suggested by Jensen and Lowry (1997). After 3 months, the patient came to our clinic and was found to have recurrent incontinence. Surprisingly, we found out that she had not complied with any of the rehabilitation measures and had self-digitated regularly. When questioned by our psychologist, she admitted that, after having been cured, her relatives did not take care of her any more as she was no longer incontinent, such that she felt abandoned. Therefore, she preferred her disabling condition and the assistance of her family. We realized that the psychosomatic component of her disease had not been properly investigated prior to surgery, but that it was the main cause of failure. It is for this and similar reasons that Chatoor et al. (2007), as already mentioned in the Introduction, underlined the importance of a holistic approach.

9.5 Sacral Neuromodulation

The role of sacral nerve stimulation in treating fecal incontinence and refractory constipation was fully detailed in the Supplement of Colorectal Disease, March 2011. According to Matzel (2011) and Melenhorst et al. (2007), the spectrum of indications has expanded based on the improved results of test stimulation: a 77% improvement in idiopathic fecal incontinence, 76% in sphincter rupture/episiotomy, 78% after anal repair, and 73% in neurological injury. Klaus Matzel, who is a consultant of Medtronic, reported a complication rate of 20% after permanent implantation of the pacemaker (2004) in 171 patients. Pain, infection, and pacemaker dislocation were the most frequent complications. By contrast, infection was negligible in a large series published by Wexner et al. in 2010. Electrostimulation had to be interrupted in 15 patients: temporarily in ten, permanently in five. Van Wunnik et al. (2010) reported pain at the pacemaker site in 52% of their patients.

Faucheron et al. (2010) performed 36 re-interventions in their 84 patients, mainly for sepsis and either dislocation or rupture of the electrode/pacemaker. Murphy et al. (2010), however, reported a much lower re-operation rate (12%). Only eight out of the 60 patients operated upon by Altomare et al. (2009) required re-operation for electrode explantation, but none of them had the newer type of electrode (recently constructed by the Italian urologist Spinelli), which is softer, more resistant, and less traumatizing. Lieske et al. (2010) had to explant either the electrode or the pacemaker in 12% of their patients. Fortunately, a delayed re-implantation of the electrode/pace-maker is likely to work after either complication (Malouf et al., 2010).

Sacral neuromodulation is costly, but in a paper focusing on the cost/benefits ratio it appears to be financially acceptable (Indinnimeo et al., 2000). The authors, of whom two work for Medtronic, reported that the budgeted cost for sacral neuromodulation represents only 0.6% of the money spent for patients with fecal incontinence in 5 years. As I work in a private hospital and the patients must be able to assume the high cost of the device, the use of sacral neuromodulation is limited. I performed a temporary implant in a patient with traumatic lesions to the sphincter, who did not receive a permanent implant due to a poor functional response. In my private practice, I have referred a number of incontinent patients who were candidates for neuromodulation to public hospitals, where patients' expenses are covered by the National Health Service (Bondurri et al., 2011). However, even if expensive, sacral neuromodulation is minimally invasive and effective, accounting for its increasing use. Moreover, it is indicated also for other functional disorders, such as chronic proctalgia and constipation.

The first report on the use of spinal cord electrostimulation in two constipated neurological patients treated in Rome was published by our multidisciplinary group (proctologist, radiologists and neurosurgeons) in the Proceedings of the GI Motility Symposium, held in Konigstein (Pescatori et al., 1982; available on my website: www.ucp-club.it/medici_articolo.asp). Kamm, who has written extensively on neuromodulation, encouraged me to summarize and comment on my experience, resulting in two reports, in the British Journal of Surgery (2006) and in Dis Colon Rectum (2009), on neuromodulation's mechanism of action, as illustrated by myoelectrical motor tracings recorded at the level of the distal sigmoid. The method has since been improved, with a dedicated procedure and device, and commercialized. The respective results were summarized in papers published after 2000 by several authors, as reported in Colorectal Disease, 2011, among them Matzel and Leroi.

9.5.1 Radiofrequency Energy

Here, we briefly discuss the Secca procedure. The heat released by radiofrequency energy can generate an anatomically advantageous modification of the anal canal. The result is a rapid contraction of the collagenous tissue followed by fibrosis and some degree of tightening of the anal canal itself. A few papers have reported moderate improvement in the short-term, among them the one by Felt-Bersma et al. (2007). By contrast, Kim et al. (2009) did not find any positive change in anal continence and reported complications such as anal ulcerations, bleeding, pain, and discharge. Efron et al. (2003) reported similar complications, namely, bleeding ulcers. I have no personal experience with this procedure, which has not gained popularity among coloproctologists.

9.6 Dynamic Graciloplasty and Gluteoplasty

9.6.1 Graciloplasty

Postoperative complications have been reported in more than half of the patients treated with this procedure in Maastricht, where Cor Baeten and coworkers nonetheless have extensive expertise (1988-2011). Therefore, in the hands of others, the operation is likely to be at even higher risk of complications. In one-third of the cases, the pacemaker had to be explanted. Local sepsis, pain, rectal prolapse, and suture dehiscences may require re-intervention, including bowel resection and diverting stoma (Koch et al., 2004). The interposed gracilis muscle may cause obstructed defecation in up to 90% of the patients, in which case the Biotrol Irrimatic pump may be helpful in irrigating the bowel and managing constipation (Koch et al., 2008). Obstructed defecation, which usually occurs in 15% of the cases, is responsible for half of the conversions to colostomy. Other complications are related to the stimulator and the electrical leads, with swelling and paresthesia in the donor leg (Chapman et al., 2002).

Due to the above-mentioned complications, the use of the procedure is declining. I abandoned it after operating on six patients, three for fecal incontinence and three after abdominoperineal excision of the rectum for cancer. Three patients had gracilis muscle detachment due either to ischemia or to sepsis.

9.6.2 Gluteoplasty

Training the patient is easier after this procedure, as, unlike the gracilis, the gluteus muscle is synergistic with the anal sphincters. However, postoperative complications are frequent.

McFail and Hultman (2006) operated on 25 patients. In this group, 64% had gluteal complications, such as paresthesia, cellulitis, abscesses, and severe pain, and 56% had rectal-vaginal complications, such as fistulae and prolapses. However, Guelincks and Sinsel (1996) did not report any relevant complications in 11 patients, four of whom underwent dynamic gluteoplasty.

Manuel Devesa, who has been using this procedure since 1992, nearly abandoned it due to a high complication rate of 46% (2002) and nowadays prefers to use a novel silicone-Marlex ring, similar to a Jackson-Pratt drain, as first described in 2011. Still, this is an encirclement procedure, but it is passive rather than based on a patient's voluntary contraction, as is the case in gluteoplasty. Further details are given at the end of this chapter.

9.7 Artificial Sphincter

Among the various artificial sphincter procedures, the one that until recently had the most success was the artificial bowel sphincter (ABS). However, as with dynamic graciloplasty, its popularity has markedly declined due to the high cost and frequent postoperative complications. Studies regarding the latter are summarized in Table 9.2.

The fact that no studies on ABS were presented at the 2010 ASCRS Congress, in contrast to the seven reports on sacral neuromodulation, confirms the declining use of the artificial bowel sphincter among colorectal surgeons. Wexner et al. (2009) reported early failure in four out of ten cases, due to local sepsis. More than half of the patients who had their first defecation within two days after the operation subsequently had an infection requiring removal of the prosthesis. Late failures were due to a malfunction of the device. Overall, the prosthesis has been removed in 31 out of 51 patients, around 60%, which represents a high failure rate.

Similar concerns were raised by Altomare (2001), Devesa (2002) and others, who, after their initial enthusiasm for the device, reported negative medium and long-term results, among them the frequent need for enemas due to obstructed defecation caused by the device. Lehur, who also was a supporter of the ABS and taught many surgeons how to implant it, eventually reconsidered the efficacy of the procedure in light of the negative outcome of his patients, as reported in Table 9.2. He now recommends the use of a novel prosthesis, the magnetic sphincter (Lehur et al., 2010). Whether poor outcome is later determined also with this novel procedure remains to be seen. Meanwhile patients are undergoing surgery, with the implantation of costly devices.

Senagore et al. (1993) suggested that, given their controversial unsatisfactory results, novel and costly procedures should be tested in prospective randomized trials conducted at quality institutions prior to being introduced into clinical routine. Adequate investigations are needed to demonstrate that such procedures can achieve better outcome than less cost-intensive operations, whose efficacy has been already proven. This was not true in some cases, as underlined by Jayne and Finan (2005).

Industry contributes to medical progress, but, understandably, profit is its main interest. Some surgeons become involved based on their enthusiasm for innovations in the field. Unfortunately, patients may suffer due to the realities of these new technologies, if there are associated complications and failures.

Goligher, in the article "Skepticism in surgery" (1990), wrote that most innovations, are ultimately found to be either ineffective or dangerous. Clearly, innovations have to be invented and tested; this is inherent to eventual progress, but sometimes the price paid by healthcare budgets and in terms of patient safety are too high. Consider Wexner et al.'s report on the results obtained with ABS. The authors should be commended for their

Table 9.2 Complications following artificial sphincter implantation (ABS in all series but one study)

First author	Year	Cases (N)	Follow-up (mo.)	% Sepsis	% Re-interventions	% Explants
Altomare	2001	28	19	18	32	25
Wong	2002	112	18	25	46	37
Ortiz	2002	22	26	9	50	32
Parker	2003	37	39	34	37	40
Michot	2003	25	34	7	28	20
Da Silva	2004	11	12	12	12	0
Lehur	2007	32	26	0	53	31
Wexner	2009	51	41	40	60	60
Ruiz Carmona	2009	17[a]	68	30	65	65

[a]Acticon (AMS, Minneapolis, USA).

honesty and accuracy, but, given the 60% failure rate and the 86% rate of complications after a procedure lasting 2 hours, this means a lot of money spent not only to buy, but also to implant the costly device, and then to re-operate on patients in whom it failed. One may justifiably consider whether the costs and health risks are worthwhile.

Fortunately, in the USA, the FDA oversees of the clinical use of novel technologies. In other countries, the National Health Service carefully controls the use of novel procedures, e.g., implantation of the ABS in Spain was restricted to selected institutions run by accredited specialists. A new international Society, the ECTA (Eurasian Colorectal Technology Association, www.ectamed.org), has been founded to encourage the correct use and discourage the abuse of new technologies. A wise balance between prudence and innovation is not easy, but is urgently needed. It may help us to decide whether to carry out a novel procedure in its early stage or, better, whether to perform it at all, based on the reported outcome in many patients with long follow-up. This may well help us to decrease the postoperative complications rate.

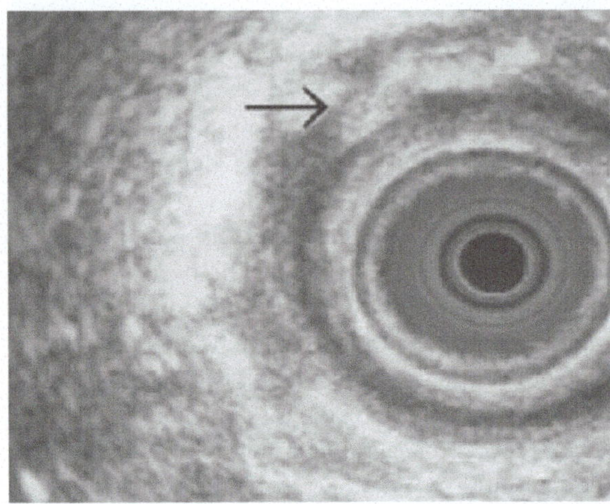

Fig. 9.3 Transanal ultrasonography with a rotating probe. Hyperechogenic spots (*arrow*) represent a bulking agent (silicone) or PTQ that has been injected in the intersphincteric space to correct mild fecal incontinence. Cases in which this or similar substances have become dislocated have been described. The complications of the procedure are rare and mild

9.8 Bulking Agents

The procedure is rather costly (at least 1500 Euros per patient) but is minimally invasive and complications are seldom. An essentially cost-free method is to perianally inject autologous fat harvested from the thigh and adequately prepared by centrifugation. Unfortunately, as happened in our patients, the fat tends to be reabsorbed and to lose its bulking effect with time (Bernardi et al., 1998). The dislocation of silicone (PTQ) was reported by de la Portilla et al. (2009), as shown in Fig. 9.3. The only negative effect of this adverse event is that it does not improve anal continence. Soerensen et al. (2009) did not report any complications following injection of silicone spherules in 33 patients, not even mild pain or soreness, but a conflict of interest disclosure was lacking at the end of their paper. Bartlett and Ho (2009) reported nine cases with minor complications out of 94 injected with PTQ: mucosal ulceration in one patient, constipation and/or diarrhea in two, pain and/or soreness in three, and local sepsis in one, requiring a cutaneous incision to remove the injected silicone. The other two patients had a late dislocation of the PTQ, which was detected at anal US.

Either during or after the injection of Durasphere, this bulking agent may penetrate into the vagina. This happened in one of my patients, without any negative consequences (Altomare et al., 2008). Ganio et al. (2008) observed only a minor adverse event in one of their 10 patients injected with Coaptite: the bulking agent was discharged through the cutaneous site of the injection. Neither toxic nor allergic complications have been reported so far.

Submucosal injection of Nasha/Dx gel was not followed by any adverse events in 34 patients treated for fecal incontinence by a Swedish group (Danielson et al., 2010) that presented an Abstract at the 2010 ASCRS Congress, in which a significant improvement in the long-term quality of life was reported. This is an interesting finding, as the prospective multicenter SICCR study of Durasphere by Altomare et al. (2008) reported an improvement in the continence score, but no improvement in quality of life.

9.9 Puborectalis Sling and Silicone Ring

9.9.1 Puborectalis Sling

Yamana et al. (2004), in Japan, operated on eight patients with idiopathic fecal incontinence, positioning a polyester sling (2 x 6 cm) with two strips at the level of the puborectalis muscle in order to narrow the anorectal angle, similar to the Angelchik prosthesis described decades ago and previously used to restore the His angle in patients with gastroesophageal reflux. Post-anal and suprapubic incisions are made, the sling is positioned to push the anorectal angle anteriorly, and the ends of the two strips are anchored to the pubic symphisis. No severe complications occurred postoperatively. One patient had sepsis of the surgical wound and another had a rectal ulceration, due to migration of the sling, which eroded the posterior wall of the rectum and was then removed.

9.9.2 Silicone Ring

Devesa et al. (2011) operated on 33 patients with fecal incontinence using a novel prosthesis consisting of a radiopaque silicone ring. The presence of multiple millimeter-size holes along its length provides additional elasticity. Mean follow-up was 3 years and all but one patient improved. Early complications included spontaneous breaking of the sling in two cases and local infection in another two. Late complications were related to skin erosion followed by infection in two patients, in one occurring 3 years after surgery, and breaking of the sling in seven patients. Synchronous or delayed reinsertion of the sling was possible in ten patients and definitive removal was required in three.

9.10 Trick of the Trade

I learned this trick from Sir Alan Parks, who used it when carrying out post-anal repair. At the beginning, when the intersphincteric plane is entered, prior to identification of the puborectalis muscle and division of the Waldeyer fascia, a wide triangle of skin, underskin, and fat tends to block the surgeon's view. An easy solution to this problem is to lift up the triangle and stitch its superior apex to the suprapubic region, above the vagina. Any kind of material may be used, as it is just a stay suture. By doing so, one achieves a better view of the operative field without the need to position a retractor. The tissues are stretched cranially, the puborectalis sling and the Waldeyer fascia become easily detectable, and the posterior wall of the distal rectum may be seen once the fascia is divided (Fig. 9.4).

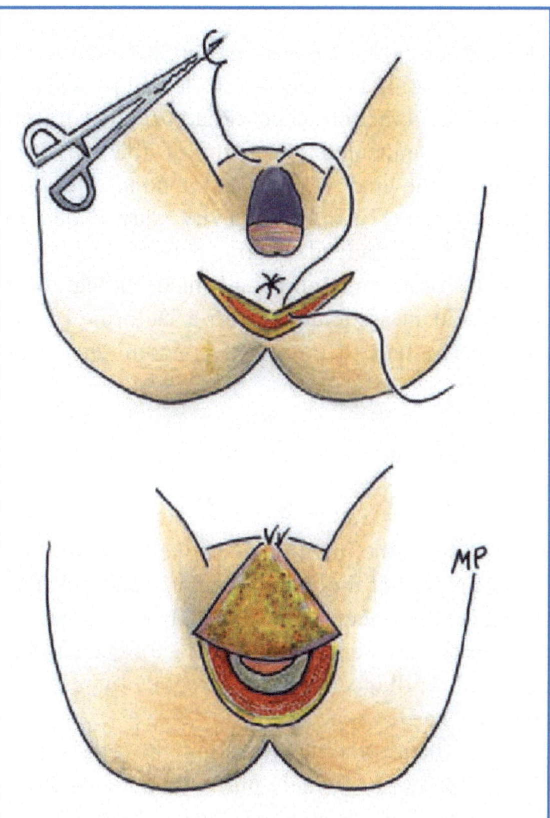

Fig. 9.4 A retro-anal skin triangle is sutured to the suprapubic area by one or two U-shaped stitches. External sphincter, puborectalis muscle, Waldeyer's fascia, and distal rectum *(pink)* are seen

9.11 Unforgettable Complications

9.11.1 The First Five

When I reviewed the first 25 post-anal repairs that I had performed, in the late 1980s, I found that five patients had local infection at the site of the surgical wound, with a severe breakdown of the sutures plicating the muscles, followed by a recurrence of fecal incontinence. It had been frustrating to see the unhealed perineum of the suffering patients, who had wide open wounds, with the sutures floating in a deep cavity, surrounded by necrotic tissue. Indeed, the five patients had something in common: sphincter plication had been carried out in association with a Delorme procedure, performed to correct a concomitant rectal prolapse.

Time for the reader to venture a hypothesis. What was the cause of failure?

I realized that the infection was likely due to fecal contamination of the intersphincteric and retrorectal spaces, as mucosectomy had been performed prior to the post-anal repair. Therefore, fecal and bacterial spillage from the rectal lumen had entered "sterile" spaces.

Since then, when performing the two procedures together, I routinely place the patients under strong antibiotic prophylaxis, using both metronidazole and kefalosporin, and clean the operative field, irrigating it with iodine and changing the towels, gloves, and instruments at the end of the Delorme. Alternatively, muscle plicating stitches might be protected prior to be knotted (Fig. 9.5) By adopting this routine, my patients have not had any of these complications.

9.11.2 The Last One

P. was a 15-year-old girl when I first operated on her, for congenital fecal incontinence. It was a demanding operation, as only part of the sphincters were present, therefore necessitating a complex sphincteroplasty. Fortunately, she did well for many years, until age 33. Since her father had left the family when she was a child and because the first operation had improved her quality of her life, P. was very attached to me. She is an intelligent young woman, suffers from chronic amenorrhea and a stammer and is cross-eyed and very shy. She has a very possessive mother.

Two years earlier I had to re-operate on her due to moderate recurrent incontinence. At surgery, carried out with the patient in the lithotomy position, fluid leaking from the vagina, with the risk of contaminating the perineum, was noted. To prevent sepsis, I filled the vagina with gauze. The maneuver was rather difficult, as she had never had sexual intercourse and thus had an intact hymen. An incomplete puborectalis sling was sutured to the residual external sphincters, the bowel was confined for a week, and P. was discharged after an uneventful postoperative course. Her anal continence improved.

Eight months later, she started to complain of constipation and lower abdominal pain. She was given antispasmodics and fiber, but the symptoms worsened. Pelvic US confirmed the presence of a mass, already detected on plane X-ray of the abdomen. MRI confirmed the dislocation of the uterus seen at US, and a teratoma was diagnosed. As the gynecologist told her that she might need a hysterectomy, I referred her to a skilled oncologic surgeon, a colleague of mine. Of course, P. was very worried and not readily reassured. After a week, she was admitted to my colleague's hospital.

What do you think of this case? Was there any relationship between the patient's symptoms and the previous operations performed for fecal incontinence?

Two months later, P. called me saying that everything had gone well, but she wanted to see me in my office. She came with her mother, as usual. P. was smiling, but had an intriguing expression on her face. The mother looked nervous. The two women sat down in front of me and P. gave me a sheet of paper, without saying anything. I started reading. It was the operation sheet, signed by my colleague's assistant. According to the report: "Prior to commencing the operation, with the patient under general anesthesia, a careful vaginal exploration was carried out, made difficult by the presence of the hymen, and a fist-like hard mass was removed, which was found to be a calcified gauze. A plane x-ray was then performed in the operating theatre, revealing no pathologic mass in the lower abdomen. The patient was awakened and sent to the ward" (Fig. 9.6).

"Bloody gauze!" I thought. "The one I had placed in the vagina prior to starting the sphincteroplasty." I remembered that I had decided not to pull it out at the end of the operation, to keep the perineal wound free of any vaginal smear contamination; but at the time I thought that my assistant had removed it when discharging the patient. But he didn't, and it was my fault not to have thought about the gauze when I saw P. at follow-up as an outpatient, or when I heard about her abdominal pain, and finally when the diagnosis of teratoma was made. As she was amenorrheic and did not have sexual intercourse, the gauze in the vagina sank into oblivion until it started to cause local pain. Fortunately, the oncologic surgeon carried out a vaginal exploration prior to opening the patient. I regretted not having stitched the outer end of the gauze with a suture, as it might have been easily removed like a menstrual tampon.

These thoughts preoccupied me for a while, and P. was exactly aware of my feelings. But she reassured me that she harbored no resentment.

After over a year, she still has some degree of incontinence and is scheduled for a trial of sacral neuromodulation. However, she has found a job and is rather happy. She e-mails me twice a month.

A brief comment is due here. Some readers might question my decision to share this complication, as there is a professional error behind it. I have chosen to do so in order to help you to avoid re-operating on a patient who underwent previous surgery and now has a pelvic mass. Or better, to remind you not to leave a gauze in the vagina of a patient in a case similar to this one.

The best instructive video I ever watched was at the Royal College of Surgeons of England. "Surgical disasters" by Professor Heald, showed the severe intraoperative complications that had happened during his experience teaching the TME procedure to surgeons around the world: dramatic injuries of the common iliac artery due to sparks caused by faulty diathermy, unexpected perforating traumas of the small bowel, almost left behind when closing the abdomen, etc. Rather than lose my respect, he earned my gratitude, for being honest enough to admit to these complications.

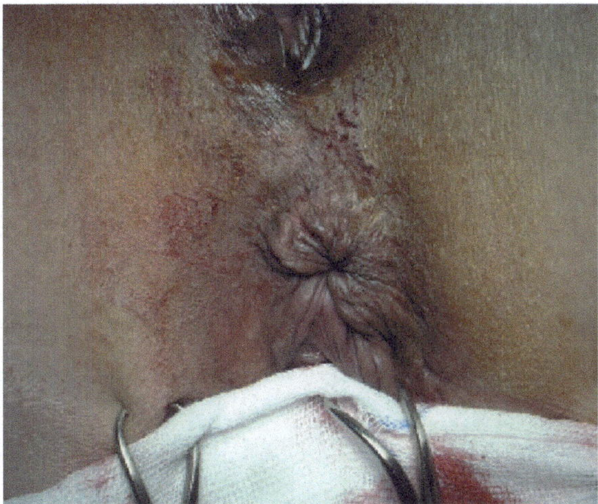

Fig. 9.5 a The cutaneous underlying surgical wound is protected

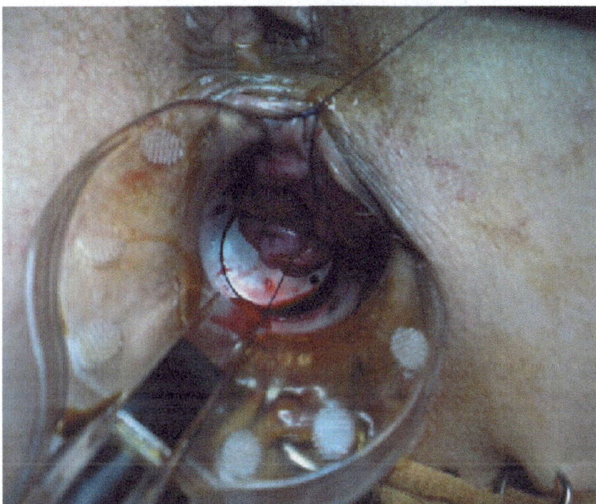

Fig. 9.5 b Block's transanal operation is performed, using an obliterative suture for rectocele and rectal internal mucosal prolapse

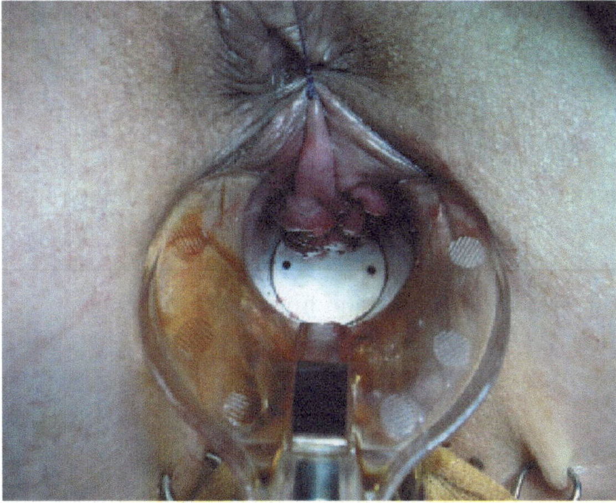

Fig. 9.5 c The Block procedure is finished

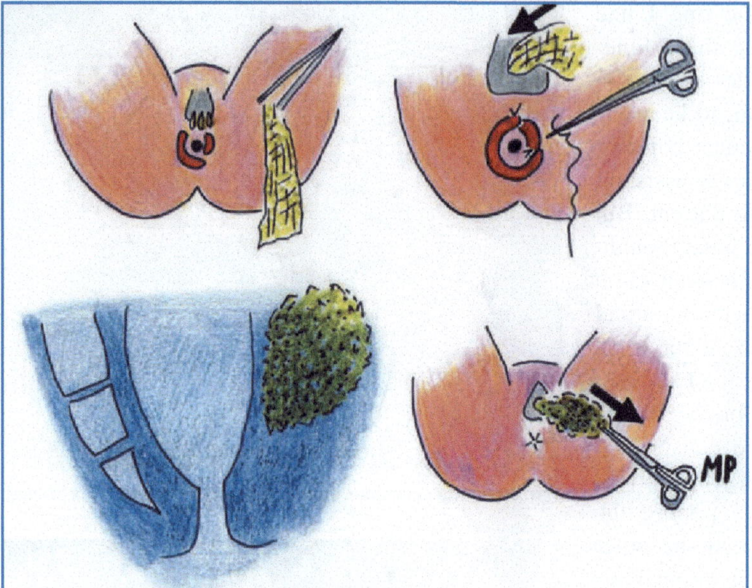

Fig. 9.6 After two sphincteroplasties for congenital fecal incontinence, pelvic teratoma was diagnosed, However, prior to its surgical removal, a vaginal exploration with the patient under anesthesia revealed a calcified gauze placed and left in the vagina during the previous operation. The gauze was removed, obviating the need for further surgery

Summary

The complication rate following post-anal repair carried out using Park's method is unlikely to be higher than 10%. Wound sepsis is more likely to occur after sphincter reconstruction, unless a diverting stoma is performed. Sphincteroplasty may be reinforced by biological meshes, without increasing the complication rate. Anterior levatorplasty may be followed by pain and dyspareunia. Bleeding is rare after any of these procedures.

More than 50% of the patients may have complications after dynamic graciloplasty and gluteoplasty. Some of these complications are severe, such as muscle detachment due to local sepsis, and some may require a stoma.

Artificial bowel sphincter (ABS) is a costly procedure that may cause obstructed defecation, requiring enemas in one-third of the patients and device explantation in over half. Due to the frequent complications and high costs, ABS has been nearly abandoned and the use of dynamic graciloplasty has declined. Unlike gluteoplasty, which is also less commonly used, both procedures were very popular a decade ago.

Sacral neuromodulation is minimally invasive, but it is costly and may require that patients undergo removal of either the leads or the pacemaker itself, as noted in up to one third of such cases. However, the newly constructed leads are more resistant and the success rate is nearly 80%.

Bulking agents are less costly and cause only a few minor complications, such as ulcers and dislocation, but they are less effective and should be reserved for patients whose incontinence is not severe and is due to a localized lesion of the internal sphincter.

A polyester puborectalis sling, aimed at narrowing the anorectal angle, may occasionally cause rectal erosion, whereas the novel silicone radiopaque ring is effective in most patients, but the sling must be re-inserted in 30% of the cases and definitive sling removal is needed in one out of ten.

Suggested Readings

Ahlberg K, Ahsgren I, Mattsson GG, Mattsson S (2010) Toilet training beneficial also in children with learning disabilities. Lakartidningen 107:2164-2168

Altomare DF, Dodi G, La Torre F et al (2001) Multicentre retrospective analysis of the outcome of artificial anal sphincter implantation for severe faecal incontinence. Br J Surg 88:1481-1486

Altomare DF, La Torre F, Rinaldi M et al (2008) Carbon-coated microbeads anal injection in outpatient treatment of minor fecal incontinence. Dis Colon Rectum 51:432-435

Altomare DF, Ratto C, Ganio E et al (2009) Long-term outcome of sacral nerve stimulation for fecal incontinence. Dis Colon Rectum 52:11-17

Altomare DF, Rinaldi M, Lobascio P et al (2011) Factors affecting the outcome of temporary sacral nerve stimulation for faecal incontinence. The value of the new tined lead electrode. Colorectal Dis 13:198-202

Baeten C, Bartolo DC, Lehur PA et al (2007) Consensus conference on faecal incontinence. Tech Coloproctol 11:225-233

Baeten C, Spaans F, Fluks A (1988) An implanted neuromuscular stimulator for fecal continence following previously implanted gracilis muscle: report of a case. Dis Colon Rectum 31:134-137

Baeten CG, Bailey HR, Bakka A et al (2000) Safety and efficacy of dynamic graciloplasty for fecal incontinence: report of a prospective, multicenter trail. Dynamic graciloplasty therapy study group. Dis Colon Rectum 43:743-751

Baeten CG, Konsten J, Spaans F et al (1991) Dynamic graciloplasty for treatment of faecal incontinence. Lancet 338:1163-1165

Bagade P, Mackenzie S (2010) Outcomes from medium term follow-up of patients with third and fourth degree perineal tears. J Obstet Gynaecol 30:609-612

Barisic GI, Krivokapic ZV, Markovic VA, Popovic MA (2006) Outcome of overlapping anal sphincter repair after 3 months and after a mean of 80 months. Int J Colorectal Dis 21:52-56

Bartlett L, Ho YH (2009) PTQ anal implants for the treatment of faecal incontinence. Br J Surg 96:1468-1475

Bharucha AE, Zinsmeister AR, Schleck CD, Melton LJ 3rd (2010) Bowel disturbances are the most important risk factors for late onset fecal incontinence: a population-based case-control study in women. Gastroenterology 139:1559-1566

Bittorf B, Ringler R, Forster C et al (2006) Cerebral representation of the anorectum using functional magnetic resonance imaging. Br J Surg 93:1251-1257

Bondurri A, Zbar AP, Tapia H et al (2011) The relationship between etiology, symptom severity and indications for surgery in cases of anal incontinence: a 25-year analysis of 1046 patients at a tertiary coloproctology practice. Tech Coloproctol 15:159-164

Brostrøm S, Due U, Lose G (2010) Pelvic floor muscle training in pregnant and parturient women—a survey of a Cochrane review. Ugeskr Laeger 172:2441-2444

Chapman AE, Geerdes B, Hewett P et al (2002) Systematic review of dynamic graciloplasty in the treatment of faecal incontinence. Br J Surg 89:138-153

Chase S, Mittal R, Jesudason MR et al (2010) Anal sphincter repair for fecal incontinence: experience from a tertiary care centre. Indian J Gastroenterol 29:162-165

Chatoor DR, Taylor SJ, Cohen CR, Emmanuel AV (2007) Faecal incontinence. Br J Surg 94:134-144

Christiansen J, Lorentzen M (1987) Implantation of artificial sphincter for anal incontinence. Lancet 2:244-245

Corman ML (1983) The management of anal incontinence. Surg Clin North Am 63:177-192

da Silva GM, Jorge JM, Belin B (2004) New surgical options for fecal incontinence in patients with imperforate anus. Dis Colon Rectum 47:204-209

Danielson J, Karlbom U, Sonnesson A, Graf W (2010) Long-term improvement in quality of life after submucous injection of-NAXA/DX for anal incontinence. Dis Colon Rectum 53:565-566

de la Portilla F, Vega J, Rada R et al (2009) Evaluation by three-dimensional anal endosonography of injectable silicone biomaterial (PTQ) implants to treat fecal incontinence: long-term localization and relation with the deterioration of the continence. Tech Coloproctol 13:195-199

Devesa JM, Hervàs PL, Vicente R et al (2011) Anal encirclement with a simple prosthetic sling for faecal incontinence. Tech Coloproctol 15:17-22

Devesa JM, Rey A, Hervas PL et al (2002) Artificial anal sphincter: complications and functional results of a large personal series. Dis Colon Rectum 45:1154-1163

Devesa JM, Vicente E, Enríquez JM et al (1992) Total fecal incontinence—a new method of gluteus maximus transposition: preliminary results and report of previous experience with similar procedures. Dis Colon Rectum 35:339-349

Di Cesare A, Leva E, Macchini F et al (2010) Anorectal malformations and neurospinal dysraphism: is this association a major risk for continence? Pediatr Surg Int 26:1077-1081

Donkol RH, Al-Nammi A (2010) Percutaneous cecostomy in the management of organic fecal incontinence in children. World J Radiol 28:463-467

Efron JE, Corman ML, Fleshman J et al (2003) Safety and effectiveness of temperature-controlled radio-frequency energy delivery to the anal canal (Secca procedure) for the treatment of fecal incontinence. Dis Colon Rectum 46:1606-1616; discussion 1616-1618

Elton C, Stoodley BJ (2002) Anterior anal sphincter repair: results in a district general hospital. Ann R Coll Surg Engl 84:321-324

Emami-Naeini P, Rahbar Z, Nejat F et al (2010) Neurological presentations, imaging, and associated anomalies in 50 patients with sacral agenesis. Neurosurgery 67:894-900; discussion 900

Engel AF, Kamm MA, Sultan AH et al (1994) Anterior anal sphincter repair in patients with obstetric trauma. Br J Surg 81:1231-1234

Evans C, Davis K, Kumar D (2006) Overlapping anal sphincter repair and anterior levatorplasty: effect of patient's age and duration of follow-up. Int J Colorectal Dis 21:795-801. Epub 2006 Mar 7

Fang DT, Nivatvongs S, Vermeulen FD et al (1984) Overlapping shinteroplasty for acquired anal incontinence. Dis Colon Rectum 27:720-722

Faucheron JL, Voirin D, Badic B (2010) Sacral nerve stimulation for fecal incontinence: causes of surgical revision from a series of 87 consecutive patients operated on in a single institution. Dis Colon Rectum 53:1501-1507

Felt-Bersma RJ, Szojda MM, Mulder CJ (2007) Temperature-controlled radiofrequency energy (SECCA) to the anal canal for the treatment of faecal incontinence offers moderate improvement. Eur J Gastreonterol Hepatol 19:575-580

Findlay J, Maxwell-Armstrong C (2010) Posterior tibial nerve stimulation for faecal incontinence. Br J Nurs 19:750-754

Findlay JM, Maxwell-Armstrong C (2011) Posterior tibial nerve stimulation and faecal incontinence: a review. Int J Colorectal Dis 26:265-273

Findlay JM, Yeung JM, Robinson R et al (2010) Peripheral neuromodulation via posterior tibial nerve stimulation - a poten-

tial treatment for faecal incontinence? Ann R Coll Surg Engl 92:385-390
Finlay IG, Richardson W, Hajivassiliou CA (2004) Outcome after implantation of a novel prosthetic anal sphincter in humans. Br J Surg 91:1485-1492
Fleshman JW, Dreznik Z, Fry RD, Kodner IJ (1991) Anal sphincter repair for obstetric injury: manometric evaluation of functional results. Dis Colon Rectum 34:1061-1067
Ganio E, Marino F, Giani I (2008) Injectable synthetic calcium hydroxylapatite ceramic microspheres (Coaptite) for passive fecal incontinence. Tech Coloproctol 12:99-102
Goligher JC (1990) Skepticism in surgery. Persp Colon Rect Surg 3:347-355
Goos M, Haberstroh J, Baumann T et al (2011) New selective endoscopic sacral nerve root stimulation - an advance in the treatment of fecal incontinence. Neurogastroenterol Motil 23:104-109
Guelincks PJ, Sinsel NK (1996) Conventional and dynamic anal sphincter plasty using the gluteus maximus muscle. Tech Coloproctol 4:89-90
Guo M, Gao C, Li D et al (2010) MRI anatomy of the anal region. Dis Colon Rectum 53:1542-1548
Halverson AL, Hull TL (2002) Long-term outcome of overlapping anal sphincter repair. Dis Colon Rectum 44:1255-1260
Hultman CS, Zenn MR, Agarwal T, Baker CC (2006) Restoration of fecal continence after functional gluteoplasty: long-term results, technical refinements, and donor-site morbidity. Ann Plast Surg 56:65-70; discussion 70-71
Indinnimeo M, Ratto C, Moschella CM et al (2010) Sacral neuromodulation for the treatment of fecal incontinence: analysis of cost-effectiveness. Dis Colon Rectum 53:1661-1669
Jarrett ME, Matzel KE, Christiansen Jet al (2005) Sacral nerve stimulation for faecal incontinence in patients with previous partial spinal injury including disc prolapse. Br J Surg 92:734-739
Jayne DG, Finan PJ (2005) Stapled transanal rectal resection for obstructed defaecation and evidence-based practice. Br J Surg 92:793-794
Jensen LL, Lowry AC (1997) Biofeedback improves functional outcome after sphincteroplasty. Dis Colon Rectum 40:197-200
Kalis V, Bednárová B, Stěpán J Jr, Rokyta Z (2010) Repair of the 3rd and 4th degree obstetric perineal tear. Ceska Gynekol 75:284-291
Karoui S, Leroi AM, Koning E et al (2000) Results of sphincteroplasy in 86 patients with anal incontinence. Dis Colon Rectum 43:813-820
Keighley MR (1991) Results of surgery in idiopathic faecal incontinence. S Afr J Surg 29:87-93
Kepenekci I, Keskinkilic B, Akinsu F et al (2011) Prevalence of pelvic floor disorders in the female population and the impact of age, mode of delivery, and parity. Dis Colon Rectum 54:85-94
Kim DW, Yoon HM, Park JS (2009) Radiofrequency energy delivery to the anal canal: is it a promising new approach to the treatment of fecal incontinence? Am J Surg 197:14-18
King VG, Boyles SH, Worstell TR et al (2010) Using the Brink score to predict postpartum anal incontinence. Am J Obstet Gynecol 203:486.e1-e5
Koch SM, Uluda O, El Naggar K et al (2008) Colonic irrigation for defecation disorders after dynamic graciloplasty. Int J Colorectal Dis 23:195-200
Koch SM, Uluda O, Rongen MJ et al (2004) Dynamic graciloplasty in patients born with an anorectal malformation. Dis Colon Rectum 47:1711-1719
Langemo D, Hanson D, Hunter S et al (2011) Incontinence and incontinence-associated dermatitis. Adv Skin Wound Care 24:126-140
Laurberg S, Swash M, Henry MM (1988) Delayed external sphincter repair for obstetric tear. Br J Surg 75:786-788
Lehur PA, McNevin S, Buntzen S et al (2010) Magnetic anal sphincter augmentation for the treatment of fecal incontinence: a preliminary report from a feasibility study. Dis Colon Rectum 53:1604-1610
Lehur PA, Zerbib F, Neunlist M et al (2002) Comparison of quality of life and anorectal function after artificial sphincter implantation. Dis Colon Rectum 45:508-513
Leroi AM (2011) The role of sacral neuromodulation in double incontinence. Colorect Dis 13(Suppl 2):15-18
Lieske B, Conaghan P, Farouk R (2010) Sacral nerve stimulation can be successful in patients with ultrasound evidence of external anal sphincter disruption. Dis Colon Rectum 53:568-569
Mackey P, Mackey L, Kennedy ML et al (2010) Postanal repair - do the long-term results justify the procedure? Colorectal Dis 12:367-372
Malouf AJ, Vaizey CJ, Nicholls RJ, Kamm MA (2000) Permanent sacral nerve stimulation for fecal incontinence. Ann Surg 232:143-148
Mander BJ, Abercromibie JF, George BD, Williams NS (1996) The electrically stimulated gracilis neosphincter incorporated as part of total anorectal reconstruction after abdominoperineal excision of the rectum. Ann Sug 224:702-711
Mander BJ, Wexner SD, Williams BS et al (1999) Preliminary results of a multicenter trial of the electrically stimulated gracilis neoanal sphincter. Br J Surg 86:543-548
Maslekar S, Gardiner AB, Duthie GS (2007) Anterior anal sphincter repair for fecal incontinence: Good longer results are possible. J Am Coll Surg 204:40-46
Matzel KE (2011) Sacral nerve stimulation for faecal incontinence: its role in the treatment algorithm. Colorect Dis 13 (Suppl 2):10-14
Matzel KE, Stadelmaier U, Gall FP (1995) Direct electrostimulation of sacral spinal nerves within the scope of the diagnosis of anorectal function. Langenbecks Arch Chir 380:184-188
Matzel KE, Stadelmaier U, Hohenberger W (2004) Innovations in fecal incontinence: sacral nerve stimulation. Dis Colon Rectum 47:1720-1728
Matzel KE, Stadelmaier U, Hohenfellner M, Gall FP (1995) Electrical stimulation of sacral spinal nerves for treatment of faecal incontinence. Lancet 346:1124-1127
Matzel KE, Stadelmaier U, Hohenfellner M, Gall FP (1995) Permanent electrostimulation of sacral spinal nerves with an implantable neurostimulator in treatment of fecal incontinence. Chirurg 66:813-817
Melenhorst J, Koch SM, Uludag O et al (2007) Sacral neuromodulations in patients with fecal incontinence: results of the first 100 permanent implantations. Colorect Dis 9:725-730

Meurette G, Rodat F, Wyart V, Lehur P (2010) Outcome and management of patients who failed sacral nerve stimulation for fecal incontinence. Dis Colon Rectum 53:567

Michot F, Costaglioli B, Leroi AM, Denis P (2003) Artificial anal sphincter in severe fecal incontinence: outcome of prospective experience with 37 patients in one institution. Ann Surg 237:52-56

Michot F, Lefebure B, Bridoux V et al (2010) Artificial anal sphincter for severe fecal incontinence implanted by a transvaginal approach: experience with 32 patients treated at one institution. Dis Colon Rectum 53:1155-1160

Miller R, Orrom WJ, Cornes H et al (1989) Anterior sphincter placation and levator plasty in the treatment of faecal incontinence. Br J Surg 76:1058-1060

Morren GL, Hallbook O, Nystrom PO et al (2001) Audit of anal sphincter repair. Colorectal Dis 3:17-22

Moscovitz, Rotholtz NA, Baig MK et al (2002) Overlapping sphincteroplasty: does the preservation of the scar influence immediate outcome? Colorect Dis 4:275-279

Murphy J, Boyle D, Prosser K et al (2010) Efficacy of sacral nerve stimulation for the treatment of fecal incontinence. Dis Colon Rectum 53:536

Nordenstam JF, Altman DH, Mellgren AF et al (2010) Impaired rectal sensation at anal manometry is associated with anal incontinence one year after primary sphincter repair in primiparous women. Dis Colon Rectum 53:1409-1414

Oberwalder M, Dinnewitzer A, Nogueras JJ et al (2008) Imbrication of the external anal sphincter may yield similar functional results as overlapping repair in selected patients. Colorectal Dis 10:800-804

Orrom WJ, Miller R, Cornes H et al (1991) Comparison of anterior sphincteroplasty and postanal repair in the treatment of idiopathic fecal incontinence. Dis Colon Rectum 34:305-310

Ortiz H, Armendariz P, DeMiguel M et al (2002) Complications and functional outcome following artificial anal sphincter implantation. Br J Surg 89:877-881

Osterberg A, Edebol Eeg-Olofsson K, Graf W (2000) Results of surgical treatment for faecal incontinence. Br J Surg 87:1546-1552

Parker SC, Spencer MP, Madoff RD et al (2003) Artificial bowel sphincter: long-term experience at a single institution. Dis Colon Rectum 46:722-729

Parks AG (1975) Royal Society of Medicine, Section of Proctology; Meeting 27 November 1974. President's Address. Anorectal incontinence. Proc R Soc Med 68:681-690

Paterson HM, Bartolo DC (2010) Surgery for faecal incontinence. Scott Med J 55:39-42

Penninckx F (2004) Belgian experience with dynamic graciloplasty for faecal incontinence. Br J Surg 91:872-878

Pescatori M (2009) Spinal cord stimulation for constipated patients. Dis Colon Rectum 52:1196

Pescatori M, Anastasio G, Bottini C, Mentasti A (1992) New grading and scoring for anal incontinence. Evaluation of 335 patients. Dis Colon Rectum 35:482-487

Pescatori M, Caracciolo F, Anastasio G (1991) Restoration of intestinal continuity after rectal excision by electrostimulated smooth and striated muscle. BAM 1:259-262

Pescatori M, Meglio M, Cioni B, Colagrande C (1982) Colonic motility in two constipated neurological patients treated by spinal cord stimulation. M. Wienbeck. ed New York: Raven Press

Pfeifer J (2004) Quality of life after sphincteroplasty. Acta Chir Iugosl 51:73-75

Pickrell KL, Broadbent TR, Masters FW, Metzger JT (1952) Construction of a rectal sphincter and restoration of anal continence by transplanting the gracilis muscle; a report of four cases in children. Ann Surg 135:853-862

Pinta T, Kylänpää-Bäck ML, Salmi T et al (2003) Delayed sphincter repair for obstetric ruptures: analysis of failure. Colorectal Dis 5:73-78

Rao SS (2010) Advances in diagnostic assessment of fecal incontinence and dyssynergic defecation. Clin Gastroenterol Hepatol 8:910-919

Richard C, Bernard D, Morgan S (1994) Results of anal sphincteroplasty for post-traumatic incontinence: with or without colostomy. Ann Chir 48:703-707

Ruiz Carmona MD, Alós Company R, Roig Vila JV et al (2009) Long-term results of artificial bowel sphincter for the treatment of severe faecal incontinence. Are they what we hoped for? Colorectal Dis 11:831-837

Rullier E, Zerbib F, Laurent C et al (2008) Morbidity and functional outcome after double dynamic graciloplasty for anorectal reconstruction. Br J Sug 87:909-913

Rygh AB, Körner H (2010) The overlap technique versus end-to-end approximation technique for primary repair of obstetric anal sphincter rupture: a randomized controlled study. Acta Obstet Gynecol Scand 89:1256-1262

Scaglia M, Delaini G, Destefano I, Hultén L (2009) Fecal incontinence treated with acupuncture—a pilot study. Auton Neurosci 145:89-92

Senagore A, Mazier WP, Luchtefeld MA et al (1993) Treatment of advanced hemorrhoidal disease: a prospective, randomized comparison of cold scalpel vs. contact Nd:YAG laser. Dis Colon Rectum 36:1042-1049

Shafik A (1993) Polytetrafluoroethylene injection for the treatment of partial fecal incontinence. Int Surg 78:159-161

Shafik A, Ahmed I, El-Sibai O, Mostafa RM (2003) Percutaneous peripheral neuromodulation in the treatment of fecal incontinence. Eur Surg Res 35:103-107

Smith K, Gonsalves S, Qureshi S et al (2010) Intra-anal permacol for the treatment of passive faecal incontinence. Dis Colon Rectum 53:566

Soerensen MM, Lundby L, Buntzen S, Laurberg S (2009) Intersphincteric injected silicone biomaterial implants: a treatment for faecal incontinence. Colorectal Dis 11:73-76

Takahashi T, Garcia-Osogobio S, Valdovinos MA et al (2002) Radio-frequency energy delivery to the anal canal for the treatment of fecal incontinence. Dis Colon Rectum 45:915-922

Tjandra JJ, Lim JF, Hiscock R, Rajendra P (2004) Injectable silicone biomaterial for fecal incontinence caused by internal anal sphincter dysfunction is effective. Dis Colon Rectum 47:2138-2146

Turell RNY (1954) The Thiersch operation for rectal prolapse and anal incontinence. State J Med 54:791-795

van Wunnik BP, Govaert B, Leong R et al (2011) Patient experience and satisfaction with sacral neuromodulation: results of a single-center sample survey. Dis Colon Rectum 54:95-100

Wexner SD, Hull T, Edden Y et al (2010) Infection rates in a large investigational trial of sacral nerve stimulation for fecal incontinence. J Gastrointest Surg 14:1081-1089

Wexner SD, Jin HY, Weiss EG et al (2009) Factors associated with failure of the artificial bowel sphincter: a study of over 50 cases from Cleveland Clinic Florida. Dis Colon Rectum 52:1550-1557

Williams JG, Wong WD, Jensen L et al (1991) Incontinence and rectal prolapse: a prospective manometric study. Dis Colon Rectum 34:209-216

Williams NS, Patel J, George BD et al (1991) Development of an electrically stimulated neoanal sphincter. Lancet 338:1166-1169

Wong WD, Congliosi SM, Spencer MP et al (2002) The safety and efficacy of the artificial bowel sphincter for fecal incontinence: results from a multicenter cohort study. Dis Colon Rectum 45:1139-1153

Yamana T, Takahashi T, Iwadare J (2004) Perineal puborectalis sling operation for fecal incontinence: preliminary report. Dis Colon Rectum 47:1982-1989

Yoshioka K, Keighley MR (1989) Sphincter repair for fecal incontinence. Dis Colon Rectum 32:39-42

Záhumenský J (2010) Severe obstetrical injuries and anal incontinence. Ceska Gynekol 75:292-296

Zailani MH, Azmi MN, Deen KI (2010) Gracilis muscle as neoanal sphincter for faecal incontinence. Med J Malaysia 65:66-67

Zorcolo L, Covotta L, Bartolo DC (2005) Outcome of anterior sphincter repair for obstetric injury: comparison of early and late results. Dis Colon Rectum 48:524-531

External Rectal Prolapse 10

10.1 Introduction

The surgical gold standard for the treatment of hemorrhoids is hemorrhoidectomy; for anal fissure, it is internal sphincterotomy; for ulcerative colitis, restorative proctocolectomy; for anal stricture, anoplasty, etc. However, for external rectal prolapse, there is no surgical gold standard, thus necessitating a tailored approach, i.e., a surgical procedure that addresses the patient's needs and his or her symptoms. This conclusion was confirmed in two recent papers, by Pescatori and Zbar (2009) and Brown et al. (2004a). While in those studies the number of patients differed (117 and 157, respectively), the surgical policy was the same, with essentially the same operations carried out in each center: Altemeier proctosigmoidectomy and a Delorme procedure (via a perineal route), sacral rectopexy and resection-rectopexy (via an abdominal route). All four were tailored to the particular patient, the nature of the prolapse, and the symptoms. These cases also underline the need for a specialist to be able to perform more than one procedure and to adapt each of them to both the patient and the disease.

To some extent, the patient with external prolapse is easy to manage, in the sense that prolapse must be treated surgically. At the same time, prolapse is difficult to manage, as the surgeon must decide which among the different procedures is the most appropriate. Since this book deals with the complications after proctological surgery, abdominal procedures will not be discussed in detail and only a limited number of operations will be considered. Nonetheless, the topic is still rather complex, as besides the above-mentioned Delorme and Altemeier operations, there are encirclement procedures, Contour Transtar resection, manual and stapled rectal mucosectomy, and transperineal and transvaginal rectopexy.

In this chapter, we discuss the potential postoperative complications, of which there are basically five: bleeding, incontinence, sepsis, dehiscence and stricture. There are also surgical failures. For example, if the patient is constipated, a sacral rectopexy is likely to worsen constipation and the consequent excessive straining might cause a recurrent prolapse. If the sphincters are weakened, a Delorme is likely to deteriorate anal continence. In elderly and fragile patients, a resection-rectopexy may be followed by a life-threatening anastomotic breakdown. If the patient has diarrhea, an Altemeier procedure is likely to worsen bowel habit following the removal of the rectal reservoir.

10.2 Postoperative Complications in Our Series

Table 10.1 provides a summary of the complications that occurred in our 75 patients treated for external rectal prolapse with perineal procedures.

A severe complication requiring a re-intervention occurred in just one patient, after an Altemeier. Another patient, a 75-year-old woman, died due to causes unrelated to the operation. When she fully recovered from the general anesthesia, she was alone on the ward, tried to get out of her bed without assistance, fell on the floor and had a fatal cranial trauma. This serves as a reminder that elderly, confused patients require a bed with lateral protection, to prevent this type of accident. None of the other complications reported, i.e., bleeding, sepsis, dehiscence, stricture, and incontinence, required surgical re-intervention. Only two patients needed dilations for an anorectal stricture following a Delorme procedure. These

M. Pescatori, *Prevention and Treatment of Complications in Proctological Surgery*,

Table 10.1 Postoperative complications among a series of 75 patients operated on for external rectal prolapse with perineal and transanal procedures, performed by a single surgeon over a period of two decades (updated from Pescatori and Zbar, 2009)

Complication	Intervention	No. of cases	Treatment	Outcome
Accidental fall and cranial trauma	Delorme-Rehn	1	-	Died
Severe rectal bleeding	Delorme-Rehn PPH	2 1	 Rectal tamponade	 Cured
Local sepsis	Delorme-Rehn PPH	4 1	Antibiotics Antibiotics	Cured Cured
Dehiscence and stricture	Delorme-Rehn	2	Dilation	Cured Improved
Sigmoid perforation	Altemeier	1	Suture and temporary stoma	Cured
Anal incontinence[a]	Delorme-Rehn Altemeier Manual mucosectomy	7 2 1	Biofeedback Biofeedback Biofeedback	Cured (3) Soiling Cured

[a]Eight patients were incontinent prior to surgery.

were performed in the office, with the patient under local anesthesia, using Hegars, up to 18 mm, then by digital exploration, and finally by gently introducing a pediatric and then a normal proctoscope (Sapimed, Alessandria, Italy), up to 26 mm. The maneuver was repeated three times at an interval of one week, with the patient instructed to self-dilate at home using either the obturator of the proctoscope or anal dilators (Dilatan), preceded by the introduction of the local anesthetic ointment Emla in the anal canal. A high-fiber diet and plenty of fluids were also prescribed.

10.3 "Live Surgery": The Prevention of Complications After a Delorme-Rehn Operation

The patient is a 68 year-old female who is continent despite being pluriparous and hysterectomized. She has been positioned on the operating table in the lithotomy position and is under spinal anesthesia. She underwent a mechanical preparation and antibiotic prophylaxis to minimize the risk of postoperative sepsis. Surgery begins with the insertion of a LoneStar retractor, which has the advantage that it does not stretch the sphincter. Using blunt rather than sharp hooks, to avoid lacerations of the anal canal, I gently pull the lower and middle prolapsed rectum through the anus using three-ring forceps, which are not completely closed, to avoid hematomas. Once the prolapse is extracted, I make a circumferential incision, using diathermy, just above the dentate line. The incision is made at this level for two reasons: 1) to preserve the sensitive, richly innervated epithelium of the lower anal canal, which is important for the sensory component of anal continence and 2) to position the recto-anal anastomosis above the lower edge of the internal sphincter and the subcutaneous part of the external sphincter, again to protect anal continence. This results in the suture being placed inside the anal canal and avoids the risk of mucosal ectropion and a "wet anus."

Prior to commencing the rectal mucosectomy, the submucosal plane should be infiltrated above the dentate line with a 1:200,000 solution of adrenaline in saline to minimize intraoperative bleeding and facilitate the dissection in the correct plane. The anesthetist should be informed of the infiltration, which in rare cases can cause side effects. I then perform the first step of the Delorme, i.e., rectal mucosectomy, using either scissors or diathermy, not directly on the tissue, but through the forceps, as described in Chap. 2 for Ferguson hemorrhoidectomy. This simple maneuver minimizes bleeding. Mucosectomy has to be carried out slowly, even though this may be tedious, because by remaining in the correct plane, between the submucosal and muscular layers, we reduce the risk of hemorrhage, which, at this stage, is usually due to inadvertent sectioning of smooth muscle fibers (Fig. 10.1). A reduction of the bleeding in turn minimizes the risk of hematoma, and thus subsequent sepsis and anastomotic dehiscence. In female patients, a particularly careful dissection is required on the anterior aspect to prevent the occurrence of postoperative vaginal fistulae, which may be due not only to a direct intraoperative vaginal lesion, but also to local ischemia, followed by loss of tissue continuity, 24-48 h after surgery. As seen in Fig. 8.11 of Chap. 8, the rectal muscle may be diastased in patients with rectocele and prolapse such that the distance between the rectum and the vagina is minimal. This is especially true in a multiparous patient, like the one we are operating on. The anterior dissection has progressed up to about 6 cm from the anal verge. The whitish fibrotic structure is not the vagina, as I easily determine by inserting a finger in the vagina (previously disinfected), but the inferior aspect of

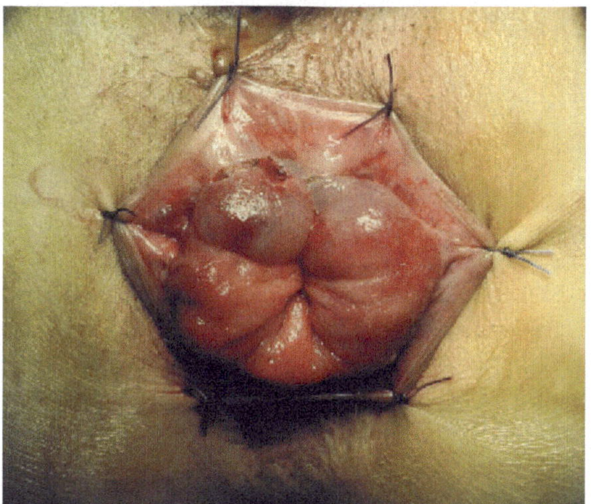

Fig. 10.1 a Rectal mucosal prolapse. Delorme's operation. The distal portion of the anal canal is fixed to the perianal skin, with an incision made just above the dentate line, to preserve the sensitive epithelium that plays a key role in maintaining continence. Patient in the lithotomy position

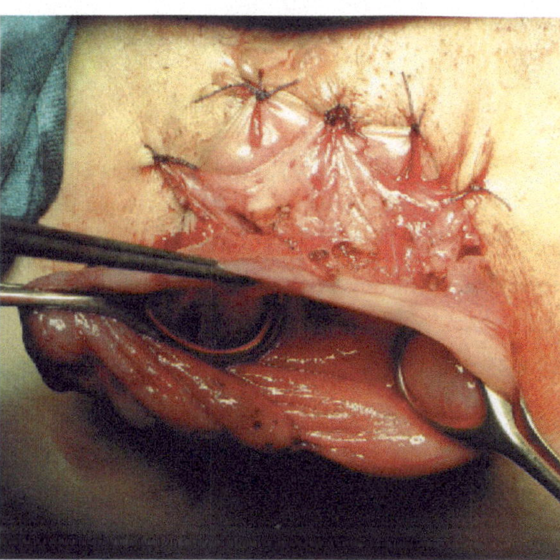

Fig. 10.1 b Beginning of the mucosal prolapsectomy

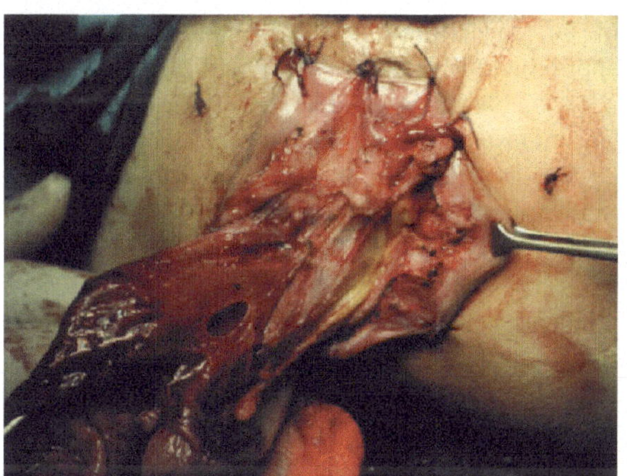

Fig. 10.1 c Mucosal cylinder of the prolapse, detached from the rectal muscle, is removed

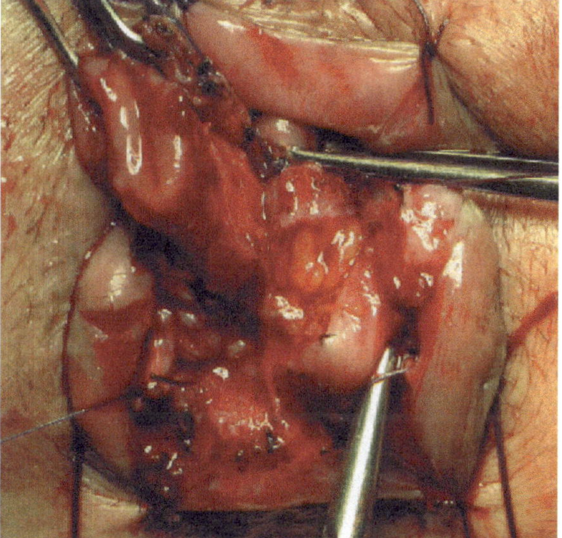

Fig. 10.1 d The rectal muscle was plicated and the middle-high rectum is prepared for suturing to the anal canal

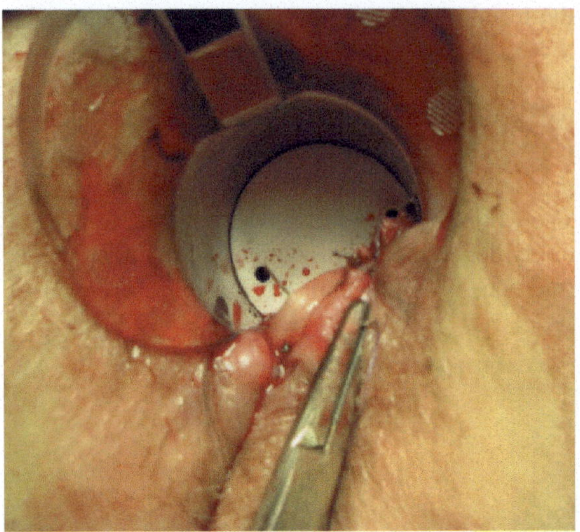

Fig. 10.1 e The rectoanal suture is finished; it is inside the anal canal to ensure continence and to avoid mucosal ectropion

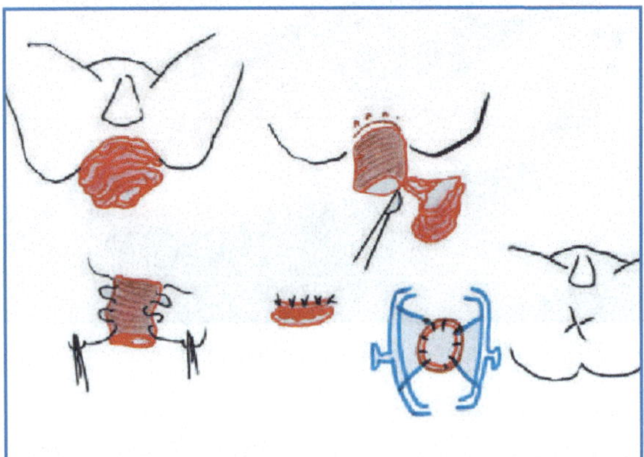

Fig. 10.1 g Operation diagram

the pouch of Douglas, which is displaced downward in this patient, due to the absence of the uterus. Again, the anatomy is well illustrated in Fig. 8.11, which is in fact a photo taken during a Delorme procedure. Therefore, injury of the peritoneal pouch should be avoided, as there might be a descended bowel loop just above it. This is similar to the risk of causing damage when performing a STARR for obstructed defecation in a patient with perineal descent and pelvic organs prolapse. The partially blind firing of the stapler might incorporate the lower extension of the pouch of Douglas. That is why Corman et al. (2006) contraindicated the use of STARR in patients with enterocele, in a "consensus paper" wisely sponsored by the stapler's manufacturer. The same precaution was recently noted by Schwandner (2011).

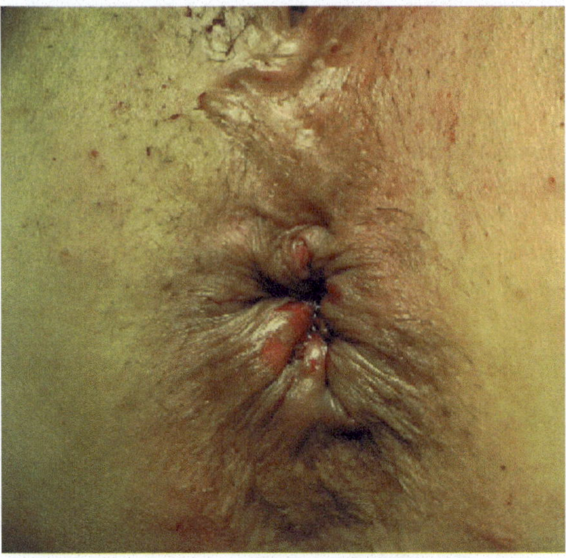

Fig. 10.1 f End of the anastomosis

Once separated from the rectal muscle, the prolapsed mucosal cylinder has to be removed from the middle rectum, using diathermy to divide the small terminal branches of the low rectal artery, possibly avoiding both intraoperative hemorrhage and deep ischemia of the proximal rectal epithelium, which might favor anastomotic breakdown. At this point, the second step of the Delorme is performed, i.e., plication of the denuded rectal muscle, avoiding excessive tightening of the sutures in order to prevent rectal muscle lacerations. Downwards displacement of the middle or upper rectum by means of the concertina-like sutures will result in the approximation of the proximal and distal epithelia, allowing the final step to be performed, a recto-anal anastomosis above the dentate line, with interrupted 2/0 vicryl sutures following removal of the Lone Star retractor (Fig. 10.2). The anastomosis, similar to a colo-anal one, should not be under tension, to minimize the risk of dehiscence. The operation is now complete. I check that the suture is intact and that, after a while, when the stretched sphincters's tone is partly restored, it has "disappeared" upwards in the anal canal, to avoid mucosal ectropion, which might cause postoperative soiling.

The postoperative mortality and anal incontinence rates following a Delorme procedure, as determined by various authors, are summarized in Table 10.2.

Most patients who complained of postoperative incontinence were incontinent prior to surgery.

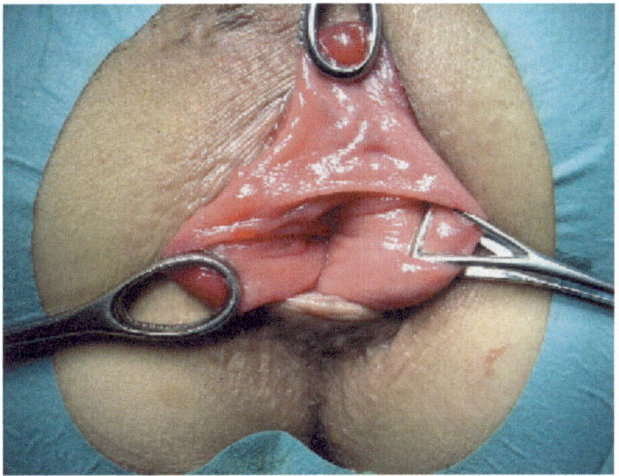

Fig. 10.2 a Rectal prolapse

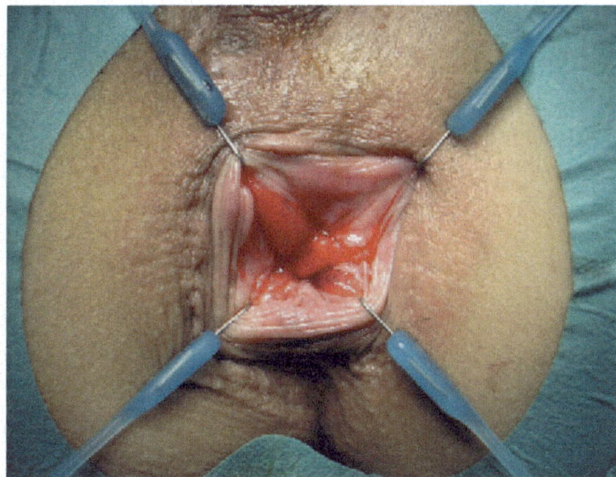

Fig. 10.2 b Positioning of the Lone Star retractor

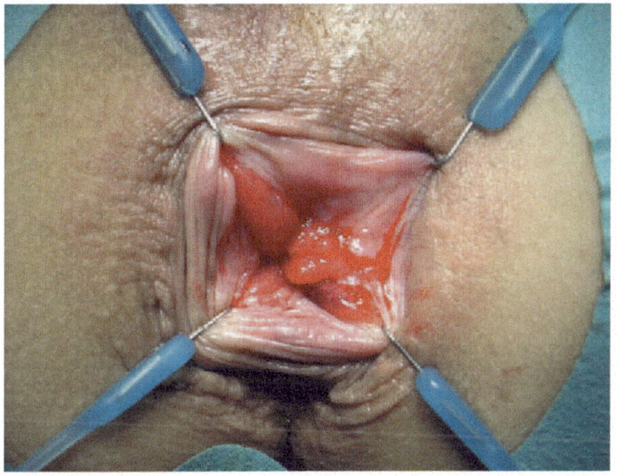

Fig. 10.2 c Polypoid lesions of a rectal solitary ulcer syndrome

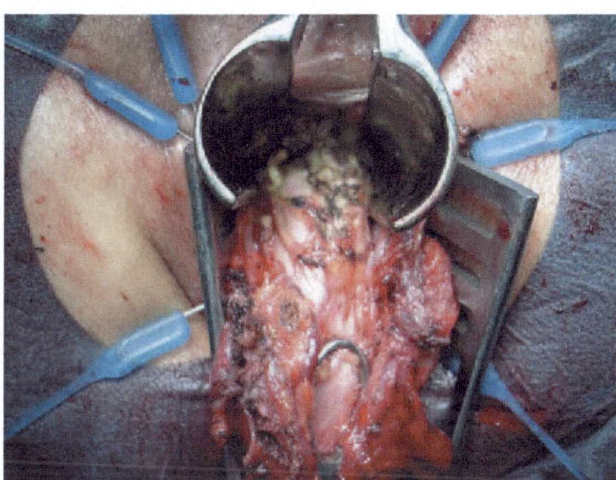

Fig. 10.2 d Altemeier's rectosigmoid resection

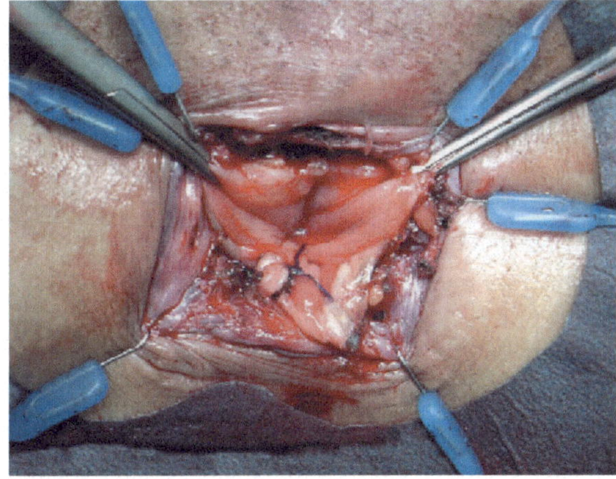

Fig. 10.2 e Colo-anal anastomosis

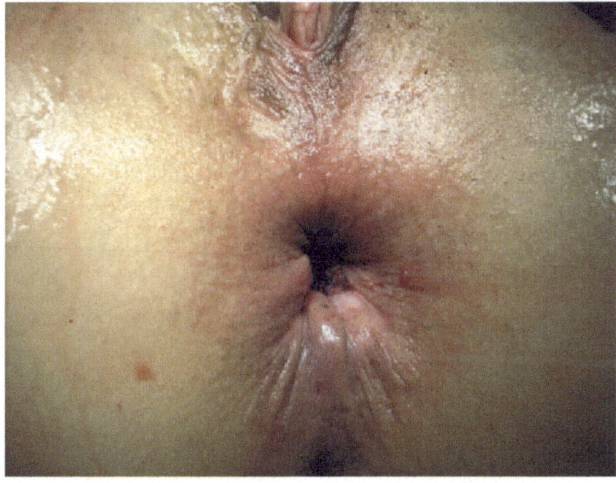

Fig. 10.2 f End of the suture

Table 10.2 Postoperative mortality and anal incontinence following a Delorme procedure

First author	Year	No. of cases	Postoperative mortality(%)	Postoperative anal incontinence (%)
Oliver	1994	41	2.4	55
Lechaux	1995	85	1.2	33
Liberman	2000	34	0	68
Watts	2000	101	4	75
Serventi	2005	21	4.8	36
Marchal	2005	60	3.3	58
Pascual	2006	21	0	13
Pescatori	2009	54	0.5[a]	13[b]
Lieberth	2009	66		
Lauretta	2010	25	0	22

[a]Not related to surgery, but to an accidental fall with cranial trauma.

[b]A post-anal repair (Pescatori) and a levatorplasty (Lechaux) were associated with the Delorme procedure in some patients with severe fecal incontinence due to defects of the striated sphincters.

Postoperative continence improved in some series; Lauretta et al. (2010) reported an improvement of anal continence in 40% of their patients.

Overall, postoperative complications, such as rectal bleeding, suture dehiscence, and anorectal stricture, occurred in 14% of the patients described in Table 10.2. In one report, by Marchal et al. (2005), the complications rate was higher (20%), with two cases of bleeding, three anastomotic dehiscences, one perirectal hematoma, two cases of perineal cellulitis, one case of peritonitis due to a small bowel perforation, one case of sepsis, one myocardial infarction, and one pulmonary embolism. Overall, out of 60 patients, there were two re-interventions and two deaths. De Nardi et al. (2006) reported a case of ischemic proctitis that required an anterior resection of the rectum with a covering stoma.

The Delorme procedure carries a low postoperative morbidity, but is likely to be followed by postoperative incontinence. Therefore, to recall the concept of tailored surgery, it should be performed in patents without severe sphincter defects. The ideal candidate is an elderly or fragile patient with respiratory problems that might indicate spinal anesthesia, a prevalently mucosal external prolapse < 8 cm in size, and satisfactory continence.

Among the patients operated on by Serventi and Binda (2005), those with postoperative complications were successfully managed by means of outpatient procedures. The authors recommended the Delorme-Rehn procedure as in patients with ascites there are fewer risks than associated with the Altemeier operation.

10.4 Complications After the Altemeier Procedure (Perineal Proctosigmoidectomy)

The results of an Italian multicentric study on 78 patients, including our own, are as follows: The mean age of the patients was 71 years, and the median length of the excised rectosigmoid was 20 cm. Patients were ASA III and IV. A levatorplasty was also carried out in 86% of the patients. There were three pelvic hematomas (3.9%), one sigmoid perforation (1.2%), and two anal strictures (2.4%). Proctalgia occurred in four patients (5%), urinary retention in two (2.4%), and worsened continence in seven (9%). Re-intervention was necessary in two patients (2.4%); there were no deaths due to the procedure. Thus, neither the complication rate nor the re-intervention rate was high (22.4 and 2.4%, respectively).

For purposes of comparison, not based on randomized prospective trials and therefore not highly scientific, the re-intervention rates due to postoperative complications following other resectional procedures for similar diseases, as reported in studies cited in the previous two chapters of this book, were: 2% after Delorme for external rectal prolapse, 4% after Delorme for rectal internal pro-

Table 10.3 Complications following Altemeier procedure as reported in an Italian series of 78 patients. Mean age, 71 years, mean specimen length 20cm, ASA III and IV, associated levatorplasty in 86% of cases

Pelvic hematoma (%)	Sigmoid perforation	Stricture	Proctalgia	Urinary retention	Worsened continence	Reinterventions	Mortality
3 (3.9)	1 (1.2)	2 (2.4)	4 (5)	2 (2.4)	7 (9)	2 (2.4)	0

lapse, and 9% after STARR for obstructed defecation due either to recto-rectal (or recto-anal) intussusception or rectocele.

Postoperative morbidity following perineal proctosigmoidectomy, as reported by the authors cited in Table 10.4, was between 5 and 24%. Most early complications were related to lung, cardiovascular, and renal diseases, such as pulmonary embolism, myocardial infarction, hypokalemia, and hypertension (Chun et al. 2004). The advanced age of the patients in Altomare's series, including one 93-year-old patient, was a significant factor. Among the complications noted in the studies cited in the table, rectovaginal fistulae and anastomotic bleeding occurred less frequently.

According to these data, perineal proctosigmoidectomy is associated with a low postoperative complication rate. Of note, patients operated on by American surgeons received local anesthesia and sedation rather than general anesthesia.

As mentioned in the "Live Surgery" section, a crucial step of the operation is when the pouch of Douglas is encountered. It is always prolapsed and often contains an enterocele, namely, a sigmoidocele. Injury to the pouch in cases in which it has to be opened and partly resected and the prolapsed bowel lifted up must be strictly avoided, in order to prevent damage to the small bowel.

It should be noted that two of the authors listed in the table had patients requiring re-operation for pelvic/presacral hematoma. Intraoperative bleeding rarely occurs when the lower sigmoid is divided; however, according Boccasanta et al. (2006) and Gravante and Venditti (2006), the risk

Table 10.4 Complications after the Altemeier procedure, as reported in the literature (732 cases)[a]

First author cases	Year	Number of patients	Mortality (n)	Anastomotic dehiscences (%)	Anal strictures (%)	Anal incontinence (%)
Agachan	1997	32	1	3	2	NR
Kimmins	2001	73	0	2	2	62
Zbar	2002	80	0	1.9[b]	0	5
Chun	2004	109	1	1.9[c]	3.8	NR[d]
Brown	2004	41	0	2	0	20[e]
Glasgow	2006	106	1	0.9[c]	0	36
Altomare	2009	78	0	1.2[f]	2.5	9[g]
Cirocco	2010	103	0	0[h]	2	15
Attuwaybi	2010	110[i]	0	NR	NR	NR

NR, Not reported.

[a]Almost all patients had preoperative incontinence. The length of the resected large bowel varied between 9 and 26 cm.

[b]With abscess.

[c]Plus one patient with pelvic hematoma who required re-operation.

[d]The incontinence score improved in 52 patients after levatorplasty ($p < 0.0001$).

[e]One-third of the patients had preoperative incontinence.

[f]One sigmoid supra-anastomotic perforation, three pelvic hematomas.

[g]Anal continence worsened after surgery.

[h]Two rectovaginal fistulae.

[i]Harmonic scalpel used in 57 patients, stapler in 61.

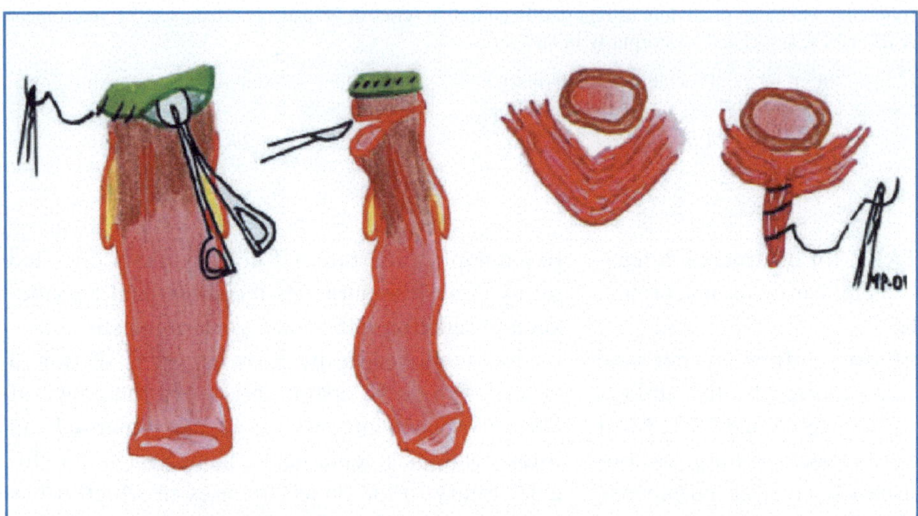

Fig. 10.3 Altemeier's proctosigmoidectomy diagram. *Left*: Opening of the pouch of Douglas and plasty for concomitant elytrocele (enterocele). *Right*: posterior levatorplasty reduces the risk of prolapse recurrence

of this complication is reduced by using a stapling device. However, Attuwaybi et al. (2010) reported less blood loss with the harmonic scalpel than with the stapler. Overall, the mean intraoperative blood loss was 48 ml. The operative time with stapled anastomosis was significantly shorter than with manual suture.

Recurrence and incontinence rates are reduced when a levatorplasty is associated with the proctosigmoidectomy (Chun et al. 2004) (Fig 10.3). Both anterior and posterior levatorplasty might cause rectal stricture and obstructed defecation. My suggestion is to modulate the tension of the levatorplasty by inserting a finger in the anorectum when tying the knots of the plasty sutures, prior to performing the colo-anal anastomosis.

A postoperative deterioration in continence can occur for several reasons. First of all, the rectum is removed. Therefore, there is no longer a reservoir for storage of the feces and to delay evacuation, normally mediated by the accommodation reflex, which is based on the intrinsic innervation of the rectum. As is the case after anterior resection of the rectum, over time, the sigmoid partly assumes some rectal functions, among them reservoir capacity by means of a progressive dilation, and absorption by means of an anatomical modification of the epithelium, including flattening of the villi. A colonic reservoir may be constructed and sutured above the anal canal at the end of the operation, as described by Williams and Keighley in their book, "Surgery of the colon, rectum and anus." This will improve continence and bowel frequency by providing for the storage of stool and by slowing colonic propulsion in the early postoperative months. Moreover, the patient who undergoes a perineal proctosigmoidectomy, e.g., an elderly multiparous female, is typically more likely to have weak sphincters and deficient sensation, with perineal descent and pudendal neuropathy. Finally, the anal sphincters are likely to be stretched during the surgical maneuvers and the stool tends to become more liquid after resection of the distal large bowel, with a partial reduction of the segmental motility of the sigmoid, whose functions include slowing the transit of the fecal stream. Some of the above-mentioned anatomical and physiological changes may be partly corrected by surgical maneuvers such as avoiding sphincter stretch and constructing a reservoir, whereas others cannot be prevented at all. Therefore, the operation is potentially harmful with respect to anal continence. However, in 30% of our patients continence improved after the Altemeier procedure, as the removal of the prolapsed rectum favors restoration of the recto-anal inhibitory reflex, which may be impaired by the presence of bulk, in turn causing soiling by permanently stimulating the relaxation of the internal sphincter.

According to a study by Wexner's group, combined Altemeier and levatorplasty carries less risk of postoperative incontinence than either Delorme or Altemeier alone (Agachan et al., 1997). In another study, out of the ten incontinent patients who had a Delorme, none became fully continent, but four improved (Lauretta et al., 2010). Use of the Lone Star retractor may well help to avoid sphincter trauma, but the device cannot be used when dealing with rectal neoplasms, as lacerations of the anal canal, which are likely to occur due to the sharp hooks of the retractor, may favor the local implantation of malignant cells.

In conclusion, the Altemeier procedure is still a valid option, as the recurrence rate of 3-19% is acceptable (Kim et al., 2010; Altomare et al., 2009), and the complication rate, as reported by many series, is not higher than 20%. There were only three deaths among a total of 732 cases (Table 10.4), with a mortality of 0.4%, even if many patients were elderly and fragile. That is why Cirocco (2010) justly defined the Altemeier as "an operation for all ages."

10.5 Complications After Other Procedures

10.5.1 Transperineal Rectopexy with the Prosthesis Fixed to the Sacrum and Posterior Levatorplasty

Kosba et al. (2010) reported the results achieved in 32 patients using a T-shaped polypropylene mesh. They had just three cases (9.3%) of superficial sepsis, all successfully treated with antibiotics. None of the male patients had sexual problems, whereas sacral rectopexy may cause a loss of ejaculation following injury of the hypogastric nerves. None of the patients had new-onset fecal incontinence, as may occur following the Delorme and Altemeier procedures since both affect or remove the rectal reservoir. Despite the rectopexy, in 80% of the patients operated upon by Kosba et al. constipation was improved, possibly because no sharp angle between the rectum and the sigmoid was created by a procedure that does not extend upward in the pelvis, and because the rectal lateral ligaments were not divided and rectal sensitivity was not impaired.

10.5.2 Transvaginal Sacrospinous Rectopexy

Gurland et al. (2010), through a vertical incision of the posterior vaginal wall, anchored the rectum to the sacrospinous ligament, bilaterally, using a Surgisis mesh. Among the seven patients who underwent a Delorme operation together with an associated urological procedure, three had complications: severe intraoperative bleeding, dynamic ileus, and urinary sepsis.

10.5.3 Manual Transanal Rectal Prolapse Excision

Beginning in the late 1970s, many patients at St Mark's Hospital underwent this procedure, which was referred to as "mucosal stripping." In 1982, Bellomo and Morganti published a paper in Coloproctology, a journal that is not indexed but for decades has nonetheless provided a forum for experts, including Mann, Nicholls, Buess, Hermanek, and Wexner, among others. Bellomo and Morganti reported an impressive series of 820 patients who underwent manual transanal excision and an internal sphincterotomy for a small rectal external mucosal prolapse. They were no recurrences or case of postoperative anal incontinence and just three cases of mild anal stricture, all successfully managed by anal dilations. These results are hard to believe and it may well have been the case that most of the patients with complications and failures were lost at follow-up, considering that other investigators, mentioned in Chap. 1, have reported a relatively high soling rate following internal sphincterotomy for anal fissure. Moreover, in none of those series was there 0 recurrences rate after either perineal or transanal surgery for rectal prolapse.

10.6 Circular Stapled Transanal Prolapsectomy

We first described this operation as belonging to the "pre-PPH era" (Pescatori et al., 1997, available at www.ucp-club.it/medici_articolo.asp), although basically it was a PPH. Only two of the 10 patients in that published series had an external prolapse,

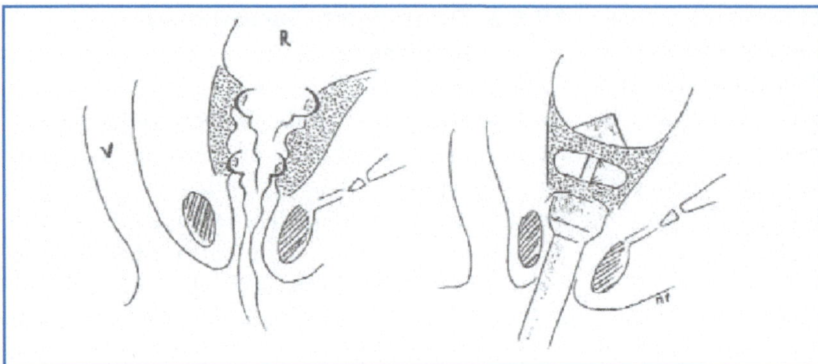

Fig. 10.4 a Circular stapled transanal prolapsectomy. A double "purse-string" suture is carried out to remove a large mucosal cylinder (rectal internal prolapse)

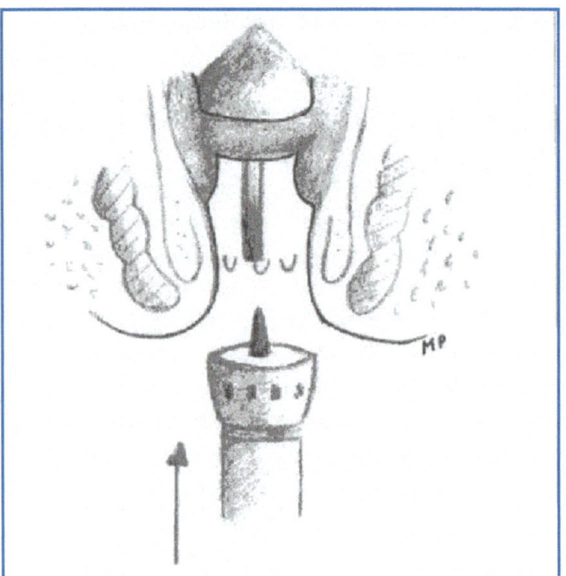

Fig. 10.4 b Stapler is inserted

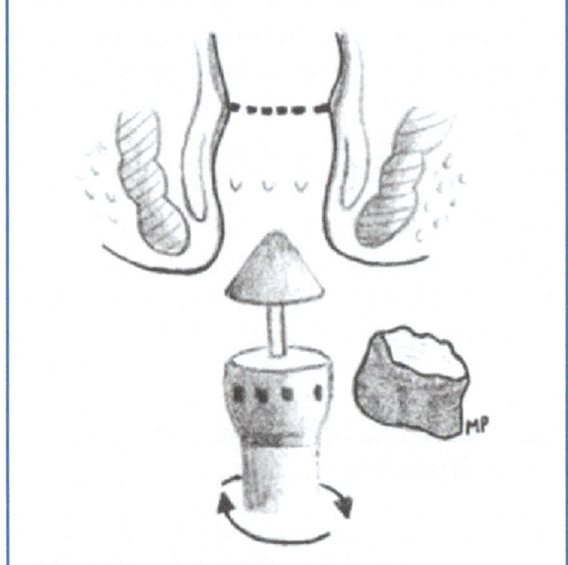

Fig. 10.4 c End of the mechanical suture

all with a size less than 3 cm. There were no postoperative complications. A double purse-string was performed in one patient to excise a larger segment of prolapsed mucosa (Fig. 10.4).

10.7 Transanal Rectal Prolapsectomy Using the Contour Stapling Device

There are only a few reports in the literature, one of them from a group in Naples, Romano et al. (2009). Those authors reported no significant complication in three patients operated on using this novel procedure. The size of the prolapse was less than 10 cm in all cases. Lieske et al. (2010) treated 20 patients using the same Transtar technique and had three cases of bleeding. In the series of nine patients of Carriero et al. (2010), there were no postoperative complications, but the authors recommended not using this procedure in patients with sphincter weakness.

The procedure is costly but has the advantage that it is minimally invasive. However, when the prolapsed bowel is divided along its anterior aspects, the surgeon is relatively "blind," as the prolapsed pouch of Douglas cannot be seen before the resection is performed. Therefore, there is the risk of injury to the peritoneal cul-de-sac, together with a descended bowel loop. Further studies on larger series with longer follow-up are needed before the "Contour-Altemeier" can be deemed as safe and effective.

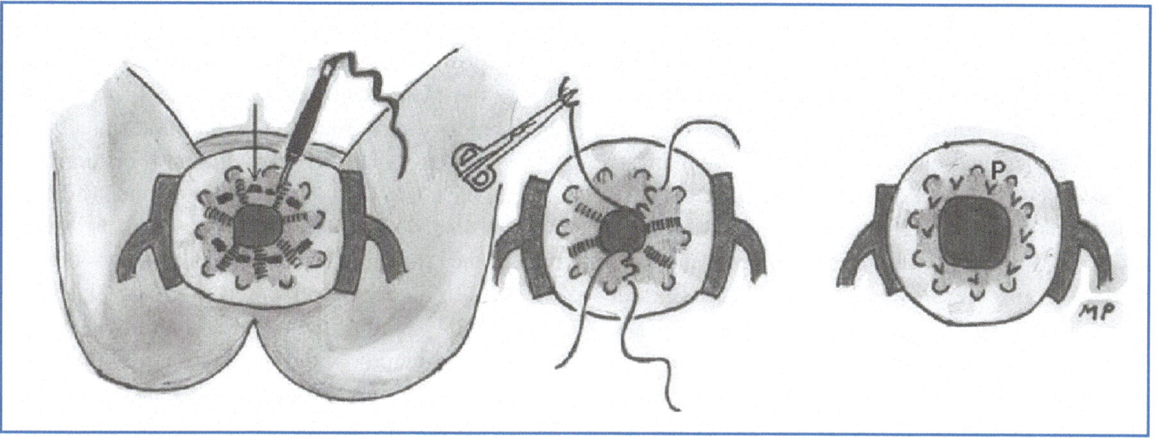

Fig. 10.5 El Sibai and Shafik's operation for prolapse: electrocauterization and plication of the rectum. Disepithelialized strips are made by electrocautery from the dentate line to the top, after which Delorme's plication is performed

10.8 Cauterization-Plication According to El-Sibai and Shafik

These two Egyptian authors reported no postoperative complications in 28 patients operated on using this technique. A postoperative improvement of anal continence was noted in 17. Based on my own, limited experience with this technique, it is a kind of mini-Delorme, without excision of the rectal mucosa. Instead several vertical strips are subjected to diathermy to disepithelialize sites where a series of concertina-like sutures will be positioned to lift up the prolapsed rectum. The operation is illustrated in Fig. 10.5. I have performed this technique in a few patients with internal rectal mucosal prolapse and obstructed defecation. One patient had severe postoperative bleeding necessitating re-operation, while another patient, with a 3-cm external mucosal prolapse, had an uneventful postoperative course.

10.9 An Unforgettable Complication

This case took place in July 2001 and involved a 37-year-old female, nulliparous and a heavy smoker, with an external rectal prolapse that, upon initial examination, was prevalently mucosal and 6 cm long. Due to the characteristics of the prolapse, a Delorme-Rehn operation was scheduled, i.e., rectal mucosectomy, rectal muscle plication, and recto-anal anastomosis. However, in the operating theatre, with the patient having been administered spinal anesthesia and the anal sphincters relaxed, the prolapse turned out to be full-thickness and double the originally determined size. Therefore, I decided to carry out an Altemeier procedure. Everything went well until the end. Once the colo-anal anastomosis and levatorplasty were completed, I noticed a bit of prolapsed mucosa protruding through the anus, just a small ectropion, which was not only aesthetically unpleasant but also a potential cause of postoperative soiling. I simply touched it with diathermy, with just the gray spot of the burned mucosa slowly retracting above the anal verge. Postoperative management consisted of intravenous fluids and nil per os for 48 hours, as the pouch of Douglas had been opened and partly resected to reduce the elytrocele and to raise a descended loop of the small bowel.

One day after starting light oral feeding, the patients had fever, crampy abdominal pain, abdominal tenderness on palpation, and a painful pouch of Douglas on digital exploration. The colo-anal anastomosis was intact. A bowel movement consisted of only a small quantity of fluid feces. Pain increased and her temperature was elevated. We realized that she was frankly peritonitic and decided to reopen her abdomen on postoperative day five.

What did we find at re-intervention?

The peritoneal cavity was full of fluid fecal matter, and, after adequate suction and irrigation with povidone iodine, a small perforation of the lower sigmoid was detected, just above the colo-anal anastomosis. No large bowel diverticula were present. The patient had been intubated under general anesthesia but had respiratory failure during the operation, due to the fact that she was a heavy smoker. After adequate lung ventilation and respiratory support, her respiratory pattern normalized. The perforation was then closed with three slowly absorbable stitches and a proximal sigmoidostomy was fashioned. The patient was discharged after an uneventful postoperative course (Fig. 10.6). The stoma was closed after 3 months and no sign of recurrent rectal prolapse was found at 2 years follow-up.

The localized sigmoid ischemia caused by the diathermy of the mucosal ectropion had caused the bowel perforation. The ectropion was at the level of the lower sigmoid sutured to the anal canal, inside the peritoneal cavity, and not protected by the levators ani, unlike in a rectal mucosal ectropion, which may be safely coagulated transanally.

I never made the mistake again of under-evaluating the size of a rectal prolapse, which had determined the change in the surgical policy, from a Delorme to an Altemeier procedure. Now, I always evaluate the extent of the rectal prolapse by performing the examination with the patient not in the Sims, but in a squatting position, as illustrated in Figure 10.7. Needless to say, after an Altemeier procedure, I no longer use diathermy nor do I resect any piece of mucosa above the colo-anal suture.

For those of you who are superstitious, let me finish by saying that the unfortunate patient was my thirteenth Altemeier!

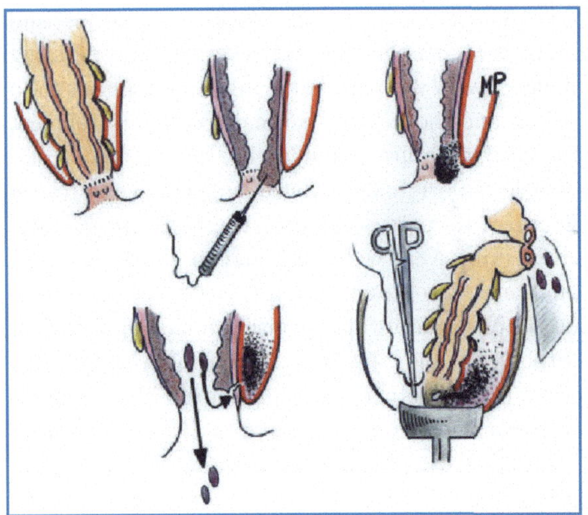

Fig. 10.6 Sigmoid perforation mechanism after Altemeier's operation, as described in "An Unforgettable Complication." The pouch of Douglas is shown in red. The seemingly trivial electrocauterization of a small mucosal prolapse of the sigmoid induced a wall ischemia. At first bowel movement (*arrows*), a perforation occurred in the pouch of Douglas, pulled down almost to the perineal plane. The consequence was peritonitis requiring urgent re-operation of the patient. Last image: suture of the intestinal defect and temporary colostomy

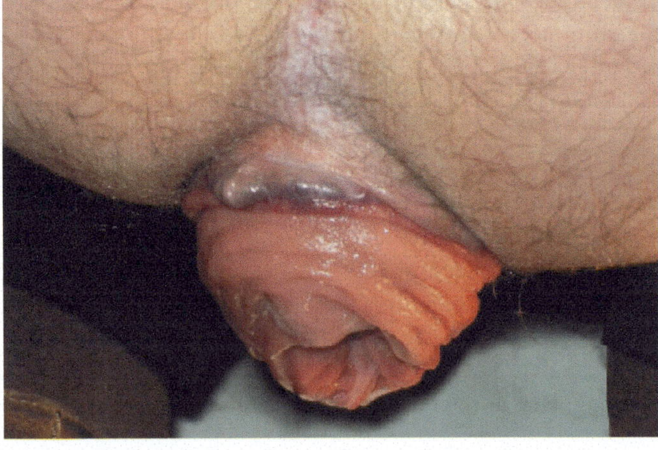

Fig. 10.7 With the patient straining while in squatting position, the size of the rectal prolapse can be precisely evaluated

Summary

Different transanal and transperineal surgeries may be performed in patients with external rectal prolapse, the most commonly used being the Delorme and Altemeier procedures. Both may traumatize the sphincters and affect or involve the excision of the rectal reservoir, thus causing postoperative incontinence, which is unlikely to occur following abdominal sacral rectopexy. Complications after Delorme and Altemeier occur in around 20% of the cases. Sacral pelvic hematoma and anastomotic dehiscence, possibly followed by anorectal stricture, are likely to require a re-intervention. Sepsis and bleeding can usually be managed with conservative management. Proctalgia and urinary retention are rare. Complications related to heart, lung, and renal diseases are not infrequent following the Altemeier procedure, as it is often carried out in elderly and fragile patients. Nevertheless the operative mortality is as low as 0.4%.

Transvaginal and transperineal mesh rectopexies may be followed by sepsis and bleeding, but these patients seldom require re-operation.

Cauterization-plication of the rectum, transanal mucosal stripping, circular stapled prolapsectomy, and Contour Transtar are not accompanied by significant postoperative complications, but only a few small series have been published so far.

Suggested Readings

Agachan F, Pfeifer J, Joo JS, Nogueras JJ, Weiss EG, Wexner SD (1997)Results of perineal procedures for the treatment of rectal prolapse. Am Surg 63:9-12

Agachan F, Reissman P, Pfeifer J, Weiss EG, Nogueras JJ, Wexner SD (1997) Comparison of three perineal procedures for the treatment of rectal prolapse. South Med J 90:925-932

Altemeier WA 3rd (1999) Pediatric orthopedic infections: missed diagnoses. Pediatr Ann 28:718-720

Altomare DF, Binda G, Ganio E, De Nardi P, Giamundo P, Pescatori M; Rectal Prolapse Study Group (2009) Long-term outcome of Altemeier's procedure for rectal prolapse. Dis Colon Rectum 52:698-703

Altomare DF, Pucciani P (2007) Perineal approach to external rectal prolapse: the Delorme procedure. In: Altomare DF, Pucciani F (2007) Rectal prolapse: Diagnosis and Clinical Management. Springer, pp 89-95

Attuwaybi B, Visco J, Butler B, Cywinski M, Barrios G, Leberer J, Singh A (2010) The Buffalo experience with Altemeier procedure for rectal prolapse. Dis Colon Rectum 53: 596-597

Beck DE (2002) Surgical therapy for colitis cystica profunda and solitary rectal ulcer syndrome. Curr Treat Options Gastroenterol 5:231-237

Bellomo R, Morganti I (1982) Results of surgical treatment of mucosal prolapse of the rectum. Coloproctology 4:65-67

Boccasanta P, Stuto A, Naldini G, Caviglia A, Carriero A (2006) Opinions and facts on reinterventions after complicated or failed stapled hemorrhoidectomy. Dis Colon Rectum 49:690-691; author reply 691-693

Brown AJ, Anderson JH, McKee RF, Finlay IG (2004) Strategy for selection of type of operation for rectal prolapse based on clinical criteria. Dis Colon Rectum 47:103-107

Brown AJ, Anderson JH, McKee RF, Finlay IG (2004) Surgery for occult rectal prolapse. Colorectal Dis 6:176-179

Carditello A, Milone A, Stilo F, Mollo F, Basile M (2003) Surgical treatment of rectal prolapse with transanal resection according to Altemeier. Experience and results. Chir Ital 55:687-692

Carriero A, Martellucci J, Talento P (2010) Perineal stapled rectal resection with Contour tranSTARR with Lone Star retractor system. Dis Colon Rectum 53:597

Carriero A, Picchio M, Martellucci J, Talento P, Palimento D, Spaziani E (2010) Laparoscopic correction of enterocele associated to stapled transanal rectal resection for obstructed defecation syndrome. Int J Colorectal Dis 25:381-387

Christiansen J (1987) The Delorme operation with retro-anal plication of the levator muscle in treatment of total prolapse of the rectum. Ann Chir 41:507-511

Chun SW, Pikarsky AJ, You SY et al (2004) Perineal rectosigmoidectomy for rectal prolapse: role of levatorplasty. Tech Coloproctol 8:3-8

Cirocco WC (2010) The Altemeier procedure for rectal prolapse: an operation for all ages. Dis Colon Rectum 53:1618-1623

Corman ML, Carriero A, Hager T et al (2006) Consensus conference on the stapled transanal rectal resection (STARR) for disordered defaecation. Colorectal Dis 8:98-101

De Nardi P, Osman N, Viola M, Staudacher C (2006) Ischemic proctitis following Delorme procedure for external rectal prolapse. Tech Coloproctol 10:253-255

Dekel A, Rabinerson D, Rafael ZB, Kaplan B, Mislovaty B, Bayer Y (2000) Concurrent genital and rectal prolapse: two pathologies—one joint operation. BJOG 107:125-129

Dippolito A, Esser S, Reed J 3rd (2005) Anterior modification of Delorme procedure provides equivalent results to Delorme procedure in treatment of rectal outlet obstruction. Curr Surg 62:609-612

El-Sibai O, Shafik AA (2002) Cauterization-plication operation in the treatment of complete rectal prolapse. Tech Coloproctol 6:51-54

Flum AS, Golladay ES, Teitelbaum DH (2010) Recurrent rectal prolapse following primary surgical treatment. Pediatr Surg Int 26:427-431

Glasgow SC, Birnbaum EH, Kodner IJ, Fleshman JW, Dietz DW (2006) Preoperative anal manometry predicts continence after perineal proctectomy for rectal prolapse. Dis Colon Rectum 49:1052-1058

Gourgiotis S, Baratsis S (2007) Rectal prolapse. Int J Colorectal Dis 22:231-243

Gramkow CS, Lanng C, Fischer A (2005) Altemeier repair of rectal prolapse. Ugeskr Laeger 167:286-289

Gravante G, Venditti D (2006) The Altemeier procedure: new technologies for an old technique. Dis Colon Rectum 49:1801-1802. Comment on: Dis Colon Rectum 49:652-660
Gurland B, Garrett KA, Firoozi F, Goldman HB (2010) Transvaginal sacrospinous rectopexy: initial clinical experience. Tech Coloproctol 14:169-173
Kim M, Reibetanz J, Boenicke L, Germer CT, Jayne D, Isbert C (2010) Quality of life after transperineal rectosigmoidectomy. Br J Surg 97:269-272
Kimmins MH, Evetts BK, Isler J, Billingham R (2001) The Altemeier repair: outpatient treatment of rectal prolapse. Dis Colon Rectum 44:565-570
Kling KM, Rongione AJ, Evans B, McFadden DW (1996) The Delorme procedure: a useful operation for complicated rectal prolapse in the elderly. Am Surg 62:857-860
Kosba Y, Elshazly WG, Abd El Maksoud W (2010) Posterior sagittal approach for mesh rectopexy as a management of complete rectal in adults. Int J Colorectal Dis 25:881-886
Lauretta A, Bellomo R, Infantino A (2010) Which approach for complete rectal prolapse? Orr-Loygue rectopexy vs. Delorme procedure. Dis Colon Rectum 53:596
Lazorthes F, Liagre A, Iovino F (2000) Rectal prolapse. J Chir 137:76-81
Lechaux JP, Lechaux D, Perez M (1995) Results of Delorme's procedure for rectal prolapse. Advantages of a modified technique. Dis Colon Rectum 38:301-307
Lee JI, Vogel AM, Suchar AM, Glynn L, Statter MB, Liu DC (2006) Sequential linear stapling technique for perineal resection of intractable pediatric rectal prolapse. Am Surg 72:1212-1215
Lehtola A, Salo JA, Fräki O, Lempinen M (1987) Treatment of rectal prolapse. A clinical study of 50 consecutive patients. Ann Chir Gynaecol 76:150-154
Liberman H, Hughes C, Dippolito A (2000) Evaluation and outcome of the Delorme procedure in the treatment of rectal outlet obstruction. Dis Colon Rectum 43:188-192
Lieberth M, Kondylis LA, Reilly JC, Kondylis PD (2009) The Delorme repair for full-thickness rectal prolapse: a retrospective review. Am J Surg 197:418-423
Lieske B, Conaghan P, Farouk R (2010) Outcome after stapled perineal rectosigmoidectomy using tranSTARR. Dis Colon Rectum 53:581
Madiba TE, Baig MK, Wexner SD (2005) Surgical management of rectal prolapse. Arch Surg 140:63-73
Marchal F, Bresler L, Ayav A et al (2005) Long-term results of Delorme's procedure and Orr-Loygue rectopexy to treat complete rectal prolapse. Dis Colon Rectum 48:1785-1790
Martínez Hernández-Magro P, Villanueva Sáenz E, Sandoval Munro RD (2003) Surgical treatment of complete rectal prolapse. Experience at a colon and rectal surgery service. Rev Gastroenterol 68:185-191
Milito G, Cadeddu F, Selvaggio I, Grande M (2010) The Delorme repair for full-thickness rectal prolapse: a retrospective review. Am J Surg 199:581-582
Mongardini M, Iachetta RP, Cola A, Effetti ED, Custureri F (2009) Altemeier operation associated with dynamic graciloplasty: a case report. J Med Case Reports 3:9317
Müller-Lobeck H, Duschka L, Schleifer P, Henne T (1996) Rehn-Delorme operation in pelvic floor insufficiency. Zentralbl Chir 121:692-697
Oliver GC, Vachon D, Eisenstat TE, Rubin RJ, Salvati EP (1994) Delorme's procedure for complete rectal prolapse in severely debilitated patients. An analysis of 41 cases. Dis Colon Rectum 37:461-467
Pascual Montero JA, Martínez Puente MC, Pascual I et al (2006) Complete rectal prolapse clinical and functional outcome with Delorme's procedure. Rev Esp Enferm Dig 98:837-843
Pescatori M, Dodi G, Salafia C, Zbar AP (2005) Rectovaginal fistula after double-stapled transanal rectotomy (STARR) for obstructed defaecation. Int J Colorectal Dis 20:83-85
Pescatori M, Favetta U, Dedola S, Orsini S (1997) Stapled transanal excision of rectal mucosal prolapse. Tech Coloproctol 1:96-98
Pescatori M, Zbar AP (2009) Tailored surgery for internal and external rectal prolapse: functional results of 268 patients operated upon by a single surgeon over a 21-year period. Colorectal Dis 11:410-419
Regenet N, De Kerviler B, Lehur PA (2001) Perineal rectosigmoid resection for exterior rectal prolapse (Altemeier operation). J Chir 138:153-156
Romano G, Bianco F, Caggiano L (2009) Modified perineal stapled rectal resection with Contour Transtar for full-thickness rectal prolapse. Colorectal Dis 11:878-881
Sailer M, Bönicke L, Petersen S (2007) Surgical options in the treatment of rectal prolapse: indications, techniques and results. Zentralbl Chir 132:350-357
Scherer R, Marti L, Hetzer FH (2008) Perineal stapled prolapse resection: a new procedure for external rectal prolapse. Dis Colon Rectum 51:1727-1730
Sewonou A, Rioux C, Golliot F et al (2002) Incidence of surgical site infection in ambulatory surgery: results of the INCISCO surveillance network in 1999-2000. Ann Chir 127:262-267
Sielezneff I, Bulgare JC, Sastre B, Sarles JC (1995) Result of surgical treatment of exteriorized rectal prolapse in adults. Experience of 21 years. Ann Chir 49:396-4
The Altemeier repair: outpatient treatment of rectal prolapse. Kimmins MH, Evetts BK, Isler J, Billingham R (2001) Dis Colon Rectum 44:565-570
Tobin SA, Scott IH (1994) Delorme operation for rectal prolapse. Br J Surg 81:1681-1684
Voulimeneas I, Antonopoulos C, Alifierakis E, Ioannides P (2010) Perineal rectosigmoidectomy for gangrenous rectal prolapse. World J Gastroenterol 16:2689-2691
Watkins BP, Landercasper J, Belzer GE et al (2003) Long-term follow-up of the modified Delorme procedure for rectal prolapse. Arch Surg 138:498-502; discussion 502-503
Watts AM, Thompson MR (2000) Evaluation of Delorme's procedure as a treatment for full-thickness rectal prolapse 87:218-222
Zbar AP, Takashima S, Hasegawa T, Kitabayashi K (2002) Perineal rectosigmoidectomy (Altemeier's procedure): a review of physiology, technique and outcome. Tech Coloproctol 6:109-116
Zuo ZG, Song HY, Xu C et al (2010) Application of Altemeier procedure in the emergent management of acute incarcerated rectal prolapse. Zhonghua Wei Chang Wai Ke Za Zhi 13:427-429

Subject Index

A

Abdominoperineal resection of the rectum 16,
Abscess
  acute abscess 68, 70, 80, 101
  anal abscess 57-80
  liver abscess 42
  occult abscess 41
  perianal abscess 42, 78-79, 91
  supralevator abscess 75
Adenocarcinoma of the rectum 109
Adenoma 28, 45, 76, 109-111, 113-116, 118
Adipose tissue 4
Adrenaline 9, 39, 91, 111-113, 123-124, 128, 168, 184
Advanced age 64, 80, 117, 157, 189
Agrapphectomy 44, 140, 152, 160
Altemeier
  procedure 150, 156, 183, 188-191, 193-195
  proctosigmoidectomy 183
Altemeier's rectosigmoid resection 187
Anal
  condylomata 121-133
  continence 57, 65, 68, 69, 72, 80, 89, 127, 128, 131, 146, 149, 150, 166, 169, 172, 174, 176, 184, 188, 193
  fissure 1-12, 18, 22, 24, 40, 41, 57, 70, 71, 125, 128, 183, 191
  hypertonia 1, 3, 4, 6, 8-10, 12, 19, 29, 39, 41
  incontinence 1-5, 17, 20, 40, 42, 64-74, 79, 109, 144-146, 168, 188
  manometry 65, 71, 78, 109, 154, 165
  perineoplasty 61
  reflex 64, 65, 136
  retractor 5, 16, 68, 113, 121
  spasm 3, 18, 25, 124, 132
  stenosis 8, 10, 18, 19, 23, 38, 40, 46-49, 124, 125
  stretch 6, 7, 12
  surgery 6, 64, 66, 77, 80
  tampon 24, 44
  ultrasound 78, 103, 104
Anastomotic dehiscence 89, 93, 121, 127, 144, 185, 188, 195
Anismus 92, 135, 137-138, 153-155, 160
Anoplasty 2, 4, 6-8, 10, 12, 20, 40-41, 48-49, 61, 63, 115, 121, 123-128, 130, 132, 140, 160, 168, 183
Anterior levatorplasty 60-61, 88, 94, 136, 143-144, 153, 160, 166, 169, 178
Anterior resection 35, 85, 90, 109, 111, 117, 121-123, 127, 136-137, 188, 190
Antibiotic prophylaxis 16, 34, 89, 101, 110, 166, 170, 176, 184
Anus
  deformed anus 64
  gaping anus 72, 167
Anxiety 78, 93, 117, 137-139, 146, 150-151, 154, 157, 160
Ascites 34, 188

B

Balloon endoscopic dilation 126
Biofeedback 42, 49, 65, 71, 92, 109, 118, 121, 125, 136, 147, 154-155, 184
Biopsy forceps 41, 114
Bleeding
  intraoperative bleeding 9, 17, 22, 37, 47, 58, 184, 189, 191
  postoperative bleeding 18, 23, 39, 57-58, 76, 79, 90, 92, 95, 99, 102, 114, 124, 149-150, 153, 157, 170, 193
  rectal bleeding 1, 10, 17, 20-22, 25, 27-29, 38-39, 49, 58, 80, 88, 104, 111, 118, 140-141, 147, 149, 152-153, 155-157, 159, 184, 188
Block 25, 38, 140-141, 144-145, 152, 157, 175, 177
Blood transfusion 38, 43, 57, 111
Botulinum toxin A (Botox) 2, 4, 6, 12, 19, 38-40, 41, 154
Bulbo-cavernosus muscle 74, 86, 88, 90, 91, 94
Bulking agent 6, 42, 49, 72, 80, 121, 125, 140, 146, 160, 165, 168, 174, 178
Buschke-Löwenstein 130-132

C

Calcium channel blockers 2, 41
Cancer 18, 32, 57, 109-112, 115, 117, 123-124, 132, 155, 170, 172
Carcinoid 109, 111, 114
Cauterization-plication 193, 195
Chemotherapy 18, 115, 121
Coagulation 17, 38, 43-44, 46, 156, 168
Coaptite 6, 72, 174
Coccygeal muscle 115
Collagene mesh 153
Colo-anal anastomosis 117, 151, 187, 190, 193-194
Colonic
  propulsion 190
  reservoir 190
Colonoscopy 28, 78, 115-117, 157-159
Colorectal surgeon 2, 5, 34, 44, 57, 65-66, 68, 78-79, 85, 87, 123, 136-137, 148, 160, 173

Colostomy
defunctioning colostomy 33, 42-43
diverting colostomy 85, 89, 92, 95
Conflict of interest 33, 67, 149, 174
Constipation 6, 10, 17, 27, 135-137, 150, 154, 158, 171-172, 174, 176, 183, 191
Contour stapler 145, 147-148
Crohn's disease 1, 8, 10, 12, 18, 20, 59-60, 67, 78, 80, 85-86, 89-90, 95
Cryotherapy 123
CT-scan 28
Curettage 7, 9, 41, 59, 61-62, 64, 67, 69-70, 75, 102-103

D

Defecography 65, 113, 135-136, 139, 141-142, 152, 154
Dehiscence 4, 7-8, 10-12, 16, 18, 28, 33, 35, 38, 41, 49, 60-61, 64, 68-69, 74-75, 80, 88-90, 93, 95, 100-104, 106, 109-110, 112, 114-115, 117, 121, 124-128, 132-133, 140-142, 144, 148, 153, 158-159, 165, 169-170, 172, 183-186, 188-189, 195
Depezzer 68, 131
Depression 137-139, 150, 154, 160
Diabetes 8, 10, 12, 18, 43, 60, 74, 80, 114, 117
Diathermy 17, 27-28, 38, 45-47, 57, 68, 75, 77, 99, 106, 111-113, 115, 124, 128, 130, 132, 139, 152, 166, 168-169, 177, 184, 186, 193-194
Digital
exploration 78, 92, 128, 141, 143, 154, 159, 165, 167, 184, 193
rectal examination 6, 10, 27, 30
Digitoclasia 7
Dilatation 7-10, 25, 38, 40-41, 43, 47-49, 122, 140, 158
Diltiazem 2, 4, 38-39
Diverticulum 10-12, 30, 32, 44-45, 121, 136, 147
Dog's ears 16
Draw-the-family test 3
Dynamic MRI 26
Dynamic perineal ultrasound 65
Dyspareunia 88, 95, 152-153, 160, 169, 178
Dysplasia 32, 36, 115, 123

E

Electrostimulation
electrostimulated acupuncture 62
of the posterior tibial nerve 6, 72, 147
tibial nerve electrostimulation 42, 168
transanal electrostimulation 6, 42, 65, 71, 79, 146, 154
Elytrocele 148, 151, 190, 193
Emphysema
cervical emphysema 28, 44
Encirclement procedure 74, 172, 183
EndoGIA 114, 144, 152-153
Endoscopic stricturectomy 41
Endosponge 102
Enemas 39, 42, 171, 173, 178
Enterocele 33-34, 45, 113, 136-139, 148, 152, 160, 186, 189-190
Excision
hemorrhoid excision 16-18, 36, 76
of the fissure 4, 6, 8, 12, 41
of the fissure and injection of botulinum toxin A 6
tags excision 40
External orifice 58, 64, 76, 91, 104
External rectal prolapse 183-184, 188, 193, 195

F

False tract 58, 76
Fascio-adipose cutaneous flap 100-101
Fecal
impaction 1, 40, 111, 167
incontinence 1, 4, 24, 57, 64-65, 78, 80, 90, 95, 109, 115, 125, 137, 141, 144-145, 153-154, 165, 167, 169-172, 174-176, 178, 191
stasis 155
urgency 1, 121, 144, 149, 152-153, 160
Fecaloma 4, 20, 22, 32, 38-40
Fecoliths 30
Ferguson procedure 15-20, 23, 26, 39, 44, 47, 49
Fibrin glue 59, 64, 66-68, 80, 100, 102
Fibrosis 11, 19, 26, 63, 66, 68, 72, 79, 92, 111, 121-122, 125-128, 140-141, 156, 160, 167, 170, 172
Fissure 1-12, 15, 17-18, 21-22, 24, 40-41, 48-49, 57, 70-71, 125, 128, 166, 183, 191
Fissurectomy 2, 4, 12
Fistula
anal fistula 1, 3, 27, 38, 41, 49, 57, 59, 62-66, 68-70, 72, 76-79, 89, 91, 103
horse-shoe fistula 59
iatrogenic fistula 58
persisting fistula 67, 69
rectovaginal fistula (RVF) 31-32, 44, 50, 85, 89-91, 93, 109, 112-113, 118, 147-148, 152-153, 169, 189
recurrent fistula 69-70
trans-sphincteric fistula 57-59, 65-66, 68-71, 75, 80
Fistuloscope 69
Fistulotomy 57-59, 66-67, 69-70, 76-79, 88, 90-91, 169
Flap
cutaneous flap 8, 36-37, 63, 66, 68, 76, 80, 100-101, 115, 118
dehiscence 69, 75, 115
diamond flap 125
house flap 115, 125, 128, 132
Limberg flap 101-102
Martius flap 89-90
rectal advancement flap 59-60, 62, 64, 66-67, 69, 75, 88-89, 95, 103
rhomboid flap 100-103
skin flap 7-9, 36, 68, 77, 117, 131, 167
Torpedo flap 115
Flavonoids 38, 41
Foley
balloon 130
catheter 39, 44, 49, 57, 75-76, 92-93, 114, 130-131, 140, 157
Fournier's gangrene 16, 42-43, 118

G

Gas incontinence 4-5, 38, 42
Gastrointestinal stromal tumors 109
General surgeon 57, 85, 104, 121, 150
Gluteoplasty 86, 88, 168-169, 172, 178

Graciloplasty 44, 86, 88, 95, 165, 168-169, 172-173, 178
Granuloma 49, 79, 140, 145, 159
Granulomatous polyp 27, 29, 44, 109

H

Harmonic scalpel 113, 189-190
Hartmann procedure 23, 34-35, 44, 110, 114
Headache 9
Hegar dilator 40, 44, 47, 111, 127, 130, 159
HeLP 19, 22
Hematoma
  perianal hematoma 23, 39, 152
  retro-rectal hematoma 32
Hematuria 21
Hemodialysis 48
Hemorrhage 12, 15, 18, 21-23, 33, 38-39, 44-45, 49, 57, 92-93, 99, 106, 111, 114, 141, 149, 153, 160, 170, 184, 186
Hemorrhoidectomy
  emergency hemorrhoidectomy 20, 40
  Ferguson hemorrhoidectomy 17-19, 23, 26, 35, 40-41, 47, 49, 113, 184
  laser hemorrhoidectomy 40
Hemorrhoidopexy
  manual hemorrhoidopexy 35
  stapled hemorrhoidopexy 15, 17, 22-23, 25, 27, 30-31, 35-36, 41-42, 45, 49
Hemorrhoids 15-50
  accessory hemorrhoids 19
  hemorrhoid grade 26
  hemorrhoidal thrombosis 21, 50
  sentinel hemorrhoid 5
  thrombosed hemorrhoids 20-22, 40
Hemostasis 7, 9, 17-19, 23, 25, 35, 39, 44, 57-58, 99, 109, 113, 124, 167
Hemostatic
  suture 22, 95
  tampon 19
Hidradenitis suppurativa 74, 80
Histological analysis 9
HIV/AIDS 60, 131
Holistic approach 3, 78, 135, 137, 165, 171
HPV (human papilloma virus) 123
Hydrocolon lavage 125, 135-136
Hymen 176
Hyperbaric oxygen therapy 8
Hypertonia 1, 3-4, 6, 8-10, 12, 19, 26, 29, 38-39, 41, 143
Hypertrophied papilla 5
Hypopituitarism 1

I

Iceberg syndrome 135, 137, 139, 147, 150
Ileostomy 136, 158-159
Immunosuppression 60
Incontinence 1-6, 10, 12, 15, 17, 19-20, 22-24, 26-27, 36, 38, 40, 42, 49, 57, 59, 61, 64-71, 74, 78-80, 88, 90-91, 95, 109-110, 112-115, 117-118, 121-122, 124-125, 133, 137, 140-142, 144-147, 152-155, 157, 160, 165, 167-172, 174-178, 183-184, 186, 188-191, 195
Infected sinus 99, 101, 104
Inflammatory bowel disease 64
Internal mucosal prolapse of the rectum 10, 21, 41-42, 138
Internal orifice 59, 66, 68-69, 74-75, 80, 104, 106
Intussusception 30, 50, 114, 121, 136, 138-146, 155-156, 159, 189
Irrigation 39-40, 76, 78, 125, 143, 157, 194
Irritable bowel syndrome 64, 72, 91, 146, 150, 159
Ischemia 9, 45, 47, 63, 68, 92, 100, 112, 124-126, 128, 135, 147, 155, 172, 185-186, 194
Ischiorectal cavity 57, 76

K

Keloid 40

L

Laparoscopic-assisted PPH 23
Laser
  depilation 103
  probe 22, 64, 80
  therapy 27, 123
Lay open 5, 57-59, 63, 65-66, 68-69, 74, 76, 80, 86, 88, 91, 100, 102-103
Leiomyosarcoma 109
Levatorplasty 44, 60-61, 87-88, 93-95, 136-137, 140, 143-144, 153, 160, 166, 169, 178, 188-191, 193
LIFT (ligation of the intersphincteric fistula tract) 66, 68, 70-71, 80
LigaSure 16-17, 21
Local anesthesia 7, 22, 37, 39-42, 59, 101, 103, 158-159, 184, 189
Local infection 89-90, 160, 170, 175-176
Lone Star retractor 24, 186-187, 191

M

Magnetic resonance imaging 11, 65
Manometry 3, 6, 10, 19, 25, 65, 71, 78, 91, 109, 154, 157, 165
Marsupialization 58, 80, 100
Mediastinum 117
Metronidazole 38, 41, 110, 117, 141, 166, 176
Milligan-Morgan 15-20, 23, 26, 38-41, 43-46, 48-49, 124
Milligan-Morgan hemorrhoidectomy 18, 20, 23, 26, 38, 43, 46, 48-49, 124
Muco-cutaneous bridge 19
Mucopexy 19-22, 42, 50
Mucosal ectropion 37, 40, 115, 124, 184, 186, 194
Mucosal stripping 141, 191, 195
Mucosectomy
  Delorme mucosectomy 30, 85
  rectal mucosectomy 26, 144, 156, 183, 184, 193
Multiparous patient 6, 80, 185

N

Natal cleft 99
Necrosectomy 42-43, 117-118
Necrosis 9, 22, 42-44, 77, 117
Nephrectomy 35
Nifedipine 25-26

Nitroglycerin 2, 9, 19, 38-39, 41
Non-healing wound 60, 115

O

Obesity 60, 74
Obliteration of the rectum 50, 130
Obstetric injury 90
Obstructed defecation 6, 10, 28, 92, 121, 125, 135, 138-143, 145, 148, 150, 154-157, 159-160, 165, 172-173, 178, 186, 189-190, 193
Off-midline incision 106
Open technique 99-102

P

Pacemaker 165, 171-172, 178
Pain 1-2, 5, 10-11, 16-17, 19, 21-22, 24-27, 30, 35, 38-39, 41-44, 47-49, 58, 61, 66-71, 76-79, 102, 110, 114, 116-117, 124-125, 136, 143, 147, 149-152, 156-160, 167, 169, 171-172, 174, 176-178, 193
Palliation 109
Palpation 59, 193
Parachute technique 112
Parasitological exam 63
Parks retractor 145
Pelvic descensus 113
Pelvic floor rehabilitation 65, 71, 80, 121, 135, 160, 165
Perineal
  scar 65, 71
  cellulitis 188
  descent 64, 66, 91, 110, 145, 165, 186, 190
  necrosectomy 42, 118
  necrosis 42
Peritonitis 33, 45, 110, 126-127, 158, 188, 194
Physiokinesis therapy 42
Pilonidal sinus 59, 74, 99-100, 102-104, 106
Plasma injection 69, 80
Plastic surgery 8, 36, 115, 132
Platelet concentration 69
Plug 27, 59, 66-68, 80, 86, 88, 90
PNEI system 136
Pneumatic dilatation 7
Pneumomediastinum 28, 30, 111, 116, 118, 127, 148
Pneumoperitoneum 28-29, 116, 118, 127
PNTML (pudendal nerve terminal motor latency) 65
Polypectomy snare 111
Polypropylene mesh 153, 191
Postoperative pain 2, 5, 17, 19, 21-22, 24-25, 27, 38, 41, 44, 47-48, 58, 77, 114, 147, 156, 167
Pouch of Douglas 33-34, 45, 49-50, 110, 113, 136, 139, 148, 151, 186, 189, 192-194
Pouchogram 126
PPH 15-17, 21-36, 39-45, 47-50, 112, 116-117, 130, 136, 140, 144-147, 149-150, 152, 160, 184, 191
Pregnancy 34
Primary closure 69, 102, 106
Primary suture 66, 68-69, 102
Probing 58-59, 91
Proctalgia
  chronic proctalgia 11, 26-27, 31, 48-49, 79, 149-150, 152, 160, 171
Proctoscopy 10, 20, 27, 92, 103-104, 123, 125, 136, 150, 157
Prostatitis 30
Prostheses 168
Pruritus ani 25
Psychological pattern 136-138, 150
Puborectalis sling 126, 154, 166, 168, 175-176, 178
Pudendal
  motor latency 79
  nerve block 25, 38
  neuropathy 7, 64-65, 79, 136, 138, 145, 190
Purse-string 24-26, 30, 33, 44-45, 152, 192

Q

Quality of life 3-4, 10, 50, 72, 79, 109, 136, 149, 160, 174

R

Radial incision 40-41, 125, 130
Radiofrequency energy 172
Radiotherapy 85, 115, 117-118, 121-122, 170
Radiowaves 16
Rectal
  diverticulum 10-11, 30, 32, 45, 136, 147
  hyposensation 66, 72, 79-80, 136, 138, 145
  inclusion cyst 30, 45
  laceration 33
  obliteration 30, 44, 50, 130
  perforation 34-35, 44, 110, 114, 166
  pocket 30-31, 44-45, 50
  pocket syndrome 30, 45
  resection 10, 30, 85, 144, 159
  sensation 65, 127, 146
  sensitivity 65, 78, 191
  stenosis 10, 40-41, 126-127, 158
  tamponade 49, 109, 184
  ulcer 109, 135, 138, 155-156
Recto-anal
  invagination 113
  repair 21
Rectocele 48, 85, 92, 135-136, 138-145, 147-148, 152-153, 156-157, 160, 169, 177, 185, 189
Rectopexy 156, 183, 191, 195
Re-routing of the fistula tract 69, 80
Retained staple 10-11, 27-28, 31, 42, 44, 47-48, 146, 151, 159
Retropneumoperitoneum 28-29, 41, 44, 50
Rhomboid incision 101
Route
  perineal route 85, 88, 140, 144, 183
  transanal route 88, 95, 117, 121, 144
  transcoccygeal route 88
  transvaginal route 88, 90

S

Sacral
  depilation 103
  nerve stimulation 8, 171
  neuromodulation 72, 80, 125, 136, 147, 165, 168, 171, 173, 177-178
  rectopexy 183, 191, 195

Sacrospinous ligament 191
Sarles 92, 140, 144-145, 147
Self expanding stent 127
Self-dilatation 8
Semi-closed hemorrhoidectomy 35
Septic shock 43
Seroma 18, 74, 100-102, 106
Sepsis
  anal sepsis 7, 12, 34, 41-43, 65, 70, 78, 103, 106
  local sepsis 12, 18, 20, 40, 47, 58, 66, 69, 74, 78, 88, 90, 93, 95, 100-102, 106, 112, 117-118, 127-128, 133, 155-156, 159, 165-167, 169-170, 172-174, 178, 184
  pelvic sepsis 33-35, 44, 50, 114, 126-127, 135, 140-141, 147, 160
  postoperative sepsis 18, 41, 153, 184
Seton 58-59, 61, 65-68, 70, 74-75, 80, 91
Sexual traumas 154
Sigmoidoscope 114
Sigmoidostomy 72, 78-79, 87, 89, 141, 147-148, 160, 166, 170, 194
Silicone spherules 174
Sitz bath 7, 39, 151
Skin tag 5, 20, 22, 36, 38, 40-42, 47, 143
Smoker 62, 64, 68, 74-75, 89, 193-194
Soiling 1-4, 10, 17, 23, 40, 42, 64, 66, 80, 89, 115, 124, 132, 146, 184, 186, 190, 193
Solitary rectal ulcer syndrome 135, 155-156
Spastic colon 141, 159
Sphincter
  artificial bowel sphincter 27, 74, 165, 173, 178
  external sphincter 2-3, 6-7, 20, 58-60, 64-66, 68, 72-73, 75-78, 87, 91, 93-94, 115, 122, 125, 128, 131, 166-170, 175-176, 184
  injury 65
  internal sphincter 1-10, 12-17, 19-20, 23, 25, 26, 29, 36, 41-42, 48-49, 63, 65-66, 68-69, 71-73, 75, 78, 80, 104, 106, 113-114, 121-122, 125, 128-129, 131, 136, 143, 145-146, 154, 166, 178, 183-184, 190-191
  neuropathic sphincter 80
  reconstruction 68, 72, 74, 78-80, 89-90, 95, 125, 165, 168-171, 178
  saving procedure 65, 70, 80
  weak sphincter 16, 64, 66, 68, 80, 121, 190
Sphincteroplasty 6, 42, 78-79, 88, 115, 146, 168-171, 176-178
Sphincterotomy
  closed sphincterotomy 2, 7
  internal sphincterotomy 1-9, 12, 19, 41, 48, 78, 128, 183, 191
  lateral sphincterotomy 9
  open sphincterotomy 2
  posterior sphincterotomy 2-3, 10
  standard sphincterotomy 2, 6
Spinal anesthesia 16, 24, 166, 184, 188, 193
Staple removal 26
Stapled rectotomy 92, 144
Stapler malfunction 23, 147
STARR 10-12, 32, 47, 85, 92-93, 112, 116, 135-137, 140-141, 144-152, 156, 158-160, 186, 189
Stem cell 4, 59, 66, 80, 89
Stoma
  defunctioning stoma 42-43
  diverting stoma 44, 78, 88-89, 92, 95, 110, 117, 126-128, 133, 140, 153, 158-160, 169-170, 172, 178
  irrigation 78
Submucosal hemorrhoidectomy 37
Survival rate 109
Suture
  breakdown 8, 64, 89, 92, 101, 114, 117, 121, 128, 133, 141, 159, 170
  dehiscence 8, 10-12, 16, 38, 41, 49, 60, 64, 69, 74-75, 80, 88, 90, 95, 100-104, 106, 109-110, 112, 124, 128, 132, 140-141, 158-159, 165, 169, 172, 188

T

TEM 28, 85, 88, 90, 109-111, 113-114, 116, 118, 133, 144
Tenesmus 10, 21, 25-26, 30, 39, 50, 104, 122, 141
THD/DGHAL 15, 19-21
THD-mucopexy 42, 50
Thrombosis of the inferior vena cava 35
Total parenteral nutrition 10, 43, 49, 93, 109, 114, 117-118, 131, 140, 170
Transanal
  prolapsectomy 137, 142, 191-192
  rectal prolapsectomy 143, 192
  ultrasonography 2-3, 6, 11, 27, 29, 105, 123, 146, 150, 154, 174
Transfusion 38-39, 43, 57, 109, 111, 114
Transgluteal neurolysis 49
Transsacral approach 90
Transtar 136, 145, 147-150, 152, 160, 183, 192, 195
Trauma to the penis 32

U

Ulceration 9, 115, 172, 174-175
Ultrasonic scalpel 16
Urgency 1, 22, 25-26, 50, 65, 72, 121-122, 141, 144, 146-147, 149, 152-153, 160
Urinary retention 4, 16-17, 20-22, 24, 38-39, 41, 48, 50, 69, 110-111, 136, 147, 152-153, 167, 188, 195
Urologic resectoscope 114
US (ultrasound) 6, 7, 10, 20, 22-23, 27, 41-42, 62, 65, 78, 91, 103-104, 131, 136, 154, 159, 165

V

VAAFT (video-assisted anal fistula technique) 66, 69, 80
VAC 34-35, 61, 101
Vagina 32-33, 72, 86, 91-94, 113, 138-139, 147-148, 153, 157, 168, 174-178, 185
Vaginismus 135
Verrucous cunniculans carcinoma 131

W

Waldeyer fascia 166, 175
Whitehead-Rand hemorrhoidectomy 35
Wound dehiscence 4, 125, 127
Wound healing agents 8

Y

Y-V anoplasty 7, 124

The manufacturer's authorised representative in the EU is Springer Nature Customer Service Centre GmbH, Europaplatz 3, 69115 Heidelberg, Germany. If you have any concerns regarding our products, please contact ProductSafety@springernature.com

Printed and bound by CPI Group (UK) Ltd, Croydon, CR0 4YY
15/07/2026
02167632-0008